STAFF TRAINING IN MENTAL HANDICAP

Edited by James Hogg, Hester Adrian Research Centre, and Peter Mittler, Professor of Special Education, University of Manchester

The issue of staff training for those working with children and adults with mental handicap has become a central concern to a variety of bodies responsible for the delivery of service to such individuals. Such bodies include those responsible for teacher and nurse training, residential and care staff, as well as policy-makers in this field.

In recent years there has been a growing body of research exploring models of training and their effectiveness. This book describes a number of major projects from the UK, USA and Australia that have considered both specific training techniques and models of delivering training to those responsible for people with mental handicap.

STAFF TRAINING IN MENTAL HANDICAP

Edited by
JAMES HOGG AND PETER MITTLER

CROOM HELM
London & Sydney

BROOKLINE BOOKS
Cambridge, Massachusetts

Croom Helm Ltd, Provident House, Burrell Row,
Beckenham, Kent, BR3 1AT

Croom Helm Australia, 44-50 Waterloo Road,
North Ryde, 2113, New South Wales

British Library Cataloguing in Publication Data

Staff training in mental handicap.
1. Social work with the mentally handicapped — Great Britain 2. Social workers — In-service training — Great Britain
I. Hogg, James. 1940- . II. Mittler, Peter
362.3'07'1141 HV3008.G7

ISBN 0-7099-3728-8

Brookline Books, PO Box 1046, Cambridge, MA 02238.

Library of Congress Cataloging-in-Publication Data

Staff training in mental handicap.

Includes bibliographies and index.
1. Mental retardation facilities — Great Britain — Employees. 2. Mental retardation facilities — Employees — Training of — Great Britain. 3. Mentally handicapped — Rehabilitation — Great Britain. I. Hogg, J. (James) II. Mittler, Peter J. [DNLM: 1. Allied Health Personnel — education. 2. Inservice Training. 3. Mental Health Services — Manpower. 4. Mental Retardation — rehabilitation. WM 18 S779]
HV3008.G7S73 1987 362.3'068'3 86-26391
ISBN 0-914797-35-2

Printed and bound in Great Britain by Mackays of Chatham Ltd, Kent

CONTENTS

PART III: TRAINING IN SPECIFIC SETTINGS

PART IV: METHODS OF DISSEMINATION

PREFACE

Even a cursory consideration of staff training in the field of mental handicap services will reveal a bewildering array of types of course content, methods of instruction, approaches to evaluation, and the involvement, as trainers and trainees, of a very wide range of professionals. This array has been engendered by the growth of services for people with mental handicap, particularly during the past 20 years. Many of the features of this overall picture of staff training reflect one simple assumption, i.e., that if staff are trained in appropriate techniques, they will use these in their service settings with consequent benefits to their clients. The purpose of this volume is two-fold. First, to illustrate that simple assumptions about the effects of staff training are not supported by the research evidence, and that we therefore must adopt a far more sophisticated framework if we are to be effective in our efforts. Second, to try to bring order into the array of staff training techniques by describing their use in a wide variety of settings and illustrating how different specific approaches to training are applicable in varying contexts.

Part One of this volume contains three chapters that address factors in the wider social context that are critical to success in training staff. Landesman-Dwyer and Knowles, in Chapter 1, deal with the evaluation of staff training in naturally occurring contexts, specifically in relation to residential settings. These authors argue that staff performance represents a complex and changing pattern of behaviour that is influenced by the surrounding social environment, staff characteristics, and the training and supervision provided to staff. If we are to evaluate the impact of a staff training programme, then the context in which the staff work must be analysed before and after training, in both the short and long term. In addition, both qualitative and quantitative aspects of the situation must be monitored.

Landesman-Dwyer and Knowles describe a model of staff training, arguing that the effectiveness of such training programmes will be a function of how well the content of the programme matches the perceived needs of staff in the setting. A number of factors need to be taken into account in effecting this match, notably the characteristics of the staff themselves, including attitudes, as well as features of the environment. They point out the compatibility of this ecological model with traditional behavioural methods of training, but note the approaches differ in the "...relative emphasis on the total environment and the complexity of the individual and environmental variables." (p.26). The authors describe a range of techniques of ecological evaluation and note a number of available instruments for characterising both environments and individuals.

Such a view of staff training as being embedded in a wider social context leads Landesman-Dwyer and Knowles to note the relation of staff training to the wider social context in which integration of people with mental handicap in the community is the ideal outcome. Mittler, in Chapter 2, takes up the theme of normalisation and its relevance to staff training in the United Kingdom. He notes that the majority of people with mental handicap are still in segregated institutional services, while few such children or adults are integrated in our eductional and social institutions. One of the major difficulties in staff training at the present time, he argues, is the institutional bias of the training provided for the majority of staff at a time at which we are seeking to develop a greater range of non-institutional services.

Mittler goes on to describe the implications of this state of affairs with respect to both its historical antecedents and the present policy of developing community services. He describes the isolation of specialist staff from each other in services and in initial and post-qualification training. He emphasises the need to develop interdisciplinary training as an essential precursor to interdisciplinary service delivery. Given the diversity of professions concerned with people with mental handicap, Mittler raises the question, "Who needs training?", going on to describe the range of nursing, educational, psychological, therapeutic and social service staff for whom initial and post-qualification training is needed.

Training of the scope and character envisaged by Mittler leads to a consideration of a variety of other issues. These include the content of training and the issues of managerial and organisational factors in successfully implementing the trained skills in service settings. The last issues look back to

Landesman-Dwyer and Knowles in Chapter One, and forward to more detailed analyses of organisation and management in Jones, Blunden, Coles, Evans and Porterfield's Chapter 6 and Cullen's Chapter 8 on training of residential staff, and McBrien and Foxen's consideration of organisational factors in educational settings in Chapter 9.

Mittler also raises the critical issue in any ecological perspective of the involvement of the family of the individual with mental handicap in service provision. This issue also recurs in several chapters, notably Halle and Touchette in Chapter 4 on teaching mothers communication skills; Jones, et al's on family involvement in goal planning for residential clients and particularly in Kiernan's Chapter 7 on the social worker-implemented Home Intervention Programme.

Towards the end of his chapter, Mittler lists a variety of essential staff skills (pp. 53-57). These are grouped under considerations of working with clients, with other professionals, with families; management and organisation skills and skills in learning and acquiring information. He concludes, however, by acknowledging the enormity of the task with which we are faced if we are to train staff effectively. Like Landesman-Dwyer and Knowles he emphasises that staff training is only one part of a much greater whole: "Staff training cannot compensate for poor services or ineffective management. A naive faith in more and better staff training is now being tempered by a growing realisation that courses do not necessarily lead to change in the behaviour of participants, far less to changes in clients with whom they work. Problems of generalisation of training across people, across settings and situations are common to people with mental handicap and the staff who work with them." (pp.61-62.)

It is the theme of how management practices can ensure the generalisation and maintenance of training skills acquired by staff which Anderson addresses in Chapter 3. He defines generalisation as the occurrence of trained behaviour across settings, subjects and behaviours that differ from those present during training. Maintenance is defined as the occurrence of the behaviour across time. In his chapter, the term "management" should be taken in the general sense of referring to the training, generalisation and maintenance of staff behaviour, a more restricted useage than that employed by Mittler (Chapter 2) and Cullen (Chapter 8), but similar in scope to that of Jones et al (Chapter 6).

Anderson provides an exhaustive review of a variety of staff management techniques from the standpoints of training, generalisation and maintenance, covering: instructional methods; modelling; role-playing; performance feedback; self-recording; feedback including praise; feedback plus monetary incentives; feedback plus work schedule incentives and combinations of techniques. It should be pointed out that throughout the remainder of the book other contributors refer to their use of these approaches to staff training, and Anderson's chapter provides an essential backdrop against which to view their studies.

Anderson goes on to take up the theme of evaluation introduced by Landesman-Dwyer and Knowles, and the issue of experimental design in evaluating staff management practices. Issues in the development of future research are also itemised (pp.107-109), as are his basic conclusions regarding the effectiveness of the various techniques (pp. 109-114).

Staff training can be ranged on a dimension from techniques concerned with highly specific strategies directed to a limited, but important, aspect of behaviour, through to much broader approaches involving a range of techniques targetting a variety of behaviours. This continuum is reflected in Part 2 of the volume. Halle and Touchette in Chapter 4 provide an example of how highly detailed experimental procedures can be translated into an intervention technique that may be used in the wider social environment. These authors review the literature indicating that language intervention programmes conducted in restricted teaching sessions often lead to a failure to generalise to the wider social environment. They argue that the effective response to this state of affairs is the development of techniques that can be used in the natural environment. Drawing on the basic literature from the experimental analysis of behaviour, they describe the development and use of delayed prompting techniques which lead to the learning of specific communicative stimulus-response relations in the natural context in which they were taught. Detailed descriptions and evaluations of studies of the technique and how it is taught to staff are presented. Recommendations on arranging the environment to create language learning opportunities are also offered. Though describing a highly controlled technique in which staff can be trained, this chapter reflects quite specifically the approach to ecological analysis advocated in Landesman-Dwyer and Knowles' Chapter 1.

Also concerned with training staff in specific techniques of language intervention, is Chapter 5 by Robson. This reports the methods and evaluation techniques employed to train teachers in the use of a self-instructional package in Project TASS. The central rationale for the Project was to seek ways in which the already existing research evidence on learning processes in people with mental handicap could be made accessible to teachers. This is done through a comprehensive language course presented to teachers in a handbook and through modelling videotapes. This self-instructional, multi-media package constitutes a "Minicourse". Careful evaluation of the course supports the contention that the minicourse package does assist the teachers involved to acquire the skills and techniques identified as being involved in structured teaching.

Project TASS employed an amalgam of Anderson's Combined Techniques, as did the series of studies of staff training in residential settings reported by Jones, Blunden, Coles, Evans and Porterfield in Chapter 6. In five studies these authors consider: (1) How to establish activity periods in a daycare setting; (2) and (3) The introduction of activity periods to a hospital ward; (4) The introduction of a system of prompts to maintain trained behaviour through minimal intervention procedures; and (5) The introduction of collaborative procedures between staff and clients' families to establish goals and provide feedback. These studies lead to a consideration of self-management by staff, the nature of collaborative development and the role of the supervisor in maintaining trained staff activities.

In Part III of the volume, two projects are reported in which two specific professions, working in two contrasted settings, were trained. Kiernan (Chapter 7) describes a Home Intervention Scheme for fieldwork social workers working with the families of children with mental handicap. Social workers were trained through two courses, A, "The Handicapped Person in the Family", and B, "Educational and Behavioural Approaches to Mental Handicap". Evaluation of the programme suggested that training of the sort described was feasible, with the format of management meetings acceptable and integratable into the normal working day. Similarly, the actual home visits on which the project was dependent for its realisation proved feasible in terms of carrying out general duties during the course of the social workers' day. Overall, the course shows that social service staff can be trained in home teaching, and the course was subsequently integrated into normal service provision.

In contrast, Cullen (Chapter 8) considers nurse training in hospitals for people with mental handicap, in relation to the organisational constraints that affect nurses' implementation of training skills. Cullen reviews the development and present status of nurse training, arguing that however well conceived available courses are, they are fundamentally ineffective in initiating change in hospitals because of a range of environmental and organisation constraints. He describes the assessment and analysis of such constraints, undertaken as part of the Resident's Development Project. He concludes that if the process of caring is to be improved, then there must be serious attempts to change care practices before people with mental handicap leave hospitals. It cannot be assumed that locational change will automatically lead to improved care practices, a conclusion that exemplifies the general points regarding ecological analysis made in the opening chapters of the book.

Part IV focusses on two models of staff training in which wide ranging dissemination is the key issue. In Chapter 9, McBrien and Foxen describe the Education of the Developmentally Young Project. In this, key staff such as Advisors in Special Education, were taught using a variety of combined training techniques to implement a basic course in behavioural methods in their own service settings, particularly schools. Evaluation of the success of the course with the key staff involved in the pyramid training method employed is presented, as well as evidence of the extent and success with which they implemented the EDY Course in their own Local Authorities. Up to 1984, 2,500 people had been trained as the base of the pyramid was broadened, the number now (1986) being closer to 3,000. McBrien and Foxen provide a number of Guidelines on the successful development of this dissemination strategy, covering attitudinal and organisational factors.

Involving an even broader context in which to disseminate staff training, is Linfoot's discussion of distance education. He examines recent developments in the provision of off-campus (distance) training programmes by universities and colleges and how these can lead to additional staff training opportunities for those who work with people with mental handicap. Here the separation of teacher and learner characterises a situation in which technical media are employed to unite them in order to permit the student to undertake the course. Linfoot describes a range of international developments in distance education, listing Universities specialising in this form of dissemination in Canada, People's Republic of China, Costa Rica, Federal Republic of Germany, Israel, Pakistan, Spain, United Kingdom and Venezuela. Detailed accounts of distance teaching in relation to courses on mental handicap are provided for work being undertaken in Australia. With the expansion world wide in services for people with mental handicap and the limited resources available for staff training, Linfoot's chapter points towards an important strategy in the coming years.

Throughout this volume a number of common themes emerge. The wide context of implementation of learnt skills is of critical concern, whether this be the immediate ecology of ward or classroom, or the neighborhood in which a small group is located. The organisational and managerial aspects of the ecology that will permit staff to use the skills they have acquired have to be analysed and modified in their own right. In complementary fashion, however, all papers in the book argue for the training of highly specific skills, typically based in behavioural intervention practices. It is only in the bringing together of context and technique that we will devise appropriate environments that will enhance the abilities and quality of life of people with mental handicap and create the conditions under which they can be effectively integrated into society.

JH and PM
November 1986

Acknowledgements

I would like to thank Linda Dowling for preparing the camera-ready manuscript of this book. This has been a long and arduous task, and she has dealt with the editors' continual requests for change and revision with unfailing good humour.

We are grateful, too, to Christine Houghton for the preparation of the Index.

We would also like to thank the Journal of Applied Behavior Analysis for permission to reproduce Figs 2, 3 and 4 in Chapter 4 of this Volume.

CONTRIBUTORS

ANDERSON S R — Director of Transitional Services
The May Institute
Box 703
100 Sea View Street
CHATHAM
Massachusetts 02633
USA

BLUNDEN R — Director
Mental Handicap in Wales - Applied Research Unit
St David's Hospital
CARDIFF CF1 9TZ

COLES E — Research Officer
Mental Handicap in Wales - Applied Research Unit
St David's Hospital
CARDIFF CF1 9TZ

CULLEN C — SSMH Chair of Learning Difficulties
Psychology Department
The University
ST ANDREWS
Fife KY16 9JU

EVANS G — Research Officer
Mental Handicap in Wales - Applied Research Unit
St David's Hospital
CARDIFF CF1 9TZ

FOXEN T H — Principal Clinical Psychologist
Claypenny Hospital
(York Health Athority)
EASINGWOLD
York YO6 3PR

HALLE J — Associate Professor
Department of Special Education
College of Education
288 Education Building
1310 South Sixth Street
CHAMPAIGN
Illinois 61820
USA

HOGG J	Deputy Director Hester Adrian Research Centre The University MANCHESTER M13 9PL
JONES A A	Department of Clinical Psychology Withington Hospital Nell Lane MANCHESTER M20
KIERNAN C	Director Hester Adrian Research Centre The University MANCHESTER M13 9PL
KNOWLES M	Assistant Professor Department of Psychiatry and Behavioural Sciences Child Development and Mental Retardation Center WJ-10 University of Washington SEATTLE Washington 98195 USA
LINFOOT K	Senior Lecturer in Education Mitchell College of Advanced Education BATHURST New South Wales 2795 Australia
LANDESMAN-DWYER S	Associate Professor Department of Psychiatry and Behavioral Sciences Child Development and Mental Retardation Center WJ-10 University of Washington SEATTLE Washington 98195 USA

McBRIEN J	Principal Clinical Psychologist Plymouth Health Authority Wingfield Mansions Molesworth Road Stoke PLYMOUTH PL3 4EN
MITTLER P J	Professor of Special Education Centre for Educational Guidance and Special Needs Department of Education The University MANCHESTER M13 9PL
PORTERFIELD J	Advisor Joseph Rowntree Memorial Trust c/o Policy Studies Institute 100 Park Village East LONDON NW1 3SR
ROBSON C	Professor Behavioural Sciences Department The Polytechnic Queensgate HUDDERSFIELD West Yorkshire HD1 3DH
TOUCHETTE P E	The Shriver Center 200 Trapelo Road WALTHAM Massachusetts 02254 USA

PART I: STAFF TRAINING/THE BACKGROUND

Chapter One

ECOLOGICAL ANALYSIS OF STAFF TRAINING IN RESIDENTIAL SETTINGS

S. Landesman-Dwyer and M. Knowles

Ecological assessment of staff training means evaluating staff performance within its naturally occurring contexts. The reasons for viewing the effects of staff training in a broad environmental framework are both theoretical and practical. In this chapter, we present a conceptual framework for analysing staff behaviour and its contribution to "quality of life" within a residential setting. We also present a theoretically guided strategy for assessing the effectiveness of staff training, one that considers indirect as well as direct effects, long-term as well as immediate gains, and qualitative as well as quantitative changes in individual staff members, residents, and the collective social environment.

I The Staff-Environment Relationship: Conceptual Issues

Every residential setting has an ambience of its own. In addition, most residential environments for individuals who are mentally handicapped have an extensive set of rules and regulations, both explicit and implicit, as well as a multitude of practical constraints and problems. Many of the practical problems associated with operating programmes in these facilities relate to hiring, training, monitoring, and keeping good staff. These problems often are affected by external political, financial, and social realities, all subject to change. To obtain an ecologically sensitive view of staff behaviour, the <u>social environment</u> in which staff function and the <u>characteristics of staff members</u> must be examined <u>thoroughly</u> - before, during, and

Ecological Analysis

A. The Social Environment

The social environment includes the direct care staff and the recipients of care or services. In many group care environments, however, this set must be enlarged to include supervisors, administrators, specialised professionals, case managers, and advocates. Besides the everyday or intimate social environment within the residence, the social network outside the home needs to be considered. This outside network may encompass friends, neighbours, relatives, and diverse individuals or groups in the local community. Figure 1 displays the social continuum of residential environments, identifying key elements in the social ecology. Each element (person) within the set potentially interacts with every other element. These social relationships may be described in terms of the frequency, intensity, and regularity of contact; the history and duration of the relationship; the qualitative nature of the relationship and the kinds of activities in which the individuals engage when together; and the personal satisfaction or perceived consequences associated with each relationship. These person-specific relationships within the social set may vary significantly in the extent to which they influence the ambience or quality of life within a given home.

Global features of the social environment also provide valuable information for depicting the social ecology of a residential setting. Examples of global features known to affect day-to-day quality of life are:

(1) the goals or mission of a given residence (e.g., as expressed in policy statements or employee orientation regarding the expected type of staff-resident relationships, the emphasis on independence training for residents, the nature and frequency of community integration activities, etc.);

(2) the internal organisation of the social set, including both formal and informal lines of authority or control among individuals or classes of individuals;

(3) the size and stability of the social organisation;

(4) the heterogeneity of the social group (e.g., in

Figure 1: The Social Environment of Residential Facilities

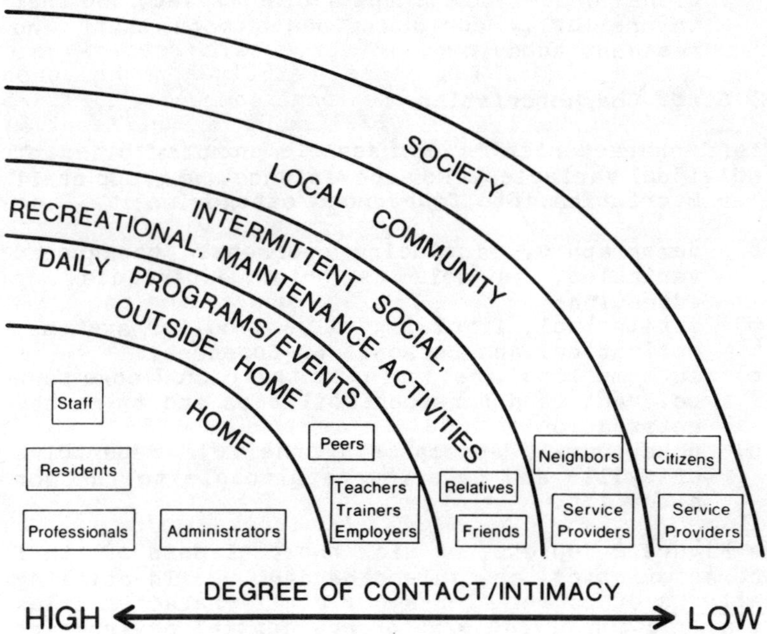

terms of prior residential experience, age, developmental level, behavioural and medical needs of residents or the demographic and attitudinal characteristics of staff members);

(5) the density of highly qualified,trained staff. Staff-resident ratio is another example of a global descriptor of the social milieu, one that theoretically could influence both staff and resident behaviour.

B. Staff Characteristics

Staff characteristics represent a complex class of individual variables. For convenience, we group staff characteristics into four broad categories:

(a) demographic, including personal background variables, as well as prior experience and education;
(b) attitudinal, involving values, belief systems, motivation, and personal preferences;
(c) informational, referring to their knowledge base relevant to job responsibilities and to mental retardation;
(d) behavioural, encompassing the full repertoire of skills and behaviour applicable to the job situation.

As Figure 2 depicts, we view these classes of staff characteristics as interdependent. Identifying patterns of correlation among staff characteristics as a function of the type of residential environment may be useful in exploring the functional consequences of particular combinations of staff variables. Similarly, idiographic analyses could provide an opportunity to identify atypical staff profiles - such as staff from a given background who deviate in their attitudes or behaviour, relative to their peers - and to assess such profiles in relation to staff performance.

The literature relating staff characteristics to actual staff behaviour in residential environments is scant - and not considerably expanded from that of two decades ago (Butterfield, 1967) despite the dramatic changes in provision of community-based residential programmes (Bruininks, Meyers, Sigford, and Lakin, 1981; Landesman-Dwyer, 1981). More importantly, no substantial theory has been proposed

Figure 2: Staff Characteristics and Behaviour

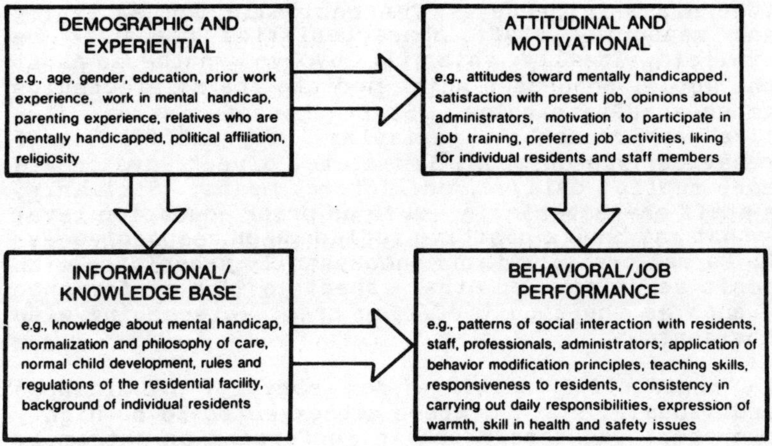

regarding the relationship of staff characteristics to job-related behaviour, although some ideas have been advanced concerning what contributes to job tenure or staff turnover (cf. Baumeister and Zaharia, in press) and to staff commitment and burnout (Cherniss, in press). The rationale for selecting and measuring staff characteristics needs to be explicit. Ideally, this will involve hypotheses about the actual processes which mediate the relationships among staff variables. Staff characteristics, just like environmental variables, may affect staff behaviour via obvious, immediate, direct ways or via more subtle, delayed, or indirect means. Similarly, a staff characteristic - such as prior education level - that may have a positive influence on responsiveness to formal training is not necessarily associated with positive effects on other aspects of job performance - such as the amount of time spent interacting with residents.

In residential settings for mentally handicapped individuals, staff members are expected to be highly competent and consistent in performing an extremely diverse set of skills, probably even greater in number and degree of specialisation than those involved in parenting or teaching non-handicapped persons. Because staff performance is likely to vary across skill areas (e.g., a person who is outstanding in his/her ability to carry out a behaviour modification programme may not be equally adept in solving unanticipated crises or in expressing spontaneous warmth and affection toward residents), it is unlikely that any simple pattern of individual characteristics will emerge to identify "optimal care providers". What is needed is a theory-based <u>functional explanation</u> of why certain staff characteristics are likely to be associated with differential job performance or responsiveness to staff training. For example, <u>if</u> older staff members were observed to interact more frequently with residents than were younger staff members, a number of questions arise regarding the reason for this. Are older individuals more social generally? More willing to interact with handicapped clients? More conscientious in fulfilling their job responsibilities than are younger individuals? Or is the variable of chronological age simply confounded with other variables, such as prior parenting experience or stronger religious beliefs about all human life? Correctly identifying which beliefs and behaviour best account for observed differences among staff members can lead to more effective strategies for promoting desired staff-client interactions, as well as prevent implementation of overly simplistic "solutions" (e.g., preferentially hiring older individuals without adequately evaluating the important behavioural qualities correlated with age).

C. Changes in Staff Performance

In our ecological paradigm for understanding staff behaviour, changes in staff behaviour theoretically can occur by altering the social environment, by modifying staff characteristics, or by a combination of both approaches. Since the topic of this volume is staff training, we will focus on the use of training technology to produce positive staff behaviour. Given our assumptions, however, about the fundamental interdependence of the social environment and the behaviour of staff (see section on "Basic assumptions" below), we do not posit that staff training is necessarily the best (i.e., most comprehensive, efficient, and durable) means for improving programme quality in all residential facilities. Quite the contrary, for some social environments, we predict that altering the individual social elements or their relationships to one another would be as effective or more so than would staff training. Even an excellent training programme that demonstrably changes staff's attitudes, motivation, knowledge base, and/or practical skills could fail to produce long term benefits for residents if the social environment does not adequately support these staff changes. At present, the belief in the value of training staff is so strong that most training programmes are designed and implemented without a careful analysis of their probable effects on the actual residential environment (Ziarnik and Bernstein, 1982). An example of such an analysis would be to estimate the cost:benefit ratio over a given period of time for training individual staff members versus providing other forms of assistance that indirectly may change staff behaviour (e.g., re-structuring the programme, altering the social composition of the staff or clients, providing new physical resources that could influence staff activities, or offering incentives for staff to behave in specified ways). Because the perceived need to provide staff training is so high, we propose an ecological or contextual assessment model to maximise understanding the influences of staff members, residents and programmes.

D. Types of Effects

Direct versus indirect effects.

Throughout the chapter, we use the terms "direct" and "indirect" to capture what we might label variously as primary versus secondary, expected versus unexpected, immediate versus delayed, or obvious versus subtle effects. If a given training programme results in significantly improved staff morale, the source of this outcome needs to be determined. Did the training programme directly deal with issues of staff morale? Were skills taught that theoretically would strengthen positive job-related attitudes? Alternatively, did staff morale improve simply because participants had time away from the difficult everyday responsibilities or took advantage of the opportunity to exchange information with trainees from other residential settings, which in turn influenced their attitudes about their job? Did trainees learn new behavioural techniques from other participants (e.g., during informal discussions)? A contextual evaluation of the change in staff morale might reveal that the improvement in morale resulted largely from a particularly negative staff member having left, which may have been an indirect result of staff training (e.g., that employee may have realised during training how unhappy or poorly suited he/she was to the job setting; alternatively, other staff members may have exerted pressure on this employee to change his/her behaviour, which in turn led to his/her resignation). The departure of this particular staff member may have influenced the morale of those who remained in the original setting; in addition, the person replacing this employee may have been an exceptionally positive, competent person who immediately influenced the morale of other staff members. The number of plausible indirect effects is large. The point is that the complexity and interdependencies inherent in these residential care settings need to be recognised when evaluating the outcome of staff training. The ecological evaluation procedures we use involve collecting information that theoretically is sensitive to both direct and indirect effects (such as those identified above), relying on multiple sources of information to maximise detecting important indirect effects.

Immediate versus long-term effects.

In the model we propose, long-term effects are treated as distinct from short-term effects. In contrast to a theory that assumes long-term effects are a straightforward retention or extension of what is initially learned during staff training, we hypothesise that different factors influence the initial acquisition versus longer term expression and maintenance of new staff knowledge, attitudes, and behaviour. Almost all staff training programmes seek to foster permanent, positive changes in staff's actual job performance. Analysing the determinants of long-term effects, as well as those related to immediate outcomes, is critical.

Qualitative versus quantitative effects.

Distinctions between qualitative and quantitative aspects of residential programmes are not clearly delineated in the literature (Landesman-Dwyer, 1985). In practice, the terms often serve as rough substitutes for "subjective" versus "objective" or for personal impressions versus formally measured aspects of programmes. We conceptualise these terms somewhat differently than this. We use qualitative to reference the ways in which programmes operate, the types of social interactions that occur, the kinds of behaviour staff exhibit, etc. Such qualitative differences may be descriptive, evaluative, or both. For example, qualitative differences between two residential facilities may include differences in type of administrative style (e.g., authoritarian, authoritative, democratic), treatment philosophy (e.g., medical model, developmental model, behaviour modification model), and geographical location (inner city, suburban, rural). These typify descriptive differences. An independent evaluation or judgement could be made regarding the actual quality of administration, treatment, or neighbourhood location, irrespective of type. That is, the administration could be judged along a continuum of overall effectiveness, just as the quality of treatment provided could be rated along a continuum from high to low or location could be evaluated as more or less integrated into a typical residential neighbourhood.

Quantitative variables include absolute and relative values (e.g., absolute frequencies versus proportions) that reflect systematic, numerically meaningful measurement obtained on some aspect of a residential programme. Examples of quantitative variables include the total time staff and residents spend in social interaction, the proportion of leisure time residents spend in social versus solitary activities, how long residents have lived in a home, the number of staff who demonstrate a particular behaviour, the ratio of resident - versus management-oriented activities, etc. Standard quantitative variables in studies of residential environments are the number of residents, the number of direct-care staff, the frequency of contact with individuals outside the home, staff and resident turnover rates, staff absenteeism, and the annual per capita cost of residential services. Although such variables appear to be quite straightforward, the actual computational procedures used vary tremendously.[1]

Both qualitative and quantitative approaches provide important information. Unfortunately, these terms have acquired connotations that we think are misleading. Qualitative and quantitative measures do not inherently differ in terms of how precise, concrete, objective, valid, easy to gather, or powerful they are. Rather, they represent different measurement strategies: one yields data more suitable for non-parametric analysis and descriptive summarisation, while the other provides information appropriate for parametric study, consistent with general assumptions underlying modern mathematical probability theories. We view quantitative measures as capable of indexing vital, warm, sensitive aspects of residential environments. Similarly, qualitative variables can refer to valid, circumscribed, and concrete facts. We strongly endorse the use of both kinds of measures to assess residential settings.

II A Theory-based Strategy for Ecological Assessment of Staff Training

A. A Model for Contextual Evaluation

1. Basic assumptions.

Our model involves five basic premises about staff-environment relations.

(i) Staff behaviour is affected, both directly and indirectly, by the social environment in which it occurs.

This implies that the behaviour of staff members is not simply a function of their skill level and commitment to the job, but also is influenced by the behaviour and expectations of others in that environment. This fundamental interdependence between individual staff members and their social millieu is the central feature of our social ecological model. The ways in which the social environment influences staff performance are admittedly complex, and include (1) bidirectional effects (i.e., a single environmental variable may have both positive and negative effects on staff), (2) interaction effect (i.e., the specific effect of a given environmental variable may be altered by the presence of one or more other variables), and (3) unrecognised influences (i.e., those not detected consciously by the participants in a given environment). The challenge is to demonstrate empirically the nature and strength of specific associations between the social environment and staff performance measures.

(ii) Staff characteristics contribute significantly to - and in some ways are inseparable from - the social environment.

The staff play a vital role in creating and maintaining the residential environment. The behavioural style, skills, attitudes, and personal preferences of staff members influence the ways in which they fulfil their job responsibilities. In residential settings, direct care staff assume a primary role in the daily social life of residents, from their interactions with residents, to fostering peer relationships, to providing opportunities for social activities in the larger community. General features of the social environment, such as staff morale and quality of communication between administrators and direct care staff, are affected in part by the personalities and past experiences of the individual staff members. This interdependency between the environment and the characteristics of the staff is demonstrated easily, yet often is overlooked in studies of staff behaviour. Even changes in physical environments can be modified significantly by those who live and work there (Knight, Weitzer and Zimring, 1978; Landesman-Dwyer,

1984; in press a).

(iii) Staff attitudes and behaviour are dynamic, rather than static, features.

This assumption has two important corollaries. The first is that staff attitudes and behaviour are amenable to change. The second is that staff attitudes and behaviour must be measured on multiple occasions, over time, to provide a valid evaluation of staff.

(iv) Staff training represents an important avenue for promoting positive changes in staff, which in turn may influence the overall social ecology of residential environments and the quality of life for individual residents.

Within this conceptual framework, the success of staff training can be determined only if staff performance is studied and analysed within its ecological context.

(v) Staff behaviour directly influences the quality of life for mentally handicapped residents.

Because staff members assume the primary responsibility for managing the programmes and activities within a residence, and because they often set the tone and level for social interactions and opportunities, they exert a powerful effect on the everyday life of residents. Many other individuals and circumstances also contribute to the residents' quality of life - such as the peer group and the social and physical resources in the surrounding community. What is important for the proposed model is the assumption that important changes in staff behaviour will result in measurable changes in resident behaviour.

2. **Formal hypotheses**.

The formal hypotheses we propose to guide evaluating staff training incorporate the fundamental ecological assumptions discussed above. We have integrated these hypotheses in a two-stage model that predicts somewhat different determinants of (or influences on) immediate versus long-term effects of staff training.

We hypothesise that the initial or immediate effects of staff training will be a function of four primary aspects of the training programme:

(i) how <u>relevant</u> the trainees perceive the content of the training programme to be, ("subjective relevance").

(ii) how <u>applicable</u> the new knowledge, skills, and/or attitudes will be to the actual job situation, as estimated by external review of the training curriculum and the job demands, ("objectively validated relevance").

(iii) the <u>effectiveness of the presentation format and style</u> - that is, how clearly the content of training is conveyed; whether the information is delivered in a manner appropriate to the entry level of knowledge of the participants and sensitive to the values and attitudes of the trainees; the extent to which practical applications are demonstrated etc. The role of the trainers or teachers is critical here.

(iv) the amount of <u>opportunity</u> provided for trainees to study, practise, and explore the new concepts and skills presented; to evaluate their own progress during training (intensity of exposure and active engagement in the learning process); and to receive individual follow-up in how effectively they can apply their new knowledge to their day-to-day work environment (individualised feedback, ("trainee specific learning opportunities").

The longer term effects of training - as detected in observable improvement in staff job performance, more frequent and appropriate patterns of social interaction, and increased opportunities for both staff and residents to derive satisfaction from their environment - will be influenced in part by the training programme elements listed above. We hypothesise that a somewhat different set of variables, however, assumes primary importance in determining the longer term changes associated with staff training.

Specifically, we predict that <u>longer term effects are influenced most strongly by three key environmental features</u>:

(i) the degree to which the demands of the job are consistent with or complement the goals of the staff training programme.

(ii) the density of trained staff - that is, the proportion of employees within a given setting who share similar knowledge, attitudes, and behavioural skills.

(iii) the appropriateness and importance of the staff training goals for the particular environment in which staff work, taking into account the needs and abilities of residents, as well as the broader administrative and social context in which a residential facility operates. This latter variable, similar to that labelled "objectively validated relevance" above, can be measured by the degree to which the goals of staff training address the major weaknesses or problems in the social ecology, build upon the natural strengths or advantages in the environment, and seek to provide residential programmes adapted to the actual needs and preferences of the individual staff and residents.

3. **Summary of model**.

Figure 3 schematically represents the relationships among the major groups of variables in our model. To summarise, this contextual evaluation model is predicated on a set of fundamental assumptions about the interdependence among social ecological variables, staff characteristics, actual staff performance, and residents' quality of life and developmental achievements. Initially, changes in staff as a result of participation in a training programme will be related to specific aspects of the training programme itself, as interpreted subjectively by the trainees and objectively by formal criteria. Subsequently, the degree to which the job environment supports the goals of training - via implicit and explicit job demands, support from other knowledgeable (trained) staff, and demonstrated utility of the training materials to the residential environment - will influence the long-term success of the programme. The success of staff training - i.e., the strength and durability of training-related changes in staff performance - is predicted to be a function of the degree to which these elements are present. Some independence between short-term and long-term effects is hypothesised, leading to the

Figure 3: General Schematic Model for Ecological Assessment of Staff Training Practices

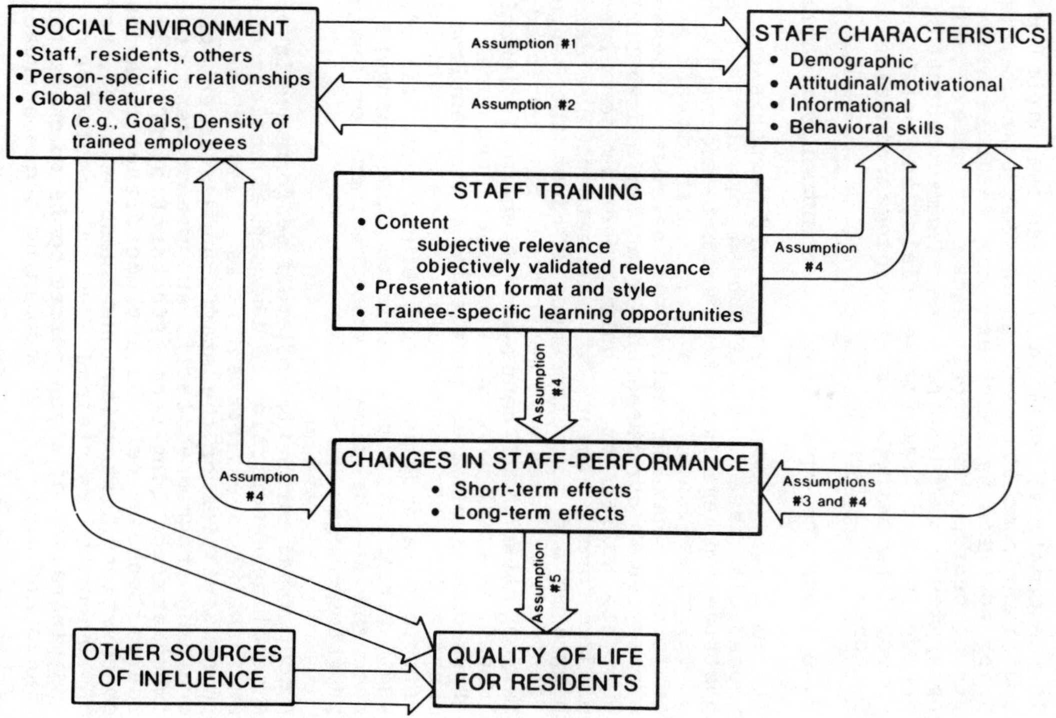

prediction that some longer term benefits could emerge in a delayed manner, even when short-term gains appear only minimal. This could occur as a result of major changes in the density of trained staff, shifts in job demands that better match the goals of the staff training programme, changes in residents served (e.g., making techniques learned during training more relevant to the new group of residents), etc.

At the practical level, a thorough evaluation of the social environment as well as of staff characteristics prior to training is viewed as a valuable means for strengthening the relevance of the training programme, influencing the format adopted for presenting the training materials, and establishing appropriate methods for providing trainee-specific feedback.

B. Methods for Conducting a Contextual Evaluation

In our own research and field experiences, we repeatedly have been astounded by changes, both positive and negative, that were not expected to occur as a consequence of a particular treatment or training. Had we relied on narrower assessment strategies in our research - that is, had we limited our data collection to only objective descriptions of the formal aspects of a treatment or training programme and to measurement of just the targeted (desired) outcomes - we never could have detected the larger pattern of cause-and-effect relationships. Indeed, we would have made some incorrect conclusions about the merits of particular interventions, by missing important beneficial or detrimental side-effects of a programme or by simply not identifying what variables truly mediated the changes that occurred at the time a new treatment or training programme began.

A contextual evaluation of staff performance involves a baseline description of the social ecology of the residential environment as well as the characteristics of the staff, an assessment of the training programme itself, and measurement of both immediate and long-term effects of staff training. The methods we rely on include direct behavioural observations, interviews and questionnaires, review of records maintained by a residence, and administration of standardised tools to characterise places and people. By combining these approaches, we maximise the opportunities to consider the validity and reliability of data from diverse sources and to detect important qualitative, indirect, and interactive effects.

1. Using behavioural observations for contextual evaluation.

Historically, ethnographic research was one of the few empirical approaches that afforded a wide-angled view of an entire social unit, acknowledging the validity of combining objective (external impressions) and subjective (insiders' perspectives) data. We believe that the use of participant observation, as formally conceived by the discipline of anthropology, provides a valuable means for studying the complex patterns of interactions between people and their residential environments. A recent monograph edited by Edgerton (1984) provides excellent examples of this type of research and the sensitive insights that can be derived from ethnographic field notes.

Over the past decade, we have explored the application of highly structured, quantitative behavioural observation as a reliable means for describing and evaluating the quality of residential services or the effects of staff training (for methodological papers, see Sackett and Landesman-Dwyer, 1977; Sackett and Landesman-Dwyer, 1982; Sackett, Landesman-Dwyer, and Morin, 1981; for examples of application from our research centre, see Landesman-Dwyer, in press a; Landesman-Dwyer, and G. Butterfield, 1983; Landesman-Dwyer, Stein, and Sackett, 1978; Schinke and Landesman-Dwyer, 1981). We have been concerned as well, along with many of our colleagues, about how to provide an informative evaluation of the residential environment itself (see Landesman-Dwyer, 1985; in press b; Landesman-Dwyer, and G. Butterfield, 1983).

There are many strategies for collecting observational data. If the primary purpose is to provide a general portrayal of the social climate and staff activities, the coding system itself must consist of categories that are mutually exclusive and exhaustive. This means that a single behavioural event cannot be coded as more than one behaviour, and every behavioural event must be scored; otherwise estimates of the proportion of occurrence will be distorted. The multidimensional nature of a single behavioural event, however, can be preserved.

For instance, the Home Observation code (Landesman-Dwyer and Watts, 1979) is a multidimensional scoring system that dimensionalises a subject's behaviour into seven separate aspects. Specifically, an observer codes the behaviour of a focal subject in terms of

(i) the major activity in which the subject is engaged,

(ii) type of vocal or physical-gestural communication occurring,

(iii) the physical proximity to other individuals,

(iv) the type of affective expression (emotional tone),

(v) with whom the subject is interacting,

(vi) who initiated the social exchange, and

(vii) the nature of stereotyped or bizarre aspects of the behaviour (if applicable).

All seven dimensions of behaviour are coded each time a subject is observed. Based on an intensive methodological study, a three-minute observation period was selected, with the subject's behaviour observed and coded once every 30 seconds throughout the period. During a month, a minimum of 16 three-minute sessions per subject (i.e. 288 separate observations), distributed across morning, afternoon, and evening hours, is needed to yield a reliable behavioural profile of activities in a group residential environment for severely and profoundly retarded individuals. When the codes within any one dimension (column) are converted to percentages (frequency of each code divided by the total number of behavioural entries for a given subject), they always add to 100. By having an exhaustive coding system that is, scoring all behavioural events rather than only the presence of a few selected behaviours a true profile of the distribution of activities and social exchanges can be generated. In addition, antecedents and consequences of particular behavioural codes can be identified, as well as calculations of changes in both relative (percentage)and absolute amounts of certain behaviour.

Other important considerations in selecting or constructing an objective behavioural coding system are:

i) demonstrated inter-observer reliability, determined at repeated intervals to assess possible observer drift;

ii) a rational or empirical basis for selecting the coding interval, the length of the observation session, the sampling of contexts and times for gathering data, and the total amount of observation per subject or per living unit;

iii) procedures to minimise common sources of scoring bias, such as unequal assignment of certain observers to certain subjects, differential timing for observing certain subjects (often associated with their participation in activities outside the home) which could distort the profiles obtained for these subjects, or seasonal effects. See Sackett (1978) for a good introduction to many of these methodological issues.

An example of a considerably different approach to gathering observational data is that of a group coding strategy. We developed a code for residential and school environments in which the behaviour of all subjects is coded during a single, brief interval. The behavioural codes are entered onto a map of the physical environment, first coding the subject's identification number then entering a numerical code to capture key aspects of the ongoing behaviour.[2] Social interactions and their direction are indicated with arrows; groups of individuals participating in a common activity are circled. The time of day and other environmental information about what is occurring are included in the pre-trial data set for each group observation. This system generates a rich data set and provides a fairly simple method for gathering data on many individuals. In fact, supervisors and direct care staff themselves have learned this code within a few hours, and have used the technique for gathering their own systematic assessment of who is where and doing what at different times of the day, days of the week, etc.

A strategy such as group coding can be readily adapted to include training-specific information about staff behaviour and its anticipated effects on the activities of residents or other staff members. Recently, we modified this code for use in a large residential facility where direct care staff and management had a major dispute about staff responsibilities and about how much time staff invested in direct habilitation and interaction with residents. By gathering the subjective perceptions of both direct care staff and management, plus directly observing major activities and specified staff functions, the dispute was minimised and a constructive plan of correct, staff training, and job upgrading has been developed.

2. **Standardised environmental instruments.**

Standardised tools to describe the environment tend to be limited in scope, and are often not related closely to the objectives of staff training. Most of these instruments lack adequate reliability and validity data or comparative norms. There are, however, situations in which such instruments are suitable for measuring selected aspects of the social and physical environment. The most frequently used tools are the Revised Resident Management Practices Scale (King, Raynes, and Tizard, 1971; Raynes, Pratt, and Roses, 1979), the Moos Ward Atmosphere Scale and the Family Environment Scale (Moos, 1974 a, b), the Jackson Characteristics of the Treatment Environment (Jackson, 1969), the Wolfensberger and Glenn (1975) PASS-3, and the Caldwell Home Observation for Measurement of the Environment (HOME) (Bradley and Caldwell, 1977). Unlike tests of intelligence or adaptive behaviour, these environmental instruments were not designed to provide an estimate of a common trait or set of traits hypothesised to characterise residential environments. The HOME, for example, was designed to measure aspects of cognitive and social stimulation in the homes of very young children. The HOME scores predict children's subsequent performance on standardised intelligence tests (Elardo, Bradley, and Caldwell, 1975). In contrast, the Resident Management Scale initially characterised different hospital and community residential environments, primarily in terms of block treatment of residents, regimentation in daily routine, and opportunities for individual choice. Whether these items still have discriminative power is not certain, given the dramatic changes in treatment philosophy and residential environments over the past two decades.

A cautionary note is warranted here: Environments judged "good" according to one instrument may not be evaluated similarly by another tool. In a longitudinal study of 37 residential environments, we discovered that living units judged as highly institutional according to the Resident Management Scale were not necessarily the lowest in cognitive stimulation, as estimated by the HOME (Landesman-Dwyer, 1984, in press a). Interestingly, in the new small living units, the management practices differed so dramatically from those observed in the old institutional wards that the Resident Management Practices Scale no longer captured important differences between the living units. Nonetheless, our behavioural and qualitative data indicate that significant differences in day-to-day treatment of residents did occur - the instrument simply did not include items relevant to these new settings. This underscores the need to gather data from multiple perspectives.

PASS-3 represents a different type of assessment tool, guided entirely by the authors' values and interpretation of "normalisation ideology". The validity of the assumptions guiding the construction of this instrument has not been tested systematically (e.g., activities and interactions among peers of handicapped individuals are scored negatively, while those involving non-handicapped persons are scored positively - regardless of any evidence about the value of these social contacts as perceived by the participants or as observed by external criteria). Many programme evaluators have adopted this tool as one means of measuring the effectiveness of training staff about normalisation ideology. Although this seems reasonable, care must be exerted to gather concurrent data from other sources about the social and adaptive development of residents in programmes judged more or less "normalised".

3. User-specific environmental assessment.

We prefer to conduct ecological assessments with

descriptive tools that directly measure aspects of the treatment environment that are compatible with the goals of the programme. We have two guiding methodological principles when we generate such tools. First, we always measure important features of the environment from both an objective and a subjective perspective. Second, we also gather the subjective information from multiple informants - a minimum of two individuals who know the environment well and who theoretically may have different values and attitudes or may have access to information about different aspects of the environment. Whenever possible, we have the subjective ratings completed by the following individuals: at least two direct care workers in the home, by an administrator or supervisor (if applicable), by a case manager or professional outside the home who knows the client(s), by a parent or relative of the client(s), by an outside professional who has had no prior contact with the home, and by members of our research staff. Although gathering opinions from so many informants may seem cumbersome, the data analysis is not difficult. Far more importantly, we view the discrepancies or differences in subjective opinions as potentially valuable data in themselves, potentially identifying problems in the functional relationships among the social participants in a given environment. At the same time, we continue to remain sensitive to the different values and expertise represented by these informants. Each person has differential access to first-hand information about what occurs within a home, which can increase the validity of conclusions about the effects of staff training programmes.

In a recent study (Landesman-Dwyer and Butterfield, 1983) of 18 specialised group homes that serve severely and profoundly retarded individuals, we developed an environmental rating instrument that concerned seven different aspects of the residential programme.

Specifically, the dimensions rated (on a four-point scale from "very strong" to "very weak") were:

(i) the perceived quality of staff,

(ii) the degree to which training in the home encourages independence in the residents,

(iii) the attention provided to health needs,

(iv) the quality of social and leisure activities in the home,

(v) the pursuit of diverse recreational and social activities in the local community,

(vi) the quality of personal space and privacy within the group home,

(vii) the suitability of common living/working areas within the home.

This rating scale was completed by two direct care providers, the administrator, a parent or relative, a case manager (the person assigned from the state agency to coordinate community-based services for mentally retarded individuals), trainers or teachers from the community day programmes that served a home's residents, two visiting professionals not affiliated with the programme, and two trained research assistants. (Because more than 60 per cent of the residents were non-verbal and had IQs below 35, we did not ask residents to provide ratings. Issues related to interviewing of mentally retarded persons are discussed by Sigelman, et al., (1981) and Wyngaarden (1981).) The use of multiple informants proved to be a valuable means for measuring the strength of a programme, its inconsistencies, and problems associated with communication about and coordination of services.

III SUMMARY

Staff performance represents a complex and changing pattern of behaviour that is influenced by the surrounding social environment, the personal characteristics of the staff, and training and supervision provided to staff. To study the effects of a particular staff training programme, a contextual evaluation of staff performance needs to be conducted prior to implementing the training, followed by assessment of the immediate and longer term outcomes of training.

In this chapter, we have described a model of staff training effects. We posit that the effectiveness of staff training programmes will be a function of how well matched their content is to the actual and perceived needs of staff in a given residential setting. In addition, the individual characteristics of staff members are predicted to influence their willingness and ability to learn from particular training methods (presentation format) and the amount of trainee-specific learning opportunities (e.g., practice and direct feedback) they will need to learn new skills, attitudes, or formal knowledge. General environmental variables - most notably, the number (density) or other trained or highly competent, motivated staff and the stability of the social environment - are hypothesised to be important in determining the extent to which staff will benefit from training, as reflected in their everyday job-related behaviour.

This ecological model is highly compatible with the traditional behaviour modification paradigm in which reinforcement to staff is viewed as important for changing their behaviour. What differs is our relative emphasis on the total environment and the complexity of the individual and environmental variables - as measured from both objective and subjective perspectives - that interact to determine the outcomes of staff training. Opportunities to receive reinforcement for desired staff behaviour may come from multiple, diverse sources, including other staff members, supervisors and professionals, residents and their family members, neighbours and others in the community, and from <u>self-evaluation</u>. Formal rewards for improved staff performances also offer another environmental source of reinforcement - i.e., strengthening the probability that what is learned during staff training will result in a demonstrable improvement in the quality of life provided for those who live and work in a given environment. Gathering a rich, descriptive contextual evaluation requires applying principles of sound scientific design, data collection, and analysis. The investment in this effort yields a data set that addresses central questions related to direct versus indirect influences, qualitative versus quantitative changes, and short-term versus long-term effects related to staff training. Given the time and cost invested in staff training programmes, and their potential for improving the services provided to mentally handicapped persons, careful evaluation of their impact is warranted.

1 There are significant differences between staff-

resident ratios as they are computed by different methods. Most investigators employ the number of assigned staff or full-time equivalents without taking into account the functional presence of staff as affected by absenteeism or by the amount of time staff spend performing tasks which do not involve direct service to residents. What appears to be a rich staffing schedule may constitute a shortage of staff, depending on one's method of computation. As part of the behavioural observations in our research, we code the number of staff and residents actually present in the room at the time of observation in order to determine the functional ratio of staff to residents.

2 Copies of the Group Residential Code are available upon request from the first author.

REFERENCES

Baumeister, A. and Zaharia, E. (in press) 'Withdrawal and Commitment to Basic Care Staff in Residential Programs' in S. Landesman-Dwyer and P. Vietze (eds.), Living With Retarded People, American Association on Mental Deficiency, Washington, D.C.

Bradley, R. and Caldwell, B. (1977) 'Home Observation for Measurement of the Environment: A Validation Study of Screening Efficiency', American Journal on Mental Deficiency, 81, 417-420

Bruininks, R.H., Meyers, C.E., Sigford, B. B. and Lakin, K. C. (eds.) (1981) Deinstitutionalization and Community Adjustment of Mentally Retarded People: (Monograph No. 4), American Association on Mental Deficiency, Washington, D.C.

Butterfield, E. (1967) 'The Characteristics, Selection and Training of Institution Personnel', in A.A. Baumeister (ed.), Mental Retardation, Aldine Publishing Co., Chicago

Caldwell, B. (1979) Home Observation for Measurement of the Environment. Preschool Version: Instruction Manual, University of Arkansas, The Center for Child Development and Education, Little Rock

Cherniss, C. (in press) 'Staff Burnout: Too Much Stress or Too Little Commitment?' in S. Landesman-Dwyer and P. Vietze (eds.), Living with Retarded People, American Association on Mental Deficiency, Washington D.C.

Edgerton, R.B. (ed.) (1984) Lives in Process: Mildly Retarded Adults in a Large City, (Monograph No. 6), The American Association on Mental Deficiency, Washington, D.C.

Elardo, R., Bradley, R. and Caldwell, B. (1975) 'The Relation of Infants' Home Environments to Mental Test Performance from Six to Thirty-six Months: A Longitudinal Analysis', Child Development, 46, 71-76

Jackson, J. (1969) 'Factors of the Treatment Environment', Archives of General Psychiatry, 21 39-45

King, R.D., Raynes, N.V. and Tizard, J. (1971) Patterns of Residential Care, Routledge & Kegan Paul, London

Knight, R., Weitzer, W. and Zimring, C. (1978) Opportunity for Control and the Built Environment: The ELEMR Project, The Environmental Institute, Amherst, MA.

Landesman-Dwyer, S. (1981) 'Living in the Community', American Journal of Mental Deficiency, 86, 223-234

Landesman-Dwyer, S. (1984) 'Residential Environments and the Social Behavior of Handicapped Individuals' in M. Lewis (ed.), Beyond the Dyad, Plenum Press, New York

Landesman-Dwyer, S. (1985) 'Describing and Evaluating Residential Environments' in R.H. Bruininks and K.C. Lakin (eds.), Living and Learning in the Least Restrictive Environment, Paul H. Brookes, Baltimore

Landesman-Dwyer, S. (in press a) 'The Changing Structure and Function of Institutions: A Search for Optimal Group Care Environments' in S. Landesman-Dwyer and P. Vietze (eds.), Living with Retarded People, American Association on Mental Deficiency, Washington, D.C.

Landesman-Dwyer, S. (in press b) 'Toward a Taxonomy of Home Environments' in N.R. Ellis and N.W. Bray (eds.), International Review of Research in Mental Retardations, (Vol. 14) Academic Press, New York

Landesman-Dwyer, S. and Butterfield, E. (1983) 'Mental Retardation: Developmental Issues in Cognitive and Social Adaptation' in M. Lewis (ed.), Origins of Intelligence: Infancy and Early Childhood (2nd ed.), Plenum Press, New York

Landesman-Dwyer, S. and Butterfield, G. (1983) Evaluation of Specialized Group Homes for Developmentally Disabled Persons, Department of Social and Health Services, Olympia, WA

Landesman-Dwyer, S., Stein, J.G. and Sackett, G.P. (1978) 'A Behavioral and Ecological Study of Group Homes' in G.P. Sackett (ed.), Observing Behavior, Volume I: Theory and Application in Mental Retardation, University Park Press, Baltimore

Landesman-Dwyer, S. and Watts, G. (1979) Manual for Behavioral Observations of Severely and Profoundly Retarded Individuals, Department of Social and Health Services, Olympia, WA.

Moos, R. (1974a) Evaluating Treatment Environments: A Social Ecological Approach, Wiley, New York

Moos, R. (1974b) Ward Atmosphere Scale: Manual, Consulting Psychologists Press, Palo Alto

Raynes, N.V., Pratt, M.W. and Roses, S. (1979) Organisational Structure and the Care of the Mentally Retarded, Croom Helm, London

Sackett, G.P. (ed.) (1978) Observing Behavior, Vol. 2: Data Collection and Analysis Methods, University Park Press, Baltimore

Sackett, G.P. and Landesman-Dwyer, S. (1977) 'Toward an Ethology of Mental Retardation: Quantitative Behavioral Observation in Residential Services' in P. Mittler (ed.), Research to Practice in Mental Retardation, Vol II: Education and Training, University Park Press, Baltimore

Sackett, G.P., Landesman-Dwyer, S. and Morin, V.N. (1981) 'Naturalistic Observation in Design and

Evaluation of Special Education Programs' in T.R. Kratochwill (ed.), Advances in School Psychology, Volume I, Lawrence Erlbaum, Hillsdale, N.J.

Sackett, G.P. and Landesman-Dwyer, S. (1982) 'Data Analysis: Methods and Problems' in D.P. Hartmann (ed.), Using Observers to Study Behavior, New Directions for Methodology of Behavioral Sciences, No. 14, Jossey-Bass, San Francisco

Schinke, S.P. and Landesman-Dwyer, S. (1981) 'Training Staff in Group Homes Serving Mentally Retarded Persons' in P. Mittler (ed.), Frontiers of Knowledge in Mental Retardation, Volume I: Social, Educational, and Behavioral Aspects, University Park Press, Baltimore

Sigelman, C.K., Schoenrock, C.J., Winer, J.L., Spanhel, C.L., Hromas, S.G., Martin, P.W., Budd, E.C. and Bensberg, G.J. (1981) 'Issues in Interviewing Mentally Retarded Persons: An Empirical Study' in R.H. Bruininks, C.E. Meyers, B.B. Sigford, and K.C. Lakin (eds.), Deinstitutionalization and Community Adjustment of Mentally Retarded People, (Monograph No. 4), American Association on Mental Deficiency, Washington, D.C.

Wolfensberg, W. and Glenn, L. (1975) PASS 3: A Method for the Quantitative Evaluation of Human Services, National Institute on Mental Retardation, Toronto

Wyngaarden, M. (1981) 'Interviewing Mentally Retarded Persons: Issues and Strategies' in R.H. Bruininks, C.E. Meyers, B.B. Sigford, and K.C. Lakin (eds.), Deinstitutionalization and Community Adjustment of Mentally Retarded People (Monograph No. 4), American Association on Mental Deficiency, Washington, D.C.

Ziarnik, J.P. and Bernstein, G.S. (1982) 'A Critical Examination of the Effect of Inservice Training on Staff Performance', Mental Retardation, 20, 109-144

Chapter Two

STAFF DEVELOPMENT: CHANGING NEEDS AND SERVICE CONTEXTS IN BRITAIN

P.J. Mittler

Introduction

Imagine a young person starting to work in the field of mental handicap this year. What kind of changes will occur in the pattern of service delivery by the time this person reaches retirement age in the 2020s? How well are we preparing new staff to meet the needs of mentally handicapped people today and what opportunities will there be for them to update their knowledge and skills in the light of the changing needs of tomorrow?

There is a sense in which we are all unqualified and ill prepared even to meet today's needs. The speed and scale of change, even within the last ten years, the flood of new information on changing practice, are so great that much of what is taught to new staff is becoming dated even before they complete their training. How much greater, then, is the challenge of helping existing staff to modify their practice and attitudes in the light of the changes that have taken place since they started working in this field? How, too, do we create an awareness of the needs of people with disabilities in the countless numbers of staff working in ordinary services?

This chapter will consider the changing needs of staff against the background of rapidly changing perceptions of the needs of mentally handicapped people and ways in which services should be delivered to meet those needs. Clearly, we are going to have to make some speculative assumptions concerning the pattern of service development over the next 50 years. For example, we shall assume a continuation of the policy of moving away from institutional and segregated forms of service provision towards one which provides a greater range of choice within community alternatives, as well as opportunities for mentally handicapped people to live, learn and work in their local community and to have full access to all its resources and services.

This assumption may be proved false: it is not impossible to imagine a renewed emphasis on the advantages of institutional and segregated models, particularly if the quality of community services is shown to be inadequate, whether through lack of resources, hostility by the public or dissatisfaction shown by the consumers or their representatives.

The extent to which staff delivering the services are able to meet the needs of mentally handicapped people in a wide range of community settings is clearly one critical element in the success of current policies. This chapter will therefore summarise the changing patterns of service delivery and the strengths and weaknesses of present training arrangements in responding to the new demands that are being placed on staff.

Although our account must necessarily be concerned with the separate training arrangements of different groups of staff, we shall argue the case for a more multidisciplinary approach to training in which people from different disciplines and working for different agencies will in future need to be trained together rather than separately. We will then consider the content of training and conclude with an attempt to summarise some of the essential skills of staff working with mentally handicapped people.

CHANGING CONTEXTS AND NEEDS

Many of the assumptions underlying recent as well as current patterns of service delivery are so familiar that it will suffice to summarise them briefly.

Community-based services

The move from institutional to community-based models has already been noted but the extent to which it has actually happened should not be exaggerated. In the United Kingdom at the present time, the majority of mentally handicapped people are still congregated together in some form of segregated institutional service. In England and Wales, there are some 28,000 children attending schools for children with severe learning difficulties, over 46,000 adults in Adult Training Centres or Social Education Centres (ATCs/SECs), 42,000 in long stay hospitals and 14,000 in local authority hostels (DHSS, 1980).

Some types of institution are more highly regarded than others and there is clearly much variation in the quality of services provided both within and between specific forms of provision.

Nevertheless, very few children attend ordinary schools, very few adults who live away from their family are in ordinary houses, enjoy a stable sexual relationship, are in full time paid employment or have full access to the whole range of services and community resources available to their fellow citizens. There is general agreement that these are desirable goals both for individuals and for the service as a whole but their realisation depends on many factors, not the least of which is the motivation, competence and skills of staff to help mentally handicapped people to acquire the skills to achieve them.

The developmental and educational approach

A second, parallel set of assumptions concerns the ability of mentally handicapped people to learn and the skills of staff to teach them to do so. In the past, and perhaps to some extent in the present, services were provided on the assumption that because mentally handicapped people were by definition thought to be incapable of learning, it was appropriate to provide no more than custodial or caring environments. The shortage of staff effectively ruled out any possibility of teaching people new skills, though many staff did try to do so, often against heavy odds and with little support from management or policy makers. Even when the importance of active teaching methods was acknowledged, the nature of well established institutional practices often made it difficult to implement a regime which placed a greater emphasis on the importance of staff helping clients to acquire new skills and competencies (see Jones et al, and Cullen, this volume).

Staff Development

Institutional tradition of training

One of our difficulties at the present time, therefore, arises from the institutional bias of the training provided for the majority of staff at the very time when we are seeking to develop a greater range of non-institutional services. Training in the future will need to concentrate on helping staff to deploy their skills in a much greater variety of settings. For example, the tradition of nurse training in hospitals for people who are mentally handicapped originally emphasised the paramedical or custodial elements of care. Later revisions of the nursing syllabus in 1971 which gave much more weight to the importance of educational and developmental activities were only partially reflected in the practice of nurse training schools or in work on the wards. This led to the most recent revision of the syllabus in 1982 which is firmly behavioural in orientation, laying particular emphasis on the acquisition of skills in the 'nursing process', including the setting of clear, short term goals for each client, the analysis of the task to be taught and the use of appropriate and carefully chosen rewards (Cullen, this volume).

It remains to be seen whether this revision can be effectively incorporated into nurse training and implemented in day-to-day work with clients.

Neglect of organisational and managerial issues

A limitation of traditional training is that it has largely ignored organisational and management issues. Newly qualified staff, whether in hospitals, hostels or schools, have rarely been introduced to questions concerned with the introduction and maintenance of innovation or ways in which change can be achieved within different types of organisation. Even experienced staff who go on courses for the purpose of acquiring specific skills are rarely helped to consider the problems of becoming a change agent in their own work settings or how to confront the obstacles to change which they are likely to meet. This neglect of organisational and managerial variables could largely nullify many current approaches to staff training. It has also led to a lowering of morale among staff committed to deploying their skills.

Neglect of generic services

A further consequence of the institutional bias of staff training arises from the lack of exposure to ordinary community services and the staff who work in them. For example, nursing staff being trained in mental handicap hospitals have little exposure to the work of the primary health care team, including general practitioners, health visitors and district nurses. ATC staff have little experience of the work of other Social Services staff, such as residential care staff or field social workers, far less home helps or staff concerned with social security and welfare benefits. Until recently, teachers in special and ordinary schools knew little about one another's work or problems.

Since it is one of the cardinal elements of normalisation theory and practice that mentally handicapped people should be able to make full use of community services, it is essential that staff working in these services should have some awareness of the needs of mentally handicapped people and consider how their service can more effectively meet them. These include the whole range of services concerned with health, education, social services and social security, housing, employment, recreation and leisure, as well as the police.

Isolation of specialist staff from one another

Even more serious in the short term is the isolation of specialist staff from their colleagues in other agencies working with mentally handicapped people. How often, for example, can ATC staff gain experience in working with profoundly multiply handicapped people in hospitals or in the special needs class of their nearest school for children with severe learning difficulties? How often do special school staff have an opportunity to gain experience of working in the child development centre of their local hospital, in other special schools or in a College of Further Education? How can they learn about the work of community mental handicap teams?

The isolation of specialist staff from one another can erect unnecessary barriers to an appreciation of the distinctive contribution which other professionals and other agencies can make. These barriers can be overcome as part of a staff development strategy in which every individual member is provided with opportunities to visit and perhaps work in other agencies. Unfortunately, such opportunities are rarely available.

Isolation at initial training

Barriers between different professions and different agencies are first laid down during initial training. Despite the lip service paid to multidisciplinary teamwork, the initial training of most professionals is carried out in largely watertight compartments, with the result that few students are provided with opportunities to learn about the work of colleagues in other disciplines. Consequently, teachers, doctors, psychologists, nurses, speech therapists, physiotherapists, occupational therapists, social workers and others begin their professional careers with very limited and quite possibly erroneous stereotypes about the work of colleagues in related disciplines.

It is difficult to imagine much radical change in initial training: the syllabus is already far too crowded and new demands are always being made for new material; specialists from other disciplines are not readily available and are themselves committed to training their own profession; in short, the priority is just not high enough. On the other hand, it should be possible to move some way towards an awareness of the work of other professionals. This can be achieved not only through lectures by other specialists but by providing opportunities for students to work with other disciplines and to gain some appreciation of their distinctive skills. Ideally, students from different disciplines can attend common lectures or classes, so that personal as well as professional contacts can be developed.

Isolation at post-experience level

Although the possibilities for joint training and collaboration across professional and service boundaries are probably greatest at the level of post-experience or post-qualifying courses, these opportunities are, with significant exceptions, largely unexploited at the present time. In general, inservice courses are organised along rigid compartmentalised lines. Each of the main statutory agencies organises its own training through its own training structures. For example, teachers attend courses organised by Local Education Authority (LEA) Advisers, often at Teachers' Centres or local Colleges, as well as those organised through Education Departments of Institutions of Higher Education. Social Service Departments (SSDs) have their own training departments, though there is not much evidence of training activity directed specifically at social services staff working with mentally handicapped people. The Certificate in Social Service is exclusively for SSD employees. Similarly, the National Health Service has its own training structures which have recently been co-ordinated by the NHS Training Authority in Bristol.

Training together

The need for more interdisciplinary joint training is not confined to staff of mental handicap services; it applies equally to staff working with children in general, with elderly people, as well as those with physical and psychiatric impairments. Fortunately, there are signs of greater recognition of this need, as well as a number of examples on which to draw.

The British Institute for Mental Handicap (BIMH) has been a pioneer in the development of multi-disciplinary courses for over 15 years. Most of its short and longer courses are equally open to staff of all disciplines, although some agencies make more use of them than others. For example, its intensive one week residential courses on working with clients who are profoundly retarded and multiply handicapped attracts staff from special needs units of schools and ATC/SECs, as well as hospital and other NHS staff. The courses are taught by staff from a variety of disciplines, including teachers, psychologists, speech and physiotherapists and specialists in sensory impairments.

Extra-Mural Departments of Universities and Colleges of Adult Education also make ideal 'neutral ground' for multi-disciplinary training courses. These provide a wide range of vocational and non-vocational courses, some of which may be award bearing, for any member of the public. These courses can be attended by parents and by mentally handicapped people themselves. Indeed, there may already be examples of adult education facilities which are being attended both by mentally handicapped people and by the staff who work with them.

The use of adult education or extra-mural courses is relatively straightforward but using them as a basis for a coordinated local training strategy calls for careful planning, perhaps involving a steering committee with representatives of all the main relevant training interests and agencies. A joint planning framework is needed for training just as much as for service planning, in order to avoid duplication and to ensure that courses are as open as possible to all relevant staff in the locality.

Training the trainers

A new approach in various parts of the UK involves the development of centralised training teams whose remit is to stimulate the development of local training initiatives. This is a different form of pyramid training than that exemplified by EDY courses (McBrien and Foxen, this volume). For example, the BIMH has recently been commissioned by the Welsh Office to play a key role in stimulating staff training initiatives as part of the All Wales Strategy for the development of community services. A number of intensive two or three day workshops have been held in different counties, with a view to bringing together staff from different agencies with responsibility for the provision of services.

The South East Thames Regional Health Authority has developed joint initiatives with the University of Kent at Canterbury and the NHS Training Authority in providing workshops and courses for staff working in mental handicap services (Mansell, 1985). These have included five day PASS (Program Analysis of Service Systems) workshops, reorientation courses for staff from existing hospitals: courses for staff working with people with severe behaviour problems and courses on developing staffed housing. Some of these courses are held at local level, others involve selected teams attending courses at a central site.

The North West Regional Health Authority is also just setting up a training team, consisting of a coordinator who is a social worker, a clinical psychologist and a nurse. One of their aims will be to stimulate the development of training teams at local level, as part of the RHA's commitment to providing locally based services and to relocating hospital residents into appropriate high quality community services.

Developing training strategies

Initiatives such as these highlight the importance of developing a systematic strategy of staff development and one that will reach all staff working with mentally handicapped people. Such a systematic strategy is very different from the somewhat random, ad hoc activities which characterise the staff training scene in most areas and in the country as a whole. Such activities can certainly be of considerable benefit to those attending and may even lead to change in the individual participants and in the organisations in which they work. A strategic approach to staff training, however, involves much more than the provision of courses and training activities.

The randomness of many training activities at the present time arises from a number of sources. In the first place, the participants are either self selected or are chosen by their employers for their interest and enthusiasm. This means that courses are 'preaching to the converted'. Course providers have frequently observed that it is the same people who come to course after course and, by definition, the same people who stay away.

There is now some evidence of greater selectivity in choosing staff for secondment to long, full-time courses. In some cases, areas of specialism are negotiated between the student, the employer and the training institution. In the case of teachers, for example, discussions can take place on the aims of the secondment, on possible changes in role on return from the course, on ways in which the school and the LEA can benefit from the seconded student making a special study of an area of the curriculum or of the needs of a particular group of children.

Second, there is little information about the extent to which course participants are able to implement change or introduce new methods into the organisations in which they work. All too often, there is a lack of interest on the part of colleagues and an absence of support from management for the introduction of new methods. The person returning from a one year course experiences what has been termed a 're-entry' problem, caused in part by resentment of some colleagues and in part by the difficulty of reconciling the demands and values of two different environments.

The implication here is that training should provide opportunities for learning to be a change agent in one's own work setting. Students need to be helped to anticipate obstacles and to consider a range of ways in which such obstacles might be overcome. This calls for some discussion of organisational and management issues. Similarly, 'middle managers' such as training officers and team leaders may need help in encouraging people who return from courses to overcome obstacles in applying new knowledge and skills.

Top down or bottom up?

A distinction is sometimes drawn between 'top down' and 'bottom up' approaches to training. A classic example of a top down approach occurs when a university or polytechnic designs a course without consultation with LEAs or teachers and then provides it on a 'take it or leave it' basis. Even if a course recruits well, it does not necessarily address the particular needs of LEAs or teachers.

A variation of the 'top down' strategy is provided by the courses in behavioural methods of teaching developed by the EDY team (McBrien and Foxen, this volume). Similarly, the mini-course in structured language teaching for children with severe learning difficulties (Robson, this volume) provides a further variation on the theme: this course was designed to be self-instructional in the first place.

WHO NEEDS TRAINING?

There is a sense in which the number of people needing training is as great as the number of people in the service. To this not insubstantial number must be added family members with day-to-day contact with a mentally handicapped person, members of voluntary agencies and the whole army of generic workers who have only limited contact with mentally handicapped people but whose attitudes and behaviour are critical to their integration into the community.

On this argument, as suggested earlier, we could all be better qualified and equipped to meet the needs of mentally handicapped people today and for the rest of our and their lifetime.

Among existing groups of staff working largely with mentally handicapped people, the majority work in some form of institutional service, with the growing exception of members of community mental handicap teams.

Residential care staff

Although the number of staff working in mental handicap hospitals has increased greatly in absolute terms over the past ten years, most of the increase has been among unqualified nursing staff. Their numbers doubled in the period 1969-1977, while the number of qualified nurses increased by only a quarter. Furthermore, major improvements in working conditions and number of hours worked has lessened the impact of these increases, so that staff: resident ratios are still grossly unsatisfactory (Development Team for Mentally Handicapped People, 1985). The report to the Secretary of State by the National Development Group (NDG, 1978) made a number of recommendations for the development of training programmes for all levels of staff though little national information is available on the extent to which these have been implemented.

The majority of residential care staff employed by local authorities are also unqualified - some 78 per cent of those who work with children and 68 per cent of those who work with adults (DHSS, 1980). Approximately half of the officers in charge and their deputies were unqualified, as were nine out of every ten care staff. Of those who did have a qualification, the majority were in nursing rather than in residential social work.

The largest single group of staff specifically trained to work with mentally handicapped people are the Registered Nurses of the Mentally Handicapped (RNMH). Some 11,000 qualified nurses are employed in mental handicap hospitals (some holding qualifications other than RNMH), as well as a further 14,000 state enrolled nurses. The Jay Committee proposed that in future hospital staff should train jointly with residential care staff employed by local authorities, and that both should qualify through the Certificate of Social Service (DHSS, 1979). This proposal was strongly opposed by a section of the nursing profession and was not accepted by the government. Since then, reports prepared by a joint working party set up by the Royal College of Nursing and the Central Council for Education and Training in Social Work have recommended more joint training at local level but the extent to which these recommendations have borne fruit is not clear.

The reponse of the Royal College of Nursing and its successor the English Nursing Board to the Jay Committee's report was to undertake a radical revision of its syllabus (ENB, 1982). Although in many ways an exemplary document, three problems remain. First, it continues the tradition of separate training for nurses, rather than exploring collaborative approaches. Second, it assumes the continued existence of mental handicap hospitals as a base for nurse training schools, despite its own repeated findings that many hospitals provided totally unsatisfactory training environments both for mentally handicapped people and for students, with the result that some nurse training schools have had their recognition withdrawn and been closed. Finally, it is not clear where the new trainers are to come from, and how they themselves will be trained.

The most encouraging developments in nursing have arisen from post-qualifying courses under the auspices of the former Joint Board for Clinical Nursing Studies. Courses in community mental handicap nursing have already been mentioned: the number of community nurses has risen from less than 50 in 1979 to well over 300 in 1984, though many of these have qualified through the BIMH six week courses. Many of these nurses work as members of Community Mental Handicap Teams, and have formed a flourishing professional association. In addition, the former Joint Board has mounted highly effective courses in behaviour modification.

Day care staff

Staff of Adult Training Centres fought an unsuccessful compaign to retain the specialist diploma awarded by the former Training Council for Teachers of the Mentally Handicapped and briefly by the Central Council for the Education and Training of Social

Workers (CCETSW). In 1980 some 60 per cent of all staff had no formal qualification, including 19 per cent of managers.

Since then, an increasing number of staff have qualified in the Certificate of Social Service (CSS) on a day release basis. In the period 1977-1984, 1511 CSS students out of a total of 8,138 gave people with mental handicap as their main client group (just under one fifth) but only 415 took a mental handicap specialism. This is partly because only 11 of the 29 CSS schemes formally declared a specialism in mental handicap, though many offered relevant courses such as behavioural techniques, programme planning and social skills training. Consideration is now being given in CCETSW to the development of a single qualification for all SSD staff, thus merging the CSS with the existing certificate of qualification in social work (CQSW). This new course would be available on a part time and day release basis and would be open to staff working in day and residential services.

The CSS has some important strengths. First, it provides joint training for all SSD staff (other than field social workers) and therefore avoids the isolation of ATC and other mental handicap staff from their colleagues working with other client groups in SSDs. Second, the training arrangements are designed to make it possible for students to relate the content of their training to their day-to-day work in the service. Study supervisors are designated to work with students, tutors, field worker supervisors and employers for this purpose. Third, it provides a training route for staff who would in many cases find it difficult to attend a full time course in a distant institution of higher education and who would not necessarily be adequately qualified to do so.

At the present time, therefore, the CSS does appear to provide the main training avenue for day services staff, though it is unfortunate that more CSS schemes do not provide a major mental handicap element.

Whatever the merits of CSS, it can be argued that there is an additional need for a small group of day service staff to have advanced specialist training. This case is all the stronger now that day services are expected to meet the needs of people with more severe handicaps and behaviour disturbances and to provide for people coming out of long stay hospitals.

Furthermore, services at present concentrated into one building are likely in future to be much more widely dispersed and integrated with other community services. In practice, this would mean that ATCS/SECS would become the 'core' of a cluster of community services, including Colleges of Further Education (FE), Manpower Services Commission courses, sheltered and open employment, leisure facilities and residential services. (For more detailed accounts of these models of provision see King's Fund, 1984; National Association of Teachers of the Mentally Handicapped, 1985 and Independent Development Council, 1985.)

These are new roles and responsibilities for ATC staff, demanding an element of reorientation and retraining for all. One way to make good use of recently trained specialist courses would be to recognise and encourage the four new two year full time courses which have been set up in recent years, validated either by the Central Council for National Academic Awards or the University of Manchester. These courses are not yet recognised for secondment purposes by Social Service Departments, even though the students have little difficulty in finding employment. Graduates from these courses could play an essential leadership or supportive role in working alongside colleagues holding the former Diploma or the CSS.

The expertise released by these courses is not being effectively harnessed at the present time for reasons that no longer seem valid. At one time, these courses were regarded as "a threat to the CSS" but it is obvious that there is scope for more than one type of course. In any case, CSS is also changing.

Social workers

Social workers have a key role in helping mentally handicapped people to gain full access to community services and in providing social work support both to them and to their families. They have a vital contribution to make throughout the whole life span of people with mental handicap but perhaps particularly at points of transition - e.g., at the time of identification and assessment, entry into school, the process of reassessment and review around the time of leaving school and moving into adult services. In supporting families at these times, they help families to adapt to the different demands on their resources as their relatives become older and as dependency needs and levels change.

During the last ten years, the rapid growth of Community Mental Handicap Teams (CMHTs) has provided opportunities for social workers to specialise in this field, and to work alongside their colleagues in nursing, psychology and other professions. Many appointments as specialist social workers have been made but these have clearly highlighted the lack of specialist training available for social workers in the field of disability in general and intellectual disability in particular.

The basic CQSW training rarely includes more than a session or two on this subject. There is only one post-qualifying course in disability (at Manchester University).

Community Mental Handicap Teams

So far, we have mainly been considering staff working in traditional disciplines and institutional services. A number of new professional roles are being developed specifically for work in community settings. Members of Community Mental Handicap Teams (CMHTs) are a good case in point.

CMHTs were first recommended by the National Development Group (1976) and have since been actively promoted by the Development Team (DHSS, 1985) and endorsed as government policy. Although the majority of Health Districts now have or shortly plan to have a CMHT (Plank, 1982), their composition, number per population, methods of work and management support vary greatly from one part of the country to another. Typically, a CMHT consists of two full-time core members - a community mental handicap nurse and a specialist social worker, often supported on a part time basis by a doctor, clinical psychologist, speech and physiotherapist.

Community mental handicap nurses can be trained on six month courses through the English Nursing Board, but the preferred mode of training seems to be the intensive six week courses organised by the British Institute for Mental Handicap.

Staff Development

Teachers and educators

Offical figures on qualifications held by teachers working in special schools are not available but a recent survey of schools for children with severe learning difficulties (SLD) in South East England (Evans and Wade, 1986) can be compared with a similar survey of schools in North West England ten years earlier (Preddy and Mittler, 1981; Mittler and Preddy, 1981). Virtually all teachers in these schools have a formal qualification in teaching but the proportion of graduates in these schools has risen from five to 42 per cent since 1977, though the proportion with specialist qualifications seems to have remained constant at around 20 per cent.

The main specialist qualifications in teaching children with SLDs are likely to be held by teachers who choose to study mental handicap as a special subject during their initial training. But the government has now decided to phase out all specialist initial training (also for teachers of the hearing impaired) and insisted that all training must take place via the in-service route. These courses are likely to cover the whole field of special educational needs, and will only provide limited opportunities for specialising in the teaching of children with SLDs.

There is certainly much to be said in favour of bringing together teachers from different areas of special needs, both from ordinary and special schools. The joint learning experiences provided by such courses can lay useful foundations for collaboration at a later stage. But do teachers working with children with SLDs need to have access to specialist courses aimed largely at meeting their needs? Obvious examples include courses on work with profoundly retarded and multiply handicapped children and those with additional complex sensory or behavioural disorders. As before, the argument against such courses is that they segregate teachers and prevent them from learning from one another. On the other hand, the distinctive needs of these teachers are in danger of being overlooked in the current climate of integrated in-service work.

One way of resolving this dilemma is to develop courses which provide a firm basis of joint study in foundation areas and in relevant professional skills, while still allowing for some degree of specialist choice for teachers with specific needs. This is one aim of the North West regional modular diploma in special educational needs (Robson, 1984).

In addition to teachers, schools employ almost as many classroom assistants, many of whom hold nursery nurse or nursing qualifications. Some LEAs hold short courses for classroom assistants (sometimes strangely known as 'non-teaching assistants') either in schools or in teachers' centres. Many have succesfully completed the EDY training course (Farrell, 1985).

Finally, the needs of staff working in colleges of Further Education should not be overlooked, as an increasing number are providing for a wider range of students with special needs, including those with severe learning difficulties (Dean and Hegarty, 1984). In view of the dearth of training opportunities in this field, it would seem sensible for training courses to cover the whole range of special needs rather than separate courses for specific disabilities

CONTENT OF TRAINING

We have been considering the changing context of service planning and delivery and some of the challenges facing providers of staff training. We turn now to a brief consideration of content and curriculum.

Our account is selective because it is necessarily limited to content which is largely common to all professions. We are not concerned with specific competencies needed by any single profession.

Initial training

The future acceptance of children and adults with special needs in general and with severe learning difficulties in particular depends in the long run on the mass of 'generic workers' in the field of human services. These include the whole range of doctors and other health professionals such as nurses, therapists of all kinds and health administrators, as well as public service staff such as social workers, residential and day care staff, social security and welfare officers and all staff working in the education service.

Staff Development

It would be unrealistic to expect much more than an 'awareness element' in the training of these professions and some thought is now being given to ways in which this can be done, particularly in the case of teachers. In future, no initial teacher training course will be accredited unless it can demonstrate that all students are exposed to a special needs element. Little up-to-date information is available on the extent to which students in other disciplines are made aware of these needs, either in general or in relation to specific disabilities. It seems that students are interested in having some information on people with special need, so that even if it is only possible to cover a little ground, this can at least provide foundations for later personal and professional involvement.

Essential elements of post-experience training

However well the foundations are laid at the stage of initial training, the major task for the future is nothing less than the training or retraining of all staff to update their knowledge and skills and to reconsider their attitudes to helping mentally handicapped people to live, learn and work successfully in the community.

What are the essential elements in such a training programme? These can be considered under a number of broad headings.

A ATTITUDES AND IDEOLOGY

Given the large majority of staff whose training and experience has mainly been within the framework of institutional or segregated services, it is essential to provide opportunities for staff to examine and explore their own attitudes and belief systems. Many of these staff are not unsympathetic to the current policy of community services, but it is natural for some of them to have strong reservations that current policies may not be in the best interests of mentally handicapped people. It is perfectly understandable that, say, nurses with lifelong experience in a hospital ward, should find it difficult to imagine how many of the hospital residents whom they know could possible live in an ordinary house, even with support, attend an ATC or make use of community recreational facilities.

Similarly, it is hard for staff of ATC/SECs to imagine some of their students in open employment or attending an Adult Education College and for teachers to visualise their children attending ordinary schools.

The current ideology of integration into mainstream facilities is so powerful that some staff may find it difficult to voice their reservations openly, in case they are thought to be either reactionary or merely defending their jobs out of self interest. So many publications in the field of mental handicap are highly critical of all segregated institutions not only for what they do but for what they are. Staff working in these facilities choose to do so at a time when there are no 'valued community alternatives'. Furthermore, they know that whatever the defects of institutional provision, whether in principle or in practice, the majority of mentally handicapped people are still using them.

It should never be assumed that the staff of segregated services are automatically opposed to community developments. Indeed, it is mental handicap hospital nurses themselves who have taken initiatives in working for the relocation of their residents, who have, belatedly perhaps, adopted the Jay Committee's 'model of care' and who have pioneered developments in the training of community nurses and in joint training with social workers.

The importance of providing opportunities for staff to discuss attitudes can be met in a number of ways. Perhaps the best known is the series of 'normalisation workshops' introduced by the Community Mental Handicap Educational Research Association (CMHERA). These provide a detailed introduction to the principles of normalisation as developed by Wolfensberger (1972) and his associates, and help participants to relate these general principles to the day-to-day realities of service provision and service planning. They also provide a foundation for more detailed training in the evaluation of a service facility given in a PASS workshop (Wolfensberger and Glenn, 1975) or in its later simplified version, known as PASSING (Wolfensberger and Thomas, 1983). PASS workshops have been held in may parts of the UK but other, simpler systems should not be overlooked - e.g., the six STAMINA checklists produced by **MENCAP** (1985) and the longer checklists published by the National Development Group (NDG, 1980).

B SKILLS IN TEACHING AND REHABILITATION

Despite the dramatic progress which has been reported in helping mentally handicapped people to acquire and use a wide range of skills, we have to recognise that many staff remain relatively unaffected by these developments. They may be aware of approaches vaguely characterised as 'behaviour modification' but have never had the opportunity to attend a training workshop or receive direct instruction in their own work setting from a skilled practitioner. Consequently, many staff who are not unsympathetic to this approach but who have not themselves had even a day's training may attempt to implement behavioural approaches on the basis of only the most limited understanding of the theory or practice involved.

The importance of providing all staff with the opportunity of acquiring a working knowledge of the principles as well as the practice of behavioural methods has been recognised for may years though progress has been uneven. In the special school sector, there is reason to believe that many staff are not only reasonably proficient in behavioural methods but have now passed to the stage where they are able to use these methods in the service of the curriculum and of individual goal planning. There is less use of indiscriminate social or food reinforcers and more emphasis on a careful selection of the task to be taught, followed by a step by step task analysis. The importance of systematic teaching to help children to generalise their learning across settings, tasks and people is also well accepted. Most important of all, there is now a strong recognition in schools that it will not be possible to find the time to carry out one-to-one teaching unless some formal division of roles and responsibilities is established, similar to the 'room management' procedures described by Jones and his colleagues in this volume.

The situation in hospitals, hostels and ATCs is less clear. Many hospitals have introduced formal training programmes in behavioural methods but their implementation is often beset by severe staff shortages which make individualised treatment impossible, as well as by organisational and administrative obstacles - e.g., inconsistent policies and practices by different charge nurses or as between the ward and the various training departments in which the resident works (Cullen, this volume).

There is no shortage of guidelines and detailed, practical, illustrated training manuals written by staff with a working knowledge of UK training contexts (e.g., NDG, 1978; Capie, Taylor and Perkins, 1980; Simon, 1981). Regular courses are also held by the BIMH and other organisations. However, the impact of these developments is uncertain. Some of the larger hospitals have been able to designate one member of staff or a small training team to act as the apex of a training pyramid but this is harder to organise in smaller units.

ATCs and hostel staff seem in general to have had less access to staff training courses in general and to behaviour modification courses in particular, partly perhaps because of different training arrangements in Social Service Departments.

Training courses up to now have placed particular emphasis on the teaching of self-care skills - particularly dressing, feeding, washing and toiletting. More recently, increasing emphasis is being placed on skills needed to relate to people, including language and communication skills. Also, all schools for children with severe learning difficulties are now regularly teaching and using a signing system. Although Makaton is the most popular, schools are now eclectic in their approach and try to select the system which is most appropriate to the child's current level of development and needs. The use of signing is likely to increase in ATCs with the development of more continuity of programming for school leavers.

In addition to training in basic self care and communication skills, increasing emphasis is being placed on helping mentally handicapped people to become more proficient in activities for daily living. In particular, attention is being given to the whole range of skills needed to live in an ordinary house and to use community facilities.

Several comprehensive summaries of suggested teaching areas have now been published, some of which have been sent free of charge to facilities for mentally handicapped people. These include the guidelines prepared by the National Development Group for ATCs and hospitals (NDG, 1977, 1978). Among the published general curriculum guidelines for children are the Portage programme (Bluma et al; 1976), that published by Rectory Paddock School (1983) and by Coupe and Porter (1986). Materials more concerned with adolescents and adults include the Bereweeke Skill Teaching System (Felce et al; 1983) and the Copewell Curriculum (Whelan and Speake, 1979; Whelan et al, 1984). Guidelines for the development of a curriculum for people with profound levels of mental handicap can be found in Hogg and Sebba (1986).

These and other published curriculum guidelines call for staff with highly developed skills in curriculum planning and delivery. Clearly, the extent to which such guidelines can be implemented depends on the availability of staff not only with requisite teaching skills but also with the time to do so. This requires a high degree of management support and an organisational framework within facilities for mentally handicapped people which would provide scope for the use of programmes of this kind. The means must therefore be found not only of training managers but also of helping front line and direct care staff to become change agents and innovators in their own work settings and to become better negotiators with their own line management.

C SKILLS IN BEHAVIOUR MANAGEMENT

The emphasis in most of these materials is on helping staff to teach clients to learn new skills. Far less guidance is available on methods of working with people with severe behaviour problems. This has also been a challenge to the skills of staff but is all the more important now that we are seeking to bring people out of hospital, as well as trying to prevent admission.

Unfortunately, this challenge is largely unmet at the present time. It has to be admitted that our knowledge of how to help people with behaviour disturbances lags a long way behind our ability to teach skills concerned with activities for daily living, such as self care, communication and community living skills. The uncritical and unskilled application of behavioural techniques is rarely effective in itself. Even when some improvement is effected in the client's behaviour, the effects are notoriously short lived (Murphy and Wilson, 1985).

There is no reliable information on the number or nature of problem behaviours in schoolchildren with severe learning difficulties but there is suggestive evidence from surveys that the numbers are considerable. For example, a survey of 53 schools in the West Midlands indicated that 19 per cent of children were reported as having severe behaviour problems - including self-injurious behaviour, over-activity, attacks on other children and extreme destructiveness; milder variants were shown by a further 26 per cent (Taylor, Crawford and Throboe, 1981). Research carried out for the Jay Committee indicated that 25 per cent of adults and 50 per cent of children in mental handicap hospitals showed severe behaviour problems. The fact that the prevalence of behaviour problems is not markedly different for children and adults suggests that the higher staff ratios found in schools do not in themselves provide a solution.

Nevertheless, there is reason to believe that existing training courses are not putting anything like enough emphasis on methods of preventing and coping with difficult behaviour. The instructive account of work at Beech Tree House (Jones, 1983) cannot easily be replicated in community settings.

SOME ESSENTIAL STAFF SKILLS

In the light of the above discussion, we can now attempt a tentative summary of a selection of skills, tasks and behaviours which are important and perhaps essential in staff working in services for mentally handicapped people and their families. They are crudely presented in the form of a list in the interests of space and no attempt is made here to justify the form or content of the list. The list is necessarily selective and incomplete and occasionally expressed in personalised and subjective language.

The skills identified here are only a starting point for discussion, but it should be emphasised that they are largely common to all staff, irrespective of the service setting in which they work or the nature of their employing authority. Clearly, some staff will be more senior or more experienced than others and some will have a more direct teaching role than others. However, the skills identified should form at least an element in any service, whether that service is based in an institution or in the community.

I WORKING WITH CLIENTS

1 Understand and respect the individuality of each mentally handicapped person, provide opportunities for the growth of individuality and of the person as a whole. Avoid generalisations, stereotypes and labelling which mask or destroy the individuality of handicapped persons.

2 Encourage clients to express choices, make decisions and participate fully in discussions concerning the selection of their own teaching and rehabilitation plans.

3 Encourage clients as a group to express their point of view and to represent their interests to staff and to management and to service providers.

4 Select, use and interpret appropriate individual assessment measures and relate these to the choice of curriculum objectives which meet the needs of individuals.

5 Make and record objective observations of behaviour in a wide variety of structured and unstructured situations.

6 Design, implement and evaluate individual programme plans for each client, based on detailed assessments and recorded observations.

7 Demonstrate proficiency in the specification of behavioural objectives, goal setting, task analysis, programme writing and a range of teaching techniques including prompting, shaping, chaining and reinforcement.

8 Devise techniques for the teaching of generalisation and maintenance of learning across settings, tasks and people.

9 Develop skills in methods of working with clients with difficult behaviour and an understanding of ways in which environmental factors can cause or complicate such difficulties.

10 Develop skills in supporting and working with

clients in a wide variety of community settings - e.g., in their own homes, in community settings such as shops, public transport, work and leisure facilities.

11 Expose clients to gradually increasing demands for independence in daily living and in integrated settings, and ensure that staff assistance, aids, appliances and prosthetic devices do not unnecessarily prolong the client's dependence on others.

II WORKING WITH OTHER PROFESSIONALS

1 Learn about the work of other professions and the settings and constraints within which they work; understand their distinctive skills in working with clients and when and how to seek their help.

2 Communicate the nature of the problem in clear language.

3 Work with other professionals in devising and carrying out individual programme plans for clients and in developing joint planning of the service within an interdisciplinary framework.

4 Acquire and practice skills in working with and supporting other professionals in their own work settings - e.g., consultancy skills in helping staff in community generic services to use or adapt teaching and rehabilitative measures previously used in institutional settings.

III WORKING WITH FAMILIES

1 Learn to understand, appreciate and respect the individuality of each family and each individual member of the family; avoid all generalisations and stereotypes concerning families.

2 Develop a range of counselling skills required for working with parents - particularly listening, sharing feelings as well as information and skills; treating parents as equal partners and respecting their expertise and experience, appreciating their strengths and needs, encouraging them to voice their own opinions and reflect their own priorities.

3 Provide opportunities for parents and other family members to play a full part in assessment, in formulating teaching priorities and in decision-making in the development of individual programme plans.

4 Provide opportunities for parents to assist in the teaching of the client, if they wish to do so and respect parents' wishes not to participate if they choose not to do so.

5 Provide regular opportunities for parents to review progress by inviting them to meetings or by visiting them at home.

IV MANAGEMENT AND ORGANISATIONAL SKILLS

1 Support, encourage and cherish all members of staff by recognising and praising their work and reducing blame and criticism to the minimum.

2 Ensure that the skills and interests of all members of staff are used to best advantage and that a staff development plan has been developed for each member of staff. Work for growth and development of staff morale and for the prevention of 'burn out'.

3 Plan the most effective use of scarce resources with respect to available finance, personnel or materials etc.

4 Help to identify, disseminate and review the aims of the service or facility in discussion with all those involved, including clients and families.

5 Develop methods of continuous monitoring and evaluation of all aspects of the service but particularly measures of the quality of services, as perceived by clients and their representatives.

6 Ensure that all clients have an individual service plan, that records of progress are kept and discussed with them and with other staff.

7 Ensure that the facility establishes, maintains and develops working relationships with all the appropriate specialist and community agencies, so that clients can benefit from opportunities to receive the help of staff of these services.

8 Make a study through guided reading and visits of the process involved in introducing and maintaining organisational change and seek ways of adapting these to the needs of the service.

V SKILLS IN LEARNING AND ACQUIRING INFORMATION

1 Know where and how to obtain information on relevant developments in services, in technical developments and in research.

2 Distinguish between opinions and facts.

3 Take or create opportunities to visit a wide range of services and facilities and learn from their experiences.

4 Read and critically evaluate the relevant professional journals and books, joining appropriate organisations and attending courses and conferences.

5 Be familiar with relevant local and national policy documents concerned with the work of the service and create opportunities for discussion of such documents with colleagues and with management.

CONCLUSIONS: MORE OF THE SAME OR TRYING ANOTHER WAY?

The argument of this chapter has been that present arrangements have failed us badly. Staff training simply has not kept pace with the demands of the service, the expansion of knowledge or the development of new skills and technologies. Nor has it matched new ideas on ways in which services should be jointly planned and delivered by multidisciplinary teams working in partnership with families and with mentally handicapped people themselves.

It is inconceivable that a surgeon, a civil engineer, a manufacturer of computers, spacecraft or weapons would use techniques which had long been overtaken by advances in knowledge and research. Yet this is precisely what we allow to happen in human services where information that is available is not accessible to many of the people in direct contact with the clients with whom they work.

The value of a service to society is reflected in the

resources devoted to the training and skills of staff who work in it. Although services for people with mental handicap are much more in the public eye than in the past, the training of staff has not been seen as a high priority. Staff, clients and relatives involved in such undervalued and underfunded services have too readily accepted the low status which is accorded to their activities by their own management and by society as a whole.

In this they are by no means unique - the training of staff working with people who are elderly, mentally ill, with offenders, long term prisoners and other minority groups is no better and is probably far worse. At least in the field of mental handicap there has been an awareness of training needs and some discussion on how progress can be made. Suggestions for change such as those put forward by the Jay Committee have highlighted the obstacles but also shown that progress is possible.

At a time of rapid change in patterns of service delivery, what can be done to help staff to respond to change? Can we develop methods of training and supporting staff which will help them to adapt to assumptions and attitudes very different from those held by earlier generations?

In looking to the future, we could distinguish between specialist staff who are now working in traditionally separate and segregated services such as special schools, hospitals, hostels and ATCs, and the larger groups of generic workers. The specialists are those who come into regular face to face contact with clients, usually in a setting which claims to help them to learn skills, increase their independence and live in ordinary community settings. The generic workers have in the past only come into occasional contact with mentally handicapped people but are likely to do so much more frequently in the future, as mentally handicapped people make increasing use of ordinary community services. They include general practitioners, staff in general hospitals, social workers, housing officers, most psychologists, people working in social security, the police, recreational and leisure services.

What initial training did the specialists have for the work they are doing now? How relevant was it for today's needs? What kind of training is available for those joining the main professions today? What opportunities are there for regular updating of knowledge and skills? How can they contribute most effectively in the short and medium term to future developments, assuming a continuing shift in emphasis from institutional to community services? To what extent do we need to modify or change existing training arrangements to meet future needs?

What can be done to create a climate of awareness and support among the armies of generic workers? Now that a special education element is a compulsory component of all courses of initial teacher training, can we envisage similar tough prescriptions in the training of doctors, social workers and the police?

More fundamentally, the time has come to ask whether the pattern of training which we have inherited from the past is one which we wish to retain for the future.

We have seen that one of the major obstacles to making effective use of local training resources lies in the long established tradition of separate training for different professional groups being provided by a variety of different training organisations - e.g., at local level by Local Education Authorities, Social Services Departments and the National Health Service, as well as by different departments within institutions of higher education. Similar divisions can be found at national level in separate and largely non-communicating departments in central government and in the major professional associations.

These divisions represent obstacles to the kind of joint training initiatives which are essential in the field of mental handicap. We have argued for the development of a single locally based training strategy for all staff working in this field, no matter who their employer happens to be, and that one of the tasks of a local training consortium would be to try to ensure that all courses were open to all staff. Colleges of Adult Education or University Extra-Mural Departments might provide a suitable neutral base for such initiatives.

In the meantime, we have to consider the situation as we find it - namely one in which different professions carry out all their initial training and much of their post-experience inservice training within the framework of training arrangements provided by their own employers or professional associations.

Having inherited this segregated pattern of training, should we opt for an incremental, step by step expansion of training along traditional lines and within the traditional professional and administrative boundaries? Or should we attempt a more radical reform of the system by trying to develop a new framework which is multidisciplinary from the start, and which will seek to capitalise on similarities in the training needs of all staff who work with mentally handicapped people?

All the signs indicate that, true to the British tradition of incrementalism, we are adapting existing institutions while developing islands of innovation at the same time. The ENB course is an example of a modern, well designed course which nevertheless rests on some doubtful assumptions about the need for single discipline hospital based training. At the same time, the ENB is developing new courses for community mental handicap nursing. Neither strategy seriously addresses the problem of training the trainers.

Although social workers are supposed to be equal partners with nurses in community teams, the almost complete absence of training opportunities either at initial or post-experience level at least has the advantage of forcing them to seek training in an interdisciplinary context. Such training is likely to take the form of ad hoc short courses on a wide range of issues.

Psychologists have few grounds for complacency. Although many psychologists are playing a leading role in developing community services, the amount and quality of training given to clinical and educational psychologists is highly variable from course to course. In the clinical field, it is still difficult to fill even the most senior mental handicap positions. Few educational psychologists specialise in mental handicap and the modal input of EP time into a school for children with SLDs is one half day every two weeks.

The training of medical personnel is still largely carried out in splendid isolation. Given the shortage of mental handicap consultants, an attempt is now being made to ensure that all general psychiatrists and child psychiatrists are able to spend some time training in a mental handicap service. Even if very few psychiatrists work in mental handicap full time, it is hoped that they will provide a psychiatric service to those mentally handicapped people who require it. This model has some similarity to assumptions made in the training of educational psychologists. Clinical psychologists still provide a specialist service.

Current approaches to training emphasise the importance of interdisciplinary courses where workers from different backgrounds and disciplines learn together. One is reminded of the Warnock distinction between locational, social and functional integration. In other words, while there is some value in having staff from different disciplines sitting in the same room and mixing socially during the coffee breaks, the most valuable form of interdisiciplinary courses comes from conscious attempts to help students to share experiences and to learn from one another. Even this is of limited value if they are unable to make use of what they have learned in developing different patterns of collaboration when they return to their work settings. It is good that nurses and social workers should study together but only if this ultimately results in better joint work, whether in a community team or other setting. It is even more important that middle and top management in both hierarchies should share these understandings and support more effective collaboration.

The All Wales Strategy represents a promising example of a radical approach to service planning and delivery coupled with an innovative approach to staff development. All staff working in mental handicap services in Wales are being given the opportunity to take part in retraining designed to help them to reorientate their work to the needs of a community based comprehensive service. So far, an energetic start has been made through a series of interdisciplinary workshops in each county. Other parts of the United Kingdom are beginning to work along similar lines.

Staff training cannot compensate for poor services or ineffective management. A naive faith in more and better staff training is now being tempered by a growing realisation that courses do not necessarily lead to a change in behaviour of participants, far less to changes in the clients with whom they work. Problems of generalisation of training across people, across settings and situations are common to people with mental handicap and the staff who work with them.

REFERENCES

Advisory Council for the Supply and Education of Teachers (1984) Teacher Training and Special Educational Needs, DES, London

Bluma, S., Shearer, J., Frohman, A. and Hilliard, J. (1976) Portage Guide to Early Education, NFER/Nelson, Windsor

Capie, A., Taylor, P. and Perkins, E. (1980) Helping the Retarded, (2nd edn.), British Institute for Mental Handicap, Kidderminster

Central Council for Education and Training in Social Work (1985) Mental Handicap: Progress and Prospects in Staff Training, CCETSW, London

Coupe, J. and Porter, J. (eds.) (1986) The Education of Children with Severe Learning Difficulties: Bridging the Gap Between Theory and Practice, Croom Helm, London

Dean, A. and Hegarty, S. (eds.) (1984) Learning for Independence, Further Education Unit, Department of Education and Science, London

Department of Education and Science (1985) Better Schools, HMSO, London

Department of Health and Social Security (1979) Report of the Committee of Enquiry into Mental Handicap Nursing and Care, (Chair, P. Jay), HMSO, London

Department of Health and Social Security (1980) Mental Handicap: Progress, Problems and Priorities, DHSS, London

Department of Health and Social Security (1985) Development Team for Mentally Handicapped People 'Fourth Report 1981-1984', HMSO, London

English National Board of Nursing, Midwifery and Health Visiting (1982) A Syllabus of Training: Professional Register Part 5: (Registered Nurse for the Mentally Handicapped), ENB, London

Evans, P. and Wade, J. (1986) Helping the Last to Come In: Educational and School Provision for Children with Severe Learning Difficulties and Multiple Handicaps, NFER/Nelson, Windsor

Farrell, P. (ed.) (1985) EDY: Its Impact on Staff Training in Mental Handicap, Manchester University Press, Manchester

Felce, D., Jenkins, J., Dell, D., Flight, C. and Mansell, J. (1983) The Bereweeke Skill Teaching System, NFER/Nelson, Windsor

Hogg, J. and Sebba, J. (1986) Profound Retardation and Multiple Impairment: Vol.2, Education and Therapy, Croom Helm, London

Independent Development Council for People with Mental Handicap (1985) Living Like Other People: Next Steps in Day Services for People with Mental Handicap, IDC and King's Fund Centre, London

Jones, M. (1983) Children at Beech Tree House, Souvenir Press, London

King's Fund (1984) An Ordinary Working Life: Vocational Services for People with Mental Handicap, Project Paper 50, King's Fund, London

Mansell, J. (1985) 'Training Staff to Work in Community Based Services' in C. Heginbotham, (ed.), Campaign for People with Mental Handicaps, London (in press)

MENCAP (1985) 'STAMINA: Local Action for Services', MENCAP, London

Mittler, P. and Preddy, D. (1981) 'Mentally Handicapped Pupils and School Leavers: A Survey in North West England' in B. Cooper, (ed.), Assessing the Handicaps and Needs of Mentally Retarded Children, Academic Press, London

Murphy G. and Wilson, B (eds.) (1985) Self Injurious Behaviour, BIMH, Kidderminster

Staff Development

National Association of Teachers of the Mentally Handicapped (1985) Ways Forward, NATMH, Blackpool

National Development Group for the Mentally Handicapped (1976) Mental Handicap: Planning Together, DHSS, London

National Development Group for the Mentally Handicapped (1977) Day Services for Mentally Handicapped Adults, DHSS, London

National Development Group for the Mentally Handicapped (1978) Helping Mentally Handicapped People in Hospitals: A Report to the Secretary of State for Social Services, DHSS, London

National Development Group for the Mentally Handicapped (1980) Improving the Quality of Services for Mentally Handicapped People: A Checklist of Standards, DHSS, London

Plank, M. (1982) Teams for Mentally Handicapped People, Campaign for People with Mental Handicaps, London

Preddy, D. and Mittler, P. (1981) Children with Severe Learning Difficulties: A Survey in North West England, Final Report to Department of Education and Science, Hester Adrian Research Centre, Manchester

Rectory Paddock School (1983) In Search of a Curriculum (2nd edn.), Wren Publications, Orpington

Robson, C. (1984) 'A Modular, In-service Advanced Qualification for Teachers: Children with Special Education Needs', British Journal of In-Service Education, 11, 32-36

Simon. G. (1981) Next Step on the Ladder, BIMH, Kidderminster

Taylor, P., Crawford, N. and Thobroe, E. (1981) '"Special Care" in 44 Schools for the Mentally Handicapped', Apex, Journal of the British Institute for Mental Handicap, 9, 79-81

Whelan, E. and Speake, (1979) Learning to Cope, Souvenir Press, London

Whelan, E., Speake, B. and Strickland, T. (1984) 'The Copewell Curriculum: Content, Development and Use' in A. Dean and S. Hegarty (eds.), Learning For Independence, Further Education Unit, Department of Education and Science, London

Wolfensberger, W. (1972) The Principle of Normalization in Human Services, National Institute on Mental Retardation, Toronto

Wolfensberger, W. and Glenn, L. (1975) Program Analysis of Service Systems, (3rd edn), National Insitutute on Mental Retardation, Toronto

Wolfensberger, W. and Thomas, S. (1983) PASSING, National Institute on Mental Retardation, Toronto

Chapter Three

THE MANAGEMENT OF STAFF BEHAVIOUR IN RESIDENTIAL TREATMENT FACILITIES: A REVIEW OF TRAINING TECHNIQUES

S.R. Anderson

The ability to produce behaviour change in mentally retarded persons has become a rapidly expanding reality in recent years. Research has resulted in numerous programmes for training an array of adaptive skills (Azrin and Foxx, 1973; Barton, Guess, Garcia and Baer, 1970; Horner and Keilitz, 1975) and suppressing an array of maladaptive behaviours (Azrin and Wesolowski, 1974; Favell, McGimsey and Jones, 1978; Foxx and Azrin, 1973). This progress has contributed to the recent thrust of social and legal actions concerned with improved care and treatment of institutionalised mentally retarded persons. In spite of isolated successes in programme development, usually with a typical personnel, Kazdin (1973) argues that the effective implementation of behaviour modification programmes cannot occur unless staff performance is both developed and maintained.

Several authors have emphasised the significance of direct-care institutional staff for implementing behaviour change in residents (Iwata, Bailey, Brown, Foshee and Alpern, 1976; Pomerleau, Bobrove, and Smith, 1973). Staff are expected to monitor a variety of resident behaviours and to provide correct social contingencies at all times. If staff fail to attend to behaviour contingently or provide few occasions for interaction, it is unlikely that residents will improve. In that case, training will be needed to provide the staff with skills in handling a diversity of residents' needs.

Unfortunately, several studies indicate that staff spend very little of their time in direct contact with residents (Daily, Allen, Chinski and Veit, 1974; Harmatz, 1973). Daily et al. (1974) found that of the 7,108 interactions they observed between staff and residents, 37 per cent occurred in the context of ward routine activities, 31 per cent occurred in the context of care, 23 per cent occurred in the context of social play, and only 9 per cent involved formal training of residents. The data also indicated that those residents perceived by staff as attractive, likeable, and intellectually more competent experienced a greater number of positive interactions (cf. Grant and Moores, 1977). The average resident was engaged in either a positive or social-play interaction in fewer than one per cent of the intervals observed.

Harmatz (1973) found that staff spent 55 per cent of their time engaged in non-child-related activities, 24 per cent engaged in child-related activities of a social nature, e.g., talking with children, and 21 per cent engaged in non-social activities, e.g., physical care. Their discussion noted that housekeeping and paperwork are not necessarily more pleasant or easier than interacting with the residents; however, staff do meet certain hospital expectations, e.g., that the beds be made.

Other studies have provided similar information. Bensberg and Barnett (cited in Bensberg, 1974) reported that less than 5 per cent of the staff's time was spent teaching residents. Both Blindert (1975) and Repp and Barton (1980) concluded that the institutional setting often fails to provide sufficient engagement or educational opportunities for many residents.

Still other authors have noted that staff also reinforce and punish residents' behaviours indiscriminately (Warren and Mondy, 1971; Meseke and Anderson, Note 1). The possible adverse effects of this type of environment on the behaviour of mentally retarded persons have been noted by several authors (Butterfield, 1967; Horner, 1980). Thus staff have to be trained to implement programmes effectively.

This review will identify and discuss techniques that have been used to alter the behaviour of direct-care staff. Occasional reference will be made as well to teachers, parents, or other adults who have been responsible for implementation of behaviour modification procedures. Reference to other populations is necessary because successful demonstrations with other populations increase the generality of the technique, and because studies involving other subject populations demonstrate procedures untried before but with implication for training direct-care staff.

Several studies have shown that training staff may not in itself result in the generalisation or maintenance of their relevant behaviour changes (Katz, Johnson and Gelfand, 1972; Panyan, Boozer and Morris, 1970; Pomerleau et al., 1973). Therefore, this chapter will also discuss issues pertaining to generalisation and maintenance of staff behaviour. Generalisation will be defined as the occurrence of trained behaviour across conditions, i.e., setting, subjects, behaviours, different from those present during training (Stokes and Baer, 1977). Maintenance will be defined as the occurrence of behaviour across time. From here on, sometimes the word "management" will be used in a general sense referring to training, generalisation, and maintenance of staff behaviour.

The distinction in the literature between training, generalisation and maintenance of staff behaviour is not always clear (McInnis, 1976; cf. Kazdin, 1973). Frequently, it is difficult to determine whether the purpose of a particular study is to investigate procedures to train a new skill; retrain a previously learned, then lost skill; programme the generalisation of a newly trained skill; or maintain skill performance. Consequently, studies do not always fit neatly into the large categories of training, generalisation or maintenance.

As an example, Katz et al. (1972) trained psychiatric staff in the "therapeutic application of reinforcement principles". No additional information concerning this training was provided. At some later unspecified time, a measure of behaviour on the ward suggested that staff rarely reinforced appropriate resident behaviour. The difficulty arises when one tries to categorise the staff's inadequate performance as (a) a problem of training, i.e., staff failed to ever demonstrate a knowledge of reinforcement principles; (b) a problem of generalisation, i.e., staff failed to generalise what they learned from the training setting to the ward setting; and/or (c) a problem of maintenance, i.e., satisfactory performance was demonstrated initially on the ward, but extinguished.

However, conclusions regarding the effectiveness of a technique for managing staff behaviour need not refer to the staff's previous training history. This has been a common practice in reviews of staff-training techniques (Gardner, 1973; Kazdin, 1977; McInnis, 1978; Watson, 1976). Unfortunately, the techniques necessary on the one hand to develop behaviour and on the other hand to programme its generalisation and maintenance are not necessarily different procedures. They may be simply a change in their topography, their frequency of occurrence, or the conditions in which they are employed. For example, immediate verbal feedback may be used to train a target staff behaviour, then changed in topography, e.g., to a written memo, delivered intermittently, change in frequency, and programmed across different settings, i.e., change in conditions, to maintain the target behaviour.

The major training techniques discussed in this chapter include: (a) instructional methods, (b) modelling, (c) role-playing, (d) performance feedback, (e) praise, (f) self-recording, (g) monetary incentives, and (h) combinations of these. Following a description of studies relevant to the use of each training technique is a discussion of issues pertaining to generalisation and maintenance of staff-behaviour changes.

STAFF MANAGEMENT TECHNIQUES

Instructional Methods

Training

Instructional methods frequently have been used to train staff behaviour. Techniques include academic instruction, verbal and written instructions, staff assignments and cues.

Academic instruction

Instructional methods such as planned lectures, discussions, course work, workshops and inservice training are frequently used to train staff. This training typically occurs in a setting other than the ward. Research examining the effects of academic instruction on staff behaviour is severely limited. Most of the relevant literature simply provides descriptions of existing programmes rather than analyses of their effectiveness (Butterfield, 1967). Frequently programme effectiveness is evaluated in terms of increases in some degree of knowledge or attitude rather than behaviour demonstrated on the ward (Barnett, cited in Butterfield, 1967; Weissman-Frisch, Crowell and Inman, 1980). The few studies that have provided an analysis of ward performance following training, generally fail to support assumptions made about their effectiveness.

Parloff (cited by Butterfield, 1967) demonstrated that staff knew that the purpose of an inservice program was to change their manner of interacting with residents; however, their behaviour did not change on the ward. Klaber (1969) compared six residential facilities in as many states and found no relation between institutional effectiveness and in-service training. Montegar, Reid, Madsen and Ewell (1977) found that the effects of an inservice training programme were not maintained in the absence of social consequences provided by supervisors. Quilitch (1975) conducted a workshop to teach staff how to lead recreational activities. In spite of this training, the workshop failed to increase significantly the activity of residents on each ward, presumably because staff were not conducting activities consistently.

Verbal or written instructions

One form of instruction is simply telling staff to behave in a specific way in regard to the residents, e.g., reinforce appropriate resident behaviour. Katz et al. (1972) used instructions for prompting staff to reinforce psychiatric patients within a token economy programme. Baseline measures suggested that the staff rarely reinforced appropriate resident behaviour. The staff were informed that two of the residents were performing poorly in occupational therapy and that a third, although performing well, was receiving little positive reinforcement. Instructions included a brief explanation that appropriate resident behaviour could be increased if it produced frequent reinforcing consequences and that undesirable resident behaviour could be decreased by reinforcing incompatible behaviour. The instructions also were posted conspicuously. Instructions had little effect on the rate of staff reinforcement. Positive contacts between staff and residents decreased slightly from five per cent to less than four per cent of the intervals observed.

Panyan et al. (1970) instructed staff to conduct daily self-help training sessions and to keep performance records. The staff had previously received formal classroom training and returned to their wards to incorporate behaviour modification techniques into their daily routines. During baseline no contingencies were in effect if the staff failed to conduct or record a session; the only intervention was verbal requests from the psychologist to "do better". Following formal classroom training, the percentage of sessions was high but dropped after a few weeks to unsatisfactory levels of performance. Thus, although classroom training was effective in developing staff behaviour, instructions were not sufficient to maintain performance.

Other studies also have shown written instructions to be unsuccessful in changing staff behaviour. Wallace, Davis and Liberman (1973) found that a memo instructing staff to conduct a social-interaction hour with residents was ineffective in changing staff behaviour. Patterson, Griffin and Panyan (1976) reported similar results. A memo instructing staff to conduct a 15-minute self-help training session each day, accompanied by data sheets and graph paper, produced no appreciable change in behaviour.

Staff assignments

McInnis (1978) suggests that underlying any successful treatment programme are carefully specified staff assignments, However, when used in isolation or in combination with verbal instructions, their effects have been minimal. For example, Iwata et al. (1976) divided residents into programme groups, with each staff member receiving responsibility for four or five residents. The staff members were responsible for seeing that their respective assigned residents received daily care services. The experimenter measured the amount of time staff engaged in six predefined categories of behaviour, including stimulation activities and direct and indirect custodial work. Staff assignments produced little or no change in direct or indirect custodial work and only a small, variable effect on stimulation activities.

Review of Training Techniques

Pommer and Steedbeck (1974) investigated the effects of staff assignments on staff at a residential child-treatment facility. Public notices listing each staff member's duties and new procedures to be implemented were posted. Although the public notices produced an immediate increase in the number of jobs completed and the number of new procedures implemented, within one week of their assignment the effects were not maintained. After the third day, a slow downward trend in performance was evident. Subsequently, additional procedures were introduced (described later) to regain previously established high levels of performance, making it impossible to determine the long-term effects of staff assignments alone.

Although the data presented here are limited, they do not support the use of staff-assignments to produce behaviour change. McInnis (1978) suggests that clearly specified staff assignments can (1) serve as a lesson play for new employees: (2) prompt staff to perform necessary responsibilities; (3) indicate to staff exactly what is expected of them, and (4) inform supervisors when and where an activity will occur so that they can observe them and provide feedback on performance. The final point may identify a critical issue. In the absence of contingencies for staff behaviour, it is unlikely that assignments will develop or maintain staff performance. However, in combination with programmed consequences for staff behaviour, the isolated effects of each may be enhanced.

Cues

Cueing staff to perform desired behaviour represents a special form of instruction. Here instructions are given during ongoing staff behaviour in an attempt to elicit additional or more accurate performance. Katz et al. (1973) informed staff that since verbal instructions failed to facilitate either task-oriented resident behaviour or reinforcing contacts, one of the experimenters would now cue them to reinforce appropriate resident behaviour. The experimenter then dispensed cues as often as possible and produced a slight but variable increase in staff reinforcement of behaviour for one resident, but not for the other two residents. A slight gain in reinforcement of one resident produced a slight gain in task-oriented behaviour.

Studies conducted with other populations may provide support for the use of cues to alter performance. Van Houten and Sullivan (1975) investigated the effects of an automated cueing system on the frequency of teacher praise in one special and two normal classrooms. The teachers were instructed to praise someone in the classroom who was working each time a brief signal was presented over the school public address system. These signals, presented at a mean rate of two per minute, markedly increased the praise rates of all three teachers. Removal of the cueing system, with instructions to continue praising, did not alter the high rate of praise statements. Reintroduction of the cueing phase, with cues presented a mean rate of three per minute, further increased the rate of teacher praise. Removing the cueing system a second time again produced no reduction in the rate of teacher praise.

Moore and Bailey (1973) used an FM wireless microphone to cue the mother of a 3-year-old, possibly autistic, child to approve and disapprove of her child's behaviour. After baseline measures of pre-academic and social behaviour, the cueing system was introduced successively for each category of behaviour. Cueing consisted of precise instructions to the mother stating what behaviours to prompt, praise and punish. Cueing the mother to approve of pre-academic behaviour and disapprove of non-compliance quickly resulted in an increase in pre-academic behaviour. Similar results were obtained with social behaviour. When cueing was discontinued, the rate of both behaviours either was maintained or improved during the follow-up sessions conducted seven months later.

Unfortunately, it is impossible to determine whether the experimental effects in the two studies just described can be attributed entirely to cueing. The instructions used, although not described in detail, may have alerted subjects to what behaviours were being monitored and under what conditions. Then, the obtrusive observer may have prompted the subjects to perform in a way consistent with their knowledge of experimenter expectations. Neither study included unobtrusive measures of staff performance. Also, neither study specified whether experimenter feedback was provided.

In spite of these problems of interpretation, cueing may have important application in the management of staff behaviour. In two of the three studies just presented, instructions, including cueing, produced substantial changes in staff performance. The significance of cueing to the effects of the instructional package remains unclear. However, at the very least, cueing provides a discriminative stimulus to look and attend to resident behaviour. Otherwise, the attending adult becomes preoccupied with other activities and fails to praise desirable resident behaviour when it occurs.

In summary: instructional methods may serve to indicate the direction or magnitude of desired responding; however, they are generally ineffective unless supported by favourable consequences. One possible exception may be the use of cues for prompting staff performance. Cues include an element of feedback, i.e., repeatedly indicating to staff occasions when they have failed to respond or responded incorrectly.

Generalisation and Maintenance

After desired behaviours have been established, it is important to ensure that they generalise and are maintained when training has stopped. As previously noted, academic instruction has been associated with increases in academic performance (Weissman-Frisch et al., 1980) but has had little effect on staff performance in the ward (Quilitch, 1975; Watson, 1976).

It is often assumed that once behaviour is developed, generalisation and maintenance of behaviour will occur without actively programming either. This strategy has been referred to by Stokes and Baer (1977) as "Train and Hope". Perhaps it is assumed that naturally ocurring contingencies in the generalisation setting will maintain, supplement and make functional newly learned skills. Unfortunately, the few studies that have evaluated generalisation and maintenance often do not support such assumptions. Several descriptive studies presented previously (e.g., Harmatz, 1973) suggest that naturally occurring communities of reinforcement for desired staff behaviour either do not exist or reinforce incompatible or alternative behaviour.

When instructional training is supplemented with training in the actual setting and/or conditions in which the technique will be used, instructions may sometimes be effective (Nay, 1975; Paul, McInnis and Mariotto, 1973). Paul et al. (1973) found that subjects who received academic instructions and on-the-floor practicum training demonstrated continued performance after supervision was faded out. This strategy of training assumes that desired responses will not be demonstrated in the ward where the conditions may vary considerably. Behaviour, therefore, is modified sequentially (Stokes and Baer, 1977) in every setting in which it will be needed.

A common technique for programming generalisation is simply to instruct staff to generalise. That is, if behaviour is not initially demonstrated in the ward, then staff are instructed, e.g., through written or verbal instructions or staff assignments, to display what they have learned and failed to generalise. Unfortunately, instructions to staff to generalise have generally been ineffective (e.g., Katz et al., 1972; Wallace et al., 1973). Even when their effects are initially favourable, behaviour may not be maintained (Panyan et al., 1970). Thus, generalised behaviour may have to be reinforced.

Only one of the instructional methods discussed here produced encouraging results in the generalisation and maintenance of behaviour. In two studies, cueing produced treatment effects that were maintained after the cueing systems were removed (Van Houten and Sullivan, 1975; Moore and Bailey, 1973). However, both studies involved only the effects of cueing on classroom teachers; thus the generality of these results is limited. A similar example of cueing with direct-care staff (Katz et al., 1973) produced only slight changes in staff behaviour.

Modelling

Training

Studies investigating the effects of modelling on staff performance have been infrequent. Modelling is often included as one component of a combination of procedures designed to train staff, including classroom instruction, role-playing, feedback and others (e.g., Watson, Gardner and Sanders, 1971). The modelling component generally involves repeated demonstrations of desired behaviours; the trainee is instructed to imitate those behaviours under controlled conditions and feedback is provided concerning the accuracy of trainee performance. This training typically occurs outside of the ward setting. No studies have systematically analysed the contributing effects of modelling to the total training package and such an analysis probably would not be cost-effective.

In other cases, modelling is used directly in the ward or classroom environment in an attempt to modify staff behaviour. Wallace et al. (1973) investigated its effects on the frequency of staff participation in a social-interaction hour conducted with residents in a neuropsychiatric facility. In a reversal design, the investigators compared several experimental variables including the effects of modelling by a professional consultant versus modelling by the supervising nurse on the ward. During modelling conditions, the model announced that the social hour was beginning, set up various games and participated in the activities with residents. Such modelling by either professional staff or the supervising ward nurse was effective in increasing the number of staff involved in the activity hour. Experimentally planned absences of the supervisor did not result in a deterioration of performance, at least over several days.

Ringer (1973) investigated the effects of modelling to train an elementary-school teacher to provide verbal and token reinforcement in an attempt to decrease inappropriate student behaviour. The model circulated around the classroom and provided praise and tokens for appropriate behaviour. Eventually, both the teacher and the model administered praise and tokens. Gradually, the teacher was given greater responsibility for conducting the programme. When the model eventually withdrew from the classroom, the teacher managed the token system and maintained disruptive behaviour at lower than baseline levels. The authors note that, although the teacher was able to use the token programme to maintain reduced levels of distruptive behaviour, transfer of control from the model to the teacher was incomplete. There was some indication that control over student behaviour was being lost. Unfortunately, there were no long-term follow-up data. Furthermore, the training did not increase the teacher's attention to appropriate student behaviour.

Gladstone and Spencer (1977) evaluated the effects of modelling on the use of praise by staff while they conducted self-care training routines with severely handicapped children. Following a baseline period, each staff member was exposed to three sessions in which one of the authors modelled praise statements. During this condition, the experimenter never discussed praise or reinforcement with the staff, nor provided them with feedback regarding their performance. This exposure resulted in increased levels of response-contingent praise provided by the staff during tooth-brushing routines.

The studies just presented suggest that modelling may be an effective staff-management technique even in the absence of explicit consequences. However, it remains unclear whether implied contingencies may have augmented the effects of modelling in at least one instance. Wallace et al. (1973) reported that the most substantial effects of modelling were obtained with the supervising nurse as model. A prior history of reinforcing and punishing staff behaviour, including accurate imitations, may have made the supervisor's behaviour discriminative for appropriate staff responses. Experimental conditions possibly were indiscriminable from previous setting events in which reinforcement and punishment contingencies were operating (Stokes and Bear, 1977).

Generalisation and Maintenance

In both the Wallace et al. (1973) and Ringer (1973) studies, training occurred within the actual setting and conditions in which the newly trained behaviours were to be displayed. Thus, problems of stimulus and response generalisation were reduced. Gladstone and Spencer (1977) found that levels of staff praise showed a marked increase during hand-and-face washing sessions where no direct modelling occurred. Setting generalisation was not evaluated.

Based on the studies presented here, conclusions regarding the maintenance of behaviour change would be tenuous. Ringer (1973) suggested that teacher control of student behaviour in the absence of the model was declining near the completion of that study. Unfortunately, Wallace et al. (1973) provided a very weak analysis of maintenance in the absence of the model, i.e., only a few days. However, as long as behaviour continued to be modelled, desired levels of staff performance were maintained. An unobtrusive measure taken six weeks after completion of the study found that the supervisory nurse continued to model social interaction and that staff involvement was maintained. Gladstone and Spencer (1977) reported that a two-week follow-up analysis showed that the levels of praise maintained in the model's absence.

Role-Playing

Training

Role-playing has been used as a training technique to teach specific or general behaviour modification skills. Similar to modelling, however, there is a paucity of research concerned with a systematic analysis of the effects of role-playing.

Gardner (1972) compared the effectiveness of role-playing and lectures in the training of institutional staff. Pre- and post-test measures were obtained on the staff's knowledge of behaviour modification principles and their ability to apply behaviour modification techniques. Two groups of subjects were exposed to either role-playing or lectures, followed by the treatment not previously introduced. Role-playing was more effective in teaching behaviour modification.

Jones and Eimers (1975) provided an example of generalisation from training to the natural environment. They trained elementary school teachers in a variety of behaviour modification skills, e.g., differential reinforcement, time-out, via role-playing in a simulated classroom environment. During role-playing, participants alternated the playing of teacher and good and bad student. The experimenter also provided instructions, modelled the desired skills, and provided feedback and praise; thus, training included a combination of training techniques. This training enabled teachers to reduce disruptive behaviour in the regular classroom across a broad range of activities.

The effects of role-playing on staff performance are encouraging, although the data are insufficient. The study by Gardner (1972) indicated only that role-playing was more effective than lectures. The study by Jones and Eimers (1975) suggests that role-playing may be effective when combined with other treatment techniques. Like modelling, role-playing is fequently used as one component in a comprehensive treatment package that generally includes lectures, modelling, feedback and other techniques.

Generalisation and Maintenance

Particularly when used as one component in a treatment package, role-playing may represent a technique for programming generalisation. Role-playing often attempts to simulate conditions similar to the ward environment and allows the trainees to practise what they have learned. Programming common stimuli has been demonstrated to be an effective generalisation technique (Stokes and Baer, 1977). Unfortunately, the studies just presented provide only limited support for this position. Gardner (1972) measured only staff performance in the role-playing condition in which the trainee was observed training another trainee who assumed the role of a resident. Thus it is impossible to draw conclusions regarding any generalisation to actual conditions on the ward. Jones and Eimers (1973) provide some support for the generalised effects of role-playing across settings and conditions. However, the experimental subjects were teachers and not direct-care staff.

Maintenance of staff behaviour has not been investigated either. One may suppose, however, that staff behaviour may not be maintained in the absence of direct consequences. At the very least, it seems important that behaviour be assessed periodically to detect decreases.

Performance Feedback

Training

Feedback refers to the procedure of providing information to staff regarding their level or quality of performance. Feedback is present in virtually all forms of consequation, including delivery of praise, monetary incentives, and self-recording. However, feedback can be used independently of other consequences, simply by providing information about what a staff person is doing. This form of feedback may be presented individually, in writing or verbally, posted publicly, or observed from videotapes.

Review of Training Techniques

Written and/or verbal feedback

Panyan et al. (1970) introduced a feedback system in an attempt to re-establish high levels of self-help training by staff. A written feedback sheet noting the percentage of sessions conducted in each self-help area was given to each staff member and posted weekly. The feedback system increased the percentage of training sessions conducted by staff across three wards.

Andrasik and McNamara (1977) examined the effects of feedback on the number of errors made by staff in a psychiatric institution. An error was scored whenever a staff member awarded points for time worked by residents that was inconsistent with the residents' work contract. Each staff member received weekly feedback in the form of a written communication noting the number of points correctly and incorrectly given. Feedback produced a reduction in errors from an initial level of 62.2 to 6.2 per cent. Errors were optimally reduced when feedback was presented to line staff and first level supervisors but increased slightly when presented to second level supervisors.

No staff management studies have investigated the effects of immediate or nearly immediate feedback on staff performance. However, several investigations involving teachers emphasise the implications of immediate feedback on trainee behaviour (Cooper, Thomson and Baer, 1970; Parsonson, Baer and Baer, 1974). Both of these studies modified the attending behaviour of teachers. Approximately every three to five minutes Parsonson et al. (1974) handed the teacher a slip of paper reporting the proportion of the teacher's last five "attentions-given" to appropriate and inappropriate child behaviours. Cooper et al. (1970) delivered feedback every ten minutes reporting the frequency of attention to appropriate child responses. In both studies, feedback produced substantial increases in the proportion of attention given to appropriate child behaviour. Cooper et al. (1970) reported that the feedback procedure was less effective for one teacher who did not read her feedback note until the end of the day.

Public Posting

As described previously, Quilitch (1975) found that

instructions were ineffective in changing staff or resident behaviour. However, when feedback was also provided in the form of publicly posting the name of assigned activity leaders and the daily number of active residents, substantial increases in the number of active residents occurred.

Pomerleau et al. (1973) investigated the effects of public posting on the behaviour of staff and residents in a psychiatric hospital. Staff individually were assigned one or more residents and were instructed to carry out a pre-arranged reinforcement schedule. The dependent measure was the mean behavioural change of assigned residents as measured by the Ward Behaviour Inventory (Burdock, Hakerem, Hardesty and Zubin, 1968). When staff were ranked on the basis of performance measured as mean behavioural change in assigned residents and the results were posted, the result was a marked increase in appropriate resident performance, presumably because staff behaviour was improved. When feedback was removed, a sharp decrease in appropriate resident behaviour occurred.

Welsch, Ludwig, Radiker and Krapfl (1973) publicly posted the percentage of projects completed each day on two wards at a state institution for mentally retarded persons. They found immediate increases in the percentage of daily completed projects compared to a baseline period of instructions and staff assignments. Unfortunately, the results are at best tenuous due to an inadequate experimental design (AB) and possible reactive effects of the staff learning during treatment that their behaviour was being monitored.

Green, Willis, Levy and Bailey (1978, Experiment 1) examined the frequency with which staff conducted toilet-training sessions. Instructions to toilet the children consistently produced erratic, infrequent results. More consistent participation occurred after the experimenter posted a large figure depicting the percentage of residents participating in the programme, with the name of the staff member responsible for the day's training. However, the staff were not aware that their behaviour was being monitored until the feedback condition was introduced. Learning that they were being observed may have done more to change their behaviour than the intervention itself.

In a second experiment, Green et al. (1978) attempted to measure the effects of more effectively conducted training programmes on the behaviour of profoundly retarded subjects in an institutional environment. Success of the staff-training programme was assessed by observing changes in resident performance during daily training and by a measure of long-term resident gain. Detailed measures were developed to observe the resident's performance during the implementation of two physical therapy programmes concerned with range-of-motion and ambulation.

Improvements in both measures were slight after a condition of immediate feedback, including supervisor praise, cueing, and modelling. Substantial improvements were obtained in a subsequent condition when the performance of residents and staff pairs were publicly posted. Unfortunately, there was no experimental analysis of the feedback and public-posting condition; therefore the controlling properties of performance posting were not confirmed. However, the authors argued that the first experiment demonstrated clearly and dramatically its effects which are consistent with the literature pertaining to performance posting. Also, the results of the outcome and process evaluations were mutually corroborative.

Videotape feedback

Videotaped playback of self-performance also has been used to improve staff performance. Panyan and Patterson (1974) instructed staff to view videotaped playback of themselves conducting a training session immediately following a live session. No comments were made to staff regarding their performance. The playback condition failed to increase the percentage of contingent reinforcement delivered by staff during training sessions. Perhaps they failed to recognise examples of desirable and undesirable behaviour in the absence of experimenter feedback.

In addition to having staff view daily videotaped records of their individual training sessions, Gelfand, Elton and Harman (1972, Experiment 1) provided verbal feedback. The experimenters praised appropriate staff behaviour on the tape, ignored inappropriate behaviour and gave instructions. Videotape feedback and verbal consequences increased staff delivery of contingent consequences, decreased negative attention and was associated with changes in child behaviour. Withdrawal of the feedback did not substantially reduce the level of performance across a period of several days.

Dowrick and Johns (1976) investigated the effects of videotaped feedback and social praise on the behaviour of one staff member on a children's psychiatric ward. Immediately after the staff member had conducted a training session with four residents, she was shown a videotaped recording of the session and the experimenter made comments of praise when, on the tape, she attended to on-task behaviour. The procedure yielded increases in attention to on-task behaviour and decreases in attention to off-task behaviour. These effects were replicated in an ABAB design.

Self-modelling represents another form of videotaped feedback. In self-modelling, persons repeatedly view videotaped recordings of themselves engaged in **desired** target behaviours. Self-modelling contrasts with other applications of videotaped feedback in that only desirable target behaviours are presented. Although the use of self-modelling in the management of the behaviour of direct-care staff has not appeared in the literature, successful application of this procedure to other populations underline its implications (Dowrick and Dove, 1980; Miklich, Chida and Danker-Brown, 1977). As an example, each weekday afternoon, Miklich et al. (1977) exposed asthmatic children in a residential rehabilitation centre to edited tapes of their bed-making. For all subjects, the frequency of daily bed-making was significantly higher in the four weeks after self-modelling than in the four weeks before. These data suggest the need to evaluate self-modelling as a training technique.

In summary, providing information to staff regarding their performance has been demonstrated repeatedly to be an effective management procedure. It should be noted, however, that performance feedback typically is confounded with the effects of the instructions that precede it. Detailed instructions, including a definition of target responses and a discussion of the level of behaviour desired, may influence the efficacy of performance feedback.

Not all studies employing performance feedback have

been concerned with both the quantity and quality of staff performance. Written, including publically posted material, and verbal feedback have produced increases in the frequency of staff conducted toilet-training sessions (Green et al., 1978, Experiment 1), self-help programmes (Quilitch, 1975), and daily assigned projects (Welsch et al., 1973). In each of these studies, the experimenters were concerned mainly with increasing the rate of performance, rather than increasing its quality.

However, feedback has also been shown to produce qualitative changes in staff performance (Dowrick and Johns, 1976; Green et al., 1973, Experiment 2; Parsonson et al., 1974). By clearly specifying Individual response components, i.e., specific exercises to be conducted, of a class of responses, i.e., physical therapy sessions, and providing feedback concerning individual components, Green et al. (1973) produced marked changes in both the quantity and quality of performance. A similar strategy could have been used to produce more effective self-help sessions in the study by Quilitch (1975). Increasing the consistency with which programme are conducted certainly may influence their effectiveness, but if those programmes are conducted incompetently, little change in resident behaviour can be expected.

Several studies have used verbal feedback (Cooper et al., 1970; Parsonson et al., 1974, both involving teachers) and videotaped feedback (Dowrick and Johns, 1976; Gelfand et al., 1972) to modify attending behaviour of adults. In all these studies, the experimenters were attempting to modify the proportion of adult attention given to appropriate and inappropriate child behaviours. Thus, the goal was not only to increase the rate of child-directed adult reinforcement but also to shift its stimulus control so that a larger proportion of adult attention followed appropriate child responses, i.e., qualitative change.

It remains unclear whether any one form of performance feedback is more effective than the others for managing staff behaviour. There has been no systematic analysis of various feedback strategies. Videotaped playback without experimenter feedback (Panyan and Patterson, 1974) was ineffective in increasing contingent reinforcement rate. Also,

Green et al. (1973, Experiment 2) found that individual feedback plus praise produced small, variable changes in behaviour. However, when public posting was added, substantial changes occurred.

Generalisation and Maintenance

In most performance feedback studies, generalisation of newly produced staff performance was neither analysed nor programmed. Setting generalisation was generally not an issue because training occurred in the settings and conditions where behaviour was desired (e.g., Green et al., 1973; Panyan et al., 1970; Parsonson et al., 1974; Quilitch, 1973). In the case of videotaped feedback, the behaviour was not analysed in settings or conditions different from those viewed in the videotapes.

In only one study (Parsonson et al., 1974) was it suggested that staff learned a generalised skill that could be applied across a variety of settings, responses and conditions. In this study, teachers were taught to judge all child behaviour across a variety of situations, rather than only a few specified child responses or under tightly controlled conditions. In a sense, the teachers were trained to generalise - to apply correct social contingencies across virtually all likely forms of child behaviour (Stokes and Baer, 1977).

In few of the studies presented herein were follow-up measures provided on maintenance of behaviour change. In many of the studies (Green et al., 1978; Panyan et al., 1970; Quilitch, 1975; Welsch et al., 1973), the feedback system was never removed. Maintenance of staff performance when the feedback system remains permanently in effect is likely. Desired staff performance maintained for 32 weeks in one feedback study (Panyan et al., 1970) and 30 to 35 days in two others (Green et al., 1978; Quilitch, 1975) before the studies were stopped. Restructuring the management system so that feedback is presented intermittently may reduce its cost and possibly result in behaviour more resistant to extinction (Ferster and Skinner, 1957).

Four studies examined the maintenance of performance feedback training after the feedback systems were removed (Cooper et al., 1970; Dowrick and Johns, 1976; Gelfand et al., 1972; Parsonson et al., 1974) with mixed results. Cooper et al. (1970) found that follow-up measures of rates of teacher attention were within the range of points during training. However, the effects of training may have been declining. Thus, the question of durability remained unanswered. Gelfand et al. (1972) found that desired behaviour maintained for several days after feedback was discontinued. No long-term measures were obtained. Dowrick and Johns (1976) found that behaviour relapsed to baseline levels each time the feedback system was withdrawn. Parsonson et al. (1974) provided the most rigorous analysis of maintenance. Post-training follow-up revealed that both teacher-subjects maintained treatment levels of performance eleven weeks after training was stopped.

In summary, the long-term effects of performance feedback and procedures to reduce its cost have not been sufficiently analysed. It is also important to note that, although it has been effective in the studies reviewed above, it has produced little or no effects in a few studies involving teachers (Cossairt, Hall and Hopkins, 1973; Rule, 1972). Thus, interventions with more consistent effects on staff behaviours have been sought.

Self-Recording

Training

The technique of self-recording requires people to identify some aspect of their behaviour and maintain a record of its occurrence (Nelson, 1977). Self-recording generally is discussed as one component of self-control. However, it has been used as a treatment technique by itself because it often has a reactive effect (Kazdin, 1974b). That is, the behaviour being observed is changed in a desirable direction. Self-recording has been used to modify a variety of behaviours, including obesity (Romanczyk, Tracey, Wilson and Thorpe, 1973), smoking (Foxx and Brown, 1979) and the study behaviour of college students (Johnson and White, 1971). While the quality of these studies varies, their conclusions consistently suggest that at least under some conditions, self-recording can produce a change in the behaviour recorded. Although it has been suggested that self-recording may prove to be an effective behaviour-change technique with staff (Loeber and Weisman,

1975), that application rarely has been reported in the literature.

Burg, Reid and Lattimore (1979) employed a self-recording procedure to increase the frequency of staff attention to profoundly retarded persons in a state residential facility. Staff were instructed about what to self-record and how many interactions to initiate and a recording card with which to score their behaviour. Other staff responsibilities were maintained or showed small improvement related to area and resident cleanliness. Favourable changes also occurred in two child-behaviour categories: self-stimulation and disruptive-aggressive behaviour.

Anderson (Note 2) used instructions, modelling, role-playing and feedback to develop the use of an incidental language-teaching sequence by a teacher and two para-professionals in a special education class-room. After training, they showed a generalised use of the teaching sequence in a diversity of teaching occasions. In a second treatment condition, self-recording procedures were successfully used to increase the frequency of teaching occasions. At the beginning of each session, every teacher received 30 tokens per child. A token represented a successful teaching interaction. When an interaction occurred, the adult took one token from the ring of tokens and put it in the pocket of her apron. At the end of each session, teachers counted the number of tokens removed from the ring and graphed the total for each child. Marked increases in the frequency of teaching occasions occurred during the self-recording condition.

Not all studies using self-recording procedures have been successful. Van Houten and Sullivan (1975) instructed teachers to count each time they praised any child's work, to calculate their praise rate in responses per minute and to graph it at the end of each class session. They further instructed the teacher to maintain a praise rate of two responses per minute. Through the self-recording phase, the experimenter checked daily each teacher's graph without delivering feedback. The self-recording procedure had negligible effects on the behaviour of one teacher and no effects on the behaviour of a second.

In another study, Burgio, Whitman and Reed (1983)

evaluated the effects of a package of techniques that included staff selected goals, self-monitoring, graphing and self-praising upon staff performance. Staff in each treatment setting established a daily goal for the number of staff-child interactions, used a wrist counter to record the frequency of their interactions, graphed the level of their responding and administered self-praise after personally evaluating their performance. These methods resulted in increases in the frequency of staff-child interactions as well as appropriate child behaviour.

The efficacy of self-recording may be determined in part by the presence or absence of several reactive variables, including 1) instructions; 2) criterion performance levels; 3) protocols and equipment used to record; and 4) externally imposed contingencies (Jones, Nelson and Kazdin, 1977). Each of these factors may contribute to the overall reactivity of self-recording:

1. In each of the studies described above, the experimenter gave explicit instructions regarding what behaviour to record, how changes in the level of that behaviour may affect the child's performance, and what level of adult behaviour needed to be achieved. Although instructions have generally been shown to be ineffective in changing staff behaviour, they may augment the effects of self-recording.

2. Criterion performance levels may enhance the efficacy of self-recording. Kazdin (1974a) found that subjects given a specific number of self-reference statements to make while self-recording made more statements than a group who were not provided a specific goal.

3. The equipment used by staff to self-record may augment the reactivity of self-recording. Recording cards (Burg et al., 1979), counters (Burgio et al., 1983) and tokens (Anderson, Note 2) may prompt or remind staff to self-record. Indeed, the more obtrusive the recording device, the more likely it is to provide discriminative value. In one unsuccessful demonstration of self-recording (Van Houten and Sullivan, 1975) it was not clear whether a recording device was provided.

   Feedback provided by obtrusive recording devices

may produce greater reactivity of self-recording. Kazdin (1974a) found that subjects who were permitted to view their counters made more reference statements (the target behaviour) than subjects whose counters were covered.

4. Most self-recording programmes include some form of supervision or monitoring by an external agent who may provide contingencies for recording. Burg et al. (1979) and Burgio et al. (1983) instructed supervisors to praise staff for using the recording card or counter, but not praise the rate of performance. However, the staff may have responded to implied contingencies. The involvement of a supervisor, who had a history of reinforcing and punishing staff responses, may have indicated to staff that their performance would be evaluated. In some instances subjects may be unable to discriminate between receiving reinforcement for self-recording and receiving reinforcement for changes in the frequency of the target response (Nelson, Lipinski and Black, 1976). External monitoring by an obtrusive observer may also contribute to the reactivity of self-recording. However, Burgio et al. (1983) included a number of procedures in an attempt to minimise reactivity.

As in the case of performance-feedback studies, not all self-recording studies have been concerned with both quantitative and qualitative changes in staff performance (cf. Burg et al., 1979). Likewise, qualitative changes in performance may be produced by specifying response components and instructing staff to maintain a record of their occurrence. For example, suppose that staff are instructed to count their attention to appropriate child behaviour. A close analysis of their behaviour may reveal that although attention has increased in frequency, its diversity and topography are very restricted, e.g., always saying "Good Girl" and in the same manner. Increased diversity of attention might be achieved by specifying the diversity of reinforcers possible, e.g., physical contact, verbal praise, food, and by instructing staff to count the occurrence of each kind individually. A similar specifiction might be made of topography of attention, e.g., smiling face, eye contact, changes in voice inflection. However, it may be impractical to instruct staff to self-record these components accurately. Thus self-recording may not be appropriate when the behaviour is difficult to count or the subject does not easily recognise its occurrence.

Furthermore, when the desired performance is complex or novel, self-recording alone may not be effective. For example, teaching the concepts of shaping, differential reinforcement, time-out from positive reinforcement, etc., typically requires some combination of instructions, modelling, role-playing, and feedback. Once such behaviours are developed, then self-recording may be introduced to increase the rate of performance and in some cases to improve its quality.

Although there are some questions about the source of self-recording's effectiveness and the extent of its generality of use, it is capable of producing desired changes in staff performance at relatively little cost. Burg et al. (1979) reported that one weekly staff meeting was sufficient to instruct staff in the use of self-recording; Anderson (Note 2) found that only one session of approximately 30 minutes was required, Burgio et al. (1983) introduced training to staff during an hour-long meeting. Thus, its relatively low cost and generally favourable results suggest the need to replicate and extend these findings.

Generalisation and Maintenance

Self-recording might be used most effectively to programme the generalisation and maintenance of staff behaviour. It seems particularly useful because of its relatively low cost of implementation. Thus, when behaviour change has been accomplished by whatever combination of training techniques needed, but is displayed in only transitory forms (or not at all) in non-training conditions, it might be modified sequentially by instructing staff to count its occurrence across non-generalised conditions (e.g., Burgio et al., 1983). After such modifications, more extensive generalisation beyond two or more conditions might occur (Stokes and Baer, 1977).

Evidence relevant to long-term maintenance of the effects of self-recording is inconclusive. Burg et al. (1979) continued to ask the staff to self-record and found that treatment levels of performance were not evident at a seven-week follow-up but had returned at an eleven-week follow-up. The authors concluded that some major changes in the physical environment of the dayroom may have resulted in the decrease in performance observed at the seven-week observation. Burgio et al. (1983) reported significant inter-staff differences in the maintenance of behaviour gain, with seven staff either increasing or maintaining and three staff decreasing their levels of contingent attention.

In summary, additional research is needed to investigate the generalistion and maintenance of self-recording and its effects. No studies have determined whether the effects of self-recording will generalise to non-training conditions or whether self-recording will need to be introduced in every condition in which behaviour change is desired. It is also unclear whether behaviour developed by self-recording will maintain either in the absence or presence of continued recording. Finally, additional research is needed to evaluate the effects of intermittent self-recording.

Feedback Including Praise

Training

Montegar et al. (1977) investigated the effects of a supervisor's approval on the frequency of staff-resident interactions in an institution for multi-handicapped persons. Following a baseline period, an inservice training programme, designed to teach appropriate methods of interacting with residents, was introduced along with contingent supervisor approval. The training sessions were conducted on the ward and included didactic lectures, modelling of various instructional methods, slides illustrating suggested activities and role-playing. Beginning simultaneously with the inservice training, a system of supervisor approval was instituted. The ward director walked through the ward and praised those staff members engaged in stimulation training. Staff performance of stimulation training increased markedly when approved by supervisors during inservice training. When supervisor approval was discontinued, staff-resident interactions returned to their baseline levels. Reinstatement of supervisor approval again produced substantial increases in percentage of staff time engaged in stimulation-training activities.

Patterson et al. (1976) displayed a poster listing each staff person's name with squares in which they could record self-help training sessions that they conducted with severely retarded persons. At the end of each two-week period, the staff member who had conducted the most training sessions was labelled the "Behaviour Engineer" and a poster proclaiming that person a "Winner" was displayed prominently. Although substantial changes occurred, the effects of treatment began to decrease. A replication conducted on a second ward produced similar results, but these data were suspect due to an increasing trend evident during baseline.

Two studies involving teachers provide further evidence for the importance of praise in managing staff behaviour. Cossairt et al. (1973) met individually with two teachers after class to tell them how often their students paid attention and how much praise the teachers gave them. These procedures did not produce systematic changes in the teachers' or the students' behaviour. In the next condition, the experimenter continued to provide feedback and in addition praised the teacher for using praise in the classroom. The praise markedly increased both teachers' use of praise in their classroom. In addition, the students in each class showed dramatic increases in attending.

Rule (1972) demonstrated a procedure for providing more immediate feedback for desired behaviour. The experimenter followed teacher-trainees as they taught and continuously recorded their frequencies of on- and off-task contacts. At the end of each five-minute period, the experimenter interrupted the trainees, showed them their recording chart and praised them when they met a specified criterion. If they had not met the criterion, the experimenter replaced them and taught for three to five minutes, while they recorded in the experimenter's place. This procedure was effective in decreasing their undesirable behaviour and increasing their desirable behaviour. Unfortunately, it is impossible to ascertain the significance of praise in the total treatment package.

A developing area in the use of social consequences is to teach children to alter adult behaviour (Graubard, Rosenberg and Miller, 1971; Seymour and Stokes, 1976; Stokes, Fowler and Baer, 1978). As an example, Stokes et al. (1978) taught four normal and four deviant children to judge the quality of their own academic work and then to prompt or cue their trainer to make positive statements about it. When these skills failed to generalise spontaneously from the trainer to other teachers, the experimenter taught such generalised responding in a multiple baseline across subjects design. Positive statements by the teachers increased during this condition.

As the authors noted, these procedures enabled the children to contact a natural community of reinforcers. This increased praise is supposed to maintain the children's improved performance, and the children's cueing is supposed to maintain the teacher's praise. The generality of this technique for institutionalised mentally retarded persons and staff has not yet been investigated. It seems unlikely that many severely and profoundly retarded individuals could be taught to cue staff attention to their work.

In summary, feedback in combination with social praise has produced substantial changes in staff performance when feedback alone (Cossairt et al., 1973; Rule, 1972) and inservice training alone (Montegar et al., 1977) were ineffective. Much additional research is needed to determine the possible utility of training children to alter staff behaviour.

Generalisation and Maintenance

In none of the studies described above was generalisation assessed or programmed. Training occurred within the actual conditions (setting, responses, children, etc) where the target behaviour was to be displayed. Nevertheless, if generalisation were found to be incomplete, it could be programmed by introducing feedback plus praise in every non-generalised condition. It remains to be determined whether a reduced schedule of social reinforcement could be used to programme generalisation.

Maintenance of behaviour change produced by feedback plus praise also has not been investigated. However, previous studies involving feedback only, if the feedback system remained (e.g., Panyan et al., 1970) or was withdrawn (e.g., Parsonson et al., 1974), uniformly showed that feedback plus praise may produce long-term maintenance of behaviour change. Furthermore, changing to an intermittent schedule of reinforcement may reduce the cost of training and produce behaviour more resistant to extinction

Feedback Plus Monetary Incentives

Training

Numerous studies have described the use of monetary incentives to modify staff behaviour. Bricker, Morgan and Grabowski (1972) used trading stamps as reinforcers for staff working with mentally retarded children. Videotaped samples of the staff's performance showed that staff spent very little time interacting with the residents. During the first treatment condition, staff were shown videotapes of their performance, feedback on the quality of work was provided and trading stamps were given based on their performance. This dramatically increased the amount of time staff spent with the children. During a second intervention period, two of the training techniques, viewing the tapes and feedback on performance, were discontinued. Interaction time became highly variable, however, it did not return to its baseline levels. Thus, the trading stamps were sufficient to maintain some of the previously established levels of performance.

Katz et al. (1972) found that although instructions and verbal prompts failed to increase staff reinforcement of patients' behaviours, monetary reinforcement of staff performance resulted in substantial increases. The staff were informed that if they could increase the frequency of their reinforcing contacts with targeted residents to a level approximating 50 per cent of the intervals observed, they would receive a fifteen dollar cash bonus. They were also told that they could receive daily feedback concerning their performance if they desired. When the monetary incentives and feedback were discontinued, staff reinforcement rates returned to near baseline levels. Unfortunately, there was no return to treatment conditions, nor was there any attempt to evaluate whether feedback alone would have maintained improved staff performance.

Although Pomerleau et al. (1973) found that feedback was effective in producing desirable changes in staff behaviour, monetary incentives were shown to produce even greater effects. The dependent measure was the mean behaviour change of assigned residents as measured by the Ward Behavioural Inventory (Burdock et al., 1960; Burdock and Hardesty, 1968). When a 20 dollar reward was given to the most cooperative aide, not contingent on the behaviour of assigned residents, little change in behaviour was noted. However, when staff were given cash awards on the basis of improvement by the assigned residents, there was a marked increase in appropriate resident performance, presumably because staff behaviour was improved. As monetary awards increased in successive weeks from ten dollars to twenty dollars to thirty dollars, the behaviour of residents improved correspondingly. When the monetary awards decreased from thirty dollars to twenty dollars, there was a marked increase in inappropriate resident behaviour.

Patterson et al. (1976) investigated the use of two schedules of pay to increase the rate of daily self-help training sessions conducted by staff. First, staff were given bingo cards for every resident with whom they were conducting training sessions. The more residents one trained, the more bingo cards one could have and thus the more probable it was that the staff member could win five dollars in cash from the experimenters. This procedure failed to improve staff behaviour.

In a subsequent condition, peer competition was introduced. The person conducting the most training sessions was chosen "Behaviour Engineer" and received a five dollar cash award. This produced an initial increase in performance that was not maintained. A replication of these procedures on a second ward produced similar effects. However, this time the effects were maintained for several weeks until the money incentive was removed. Discontinuation of the cash award produced a gradual decline in performance to baseline levels.

Pommer and Steedback (1974) found that public posting of staff duties and new procedures to be implemented, although producing an initial effect, failed to maintain staff behaviour. In a subsequent condition, staff were issued tokens worth one dollar each for performing jobs and implementing procedures within one week of assignment. The tokens regained and sustained high levels of performance when used in conjunction with public notices. Discontinuation of public notices produced some reduction in performance and discontinuation and resumption of both components produced further reductions and reinstatement, respectively. These results must be interpreted with some caution: the brevity of the experimental conditions, and trends that were not allowed to stabilise, make it impossible to assess the relative effectiveness of public notices and money reinforcement.

Two studies (Hollander and Plutchik, 1972; Hollander, Plutchik and Horner, 1973) have investigated the effects of monetary incentives on the work performance of psychiatric staff. The dependent variable was the percentage of assigned and volunteer tasks completed by staff. During the treatment condition, staff were given trading stamps contingent on completion of assigned tasks. This increased the percentage of tasks completed on the ward and increased the residents' work behaviour. When the stamp contingency was removed, performance returned to baseline levels, demonstrating experimental control but failing to show maintenance of behaviour change.

In summary, investigations employing feedback plus monetary incentives as a staff management technique generally have shown substantial and consistent effects on staff behaviour. It should be noted, however, that relevant studies were concerned not with the training of new skills, but instead with increasing the occurrence of staff behaviour from undesirable levels.

The effectiveness of these procedures must be compared to their cost. Few institutional administrators have funds available for providing money bonuses. This may be evidenced by the fact that only two of the seven studies reviewed here ended in a treatment rather than a baseline condition (Bricker et al., 1970; Pommer and Streedbeck, 1974). Thus, because of practical problems, other cost-effective staff reinforcement programmes have been sought.

Generalisation and Maintenance

None of the studies presented above assessed generalisation to extra-experimental responses or conditions. Measurements were restricted to a specific class of responses, e.g., frequency of attention. It seems problematic that generalisation would occur without direct programming.

The above studies demonstrated that staff behaviour did not maintain in the absence of monetary incentives. In five of the six studies presented, treatment-obtained levels of performance quickly returned to baseline levels when feedback plus monetary incentives were removed. The sixth study (Bricker et al., 1972) never removed the monetary incentive. Removing the feedback component produced some reduction in performance in one study (Pommer and Streedbeck, 1974) and more variability in performance in a second study (Bricker et al., 1972). Unfortunately, none of the studies evaluated whether behaviour developed using a combination of feedback and monetary incentives could be maintained by feedback alone. Finally, neither of the two studies ending in a treatment condition (Bricker et al., 1972; Pommer and Streedbeck, 1974) provided a follow-up analysis of maintenance of behaviour change. In summary, research to date has contributed little information regarding the generalisation and maintenance of behaviour established using the combination of feedback plus monetary incentives.

Feedback Plus Work Schedule Incentives

Training

Allowing staff access to preferred activities contingent on desirable work behaviour represents a potentially low-cost procedure, yet one that has been investigated only rarely. Ayllon and Azrin (1964) discussed the possible use of vacation schedules and workshift preference, but did not investigate either. Other suggestions include making preferred job assignments and rearranging work or break schedules.

Iwata et al. (1976) attempted to improve daily care and training on four units of a residential facility for mentally retarded persons. Staff who met performance criteria for stimulation training and resident treatment (e.g., dental care) were eligible for a weekly lottery for the opportunity to arrange their days off the following week. The lottery produced substantial decreases in staff off-task behaviour and in the number of residents found in soiled clothing. Increases were observed in the amount of time staff engaged in stimulation and training activities with residents, the number of residents who received daily toothbrushing and the number included in daily out-of-bed activities. The procedure of granting extra weekends off did not produce potential staff shortages as one might suppose.

Watson (1976, p. 94) also reported the use of time-off from work to reinforce staff responses. Instructions to staff to collect toileting data on 19 residents had little effect. However, when a half-day off from work was given to the outstanding data collector in each of three groups and for the shift training supervisor whose shift collected the most data, substantial increases in data collection occurred. When the contingency was removed, data collection deteriorated.

In summary, rearranging work schedules or allowing time-off from work has produced substantial increases in desirable staff performance. Iwata et al. (1976) improved staff performance across a diversity of responses by making the opportunity to win weekends off contingent on meeting criteria clearly specified for each response. In spite of the success of these procedures, the fact that few demonstrations appear in the literature may indicate that they are not easily implemented. Civil service systems, which frequently employ staff and regulate hours, are generally too inflexible to allow frequent changes in work schedules.

Generalisation and Maintenance

Neither of the studies presented above provided an analysis of the generalisation and maintenance of staff behaviour. The study by Iwata et al. (1976) suggests, however, that generalisation may be programmed across settings, responses, residents, etc. by clearly specifying what responses are desired and when and where they are to be displayed. The opportunity to rearrange work schedules or get extra time-off can then be made contingent on meeting specified criteria. It is not known whether responses would eventually generalise without the benefit of direct training.

Iwata et al. (1976) reported that two of those four units continued the lottery system after the study was discontinued. However, no follow-up data were presented to evaluate long-term maintenance. Unfortunately, the study by Watson (1976) suggests that such behaviour is not likely to be maintained once the contingency is removed.

Combinations

Frequently, several techniques are introduced individually in a stepwise progression until successful modification of staff behaviour has been achieved, for example, instructions, followed by staff assignments, followed by feedback and so on, until a successful technique or combination of techniques has been found. Many examples of sequencing techniques in this manner are available (e.g., Green et al., 1978; Katz et al., 1972; Hollander and Plutchik, 1972; Iwata et al., 1976).

In other instances, several techniques are combined and introduced simultaneously with no concern for evaluating individual components. Gladstone and Sherman (1975) trained high school students to teach profoundly retarded residents to follow simple instructions. Training techniques included modelling, rehearsal of various instructional methods (e.g. fading), corrective feedback and experimenter praise. Each student was introduced to the training after a differing number of baseline sessions. Following this training, four of the seven trainees successfully taught their child to follow the instruction, "Bring ball". Furthermore, trainees, including those unsuccessful with the first child, were able to teach a second resident to follow the instructions, "Sit down" and "Come here," even though they had not been taught how to teach those skills. The authors suggest that failure with three of the first seven residents was probably due to the residents' resistance to physical prompting rather than the failure of trainees to follow procedure.

Two studies were concerned with teaching staff to complete various assigned tasks on the ward, including observing and recording resident behaviour, distributing lunch tickets and graphing the performance of each resident (Hollander and Plutchik, 1972; Hollander et al., 1973). A six-week course demonstrated the principles of operant conditioning. At the end of the course, staff participated in question-and-answer sessions, observed modelled demonstrations and role-played required target responses. These procedures resulted in less than satisfactory rates of task completion. Desirable levels of performance were established after trading stamps were delivered contingent on completion of assigned tasks as described previously in detail.

Montegar et al. (1977) found that a combination of inservice training, feedback and social praise effectively increased the staff performance of stimulation training with multihandicapped persons. In a partial component analysis, feedback plus praise was removed to show that the effects of inservice training alone could not maintain staff performance.

Ivancic, Reid, Iwata, Faw and Page (1981) incorporated a number of techniques to teach staff to increase child verbalisation during a routine care task. Procedures included an initial inservice training session consisting of lectures, modelling and feedback, followed by a number of prompting techniques i.e., publicly posted reminders, verbal instructions and modelling as well as feedback procedures. The results indicated that staff learned the necessary skills during the bathing routines and that the change did not interfere with the completion of the direct-care task. Changes in child vocalisations showed no consistent change across conditions.

In a more recent study, Kessel, Whitman and Reid (1983) taught staff using a combination of instructions, modelling and verbal and videotaped feedback. The staff were taught to use basic behaviour management skills in a toothbrushing situation with severely and profoundly handicapped residents. After training, the staff demonstrated the appropriate and consistent use of the methods in a training and two non-training situations. The training programme also produced gains in the residents' ability to complete independently the self-care routines.

Several other investigators have combined techniques as part of staff training, including classroom instruction, modelling, role-playing, feedback and others. Unfortunately, these programmes have been evaluated only in terms of producing changes in academic performance or staff attitudes (Gardner, 1972; Paul and McInnis, 1974; Watson, et al., 1971) and not actual changes in performance on the ward.

In summary, in some instances a combination of training techniques has been employed to manage staff behaviour (Gladstone and Sherman, 1975; Ivancic et al., 1981; Kessel et al., 1983; Montegar et al., 1977). Whether there exists a combination of techniques most effective for training staff has not been determined. Some techniques were common to these studies (i.e., instructions, feedback and praise) and other techniques were not (i.e., modelling, role-playing). A combination of instructions, modelling and role-playing was found to produce less than satisfactory results in two studies (Hollander and Plutchik, 1972; Hollander et al., 1973). One obvious difference between these two sets of studies is that in the two unsuccessful attempts, consequences for staff performance were not initially applied. However, eventually reinforcing staff with trading stamps produced desirable levels of staff performance.

It should also be noted that training in the studies presented above were designed to teach an individual to apply specific behaviour-modification techniques under limited conditions. In contrast, Holland and Plutchik (1972) and Hollander et al., (1973) attempted to teach staff a general skill that could be applied to a variety of ward situations. The specialised skills provided in the former case may have been easier to teach.

Generalisation and Maintenance

Gladstone and Sherman (1975) found that the combination of videotaped modelling, rehearsal, corrective feedback and praise was effective for training four of seven trainees to teach a retarded child to follow one instruction. Furthermore, the training was sufficiently general to allow all trainers to teach a second child without additional training input. Any further generalisation was not assessed. Thus, it is still not known whether the trainers would be effective across a variety of different tasks, with different children and in different settings.

Ivancic et al., (1981) found that the combination of techniques they employed resulted in generalisation to another direct care task, dressing, without the benefit of direct programming. Their improved performance also maintained across nineteen weeks of follow up observation. Maintenance occurred in spite of the fact that various components of the supervision were decreased from 47 per cent of the days during the treatment condition to 19 per cent during the maintenance phase.

Kessel et al., (1983) found that positive change in staff behaviour generalised across two different self-care routines. The authors suggested that a combination of factors may have been responsible for this generalisation, including explicit verbal prompts to use the training methods across self-care routines and common stimuli used in training and nontraining situations, e.g., same physical setting, similar self-care routines and the observers. The authors also reported that the self-control procedures, i.e., graphing child and staff behaviours and the fading of external supervision may have resulted in maintenance of treatment gains.

Other studies (Hollander and Plutchik, 1972; Hollander et al., 1973; Montegar et al., 1977) restricted their analysis to a single class of responses in a single setting or condition. These studies were concerned only with the rate of a particular target response and not with the quality of staff performance or the effect of improved staff performance on resident behaviour. While Montegar et al. (1977) reported no follow-up data, the other studies (Hollander and Plutchik, 1972; Hollander et al., 1973) found that behaviour gradually returned to pretreatment levels when experimental contingencies were removed.

DISCUSSION

Outcome and Process Evaluation

How a treatment programme is evaluated, i.e., process or outcome, has been discussed with reference to staff training (McInnis, 1978; McInnis and Kitson, 1977). Process evaluation is defined as a means by which one judges whether each of the elements of the treatment programme is present and meets appropriate standards. Outcome evaluation is a measure of actual changes in resident behaviour.

Nearly fifty per cent of the training studies presented in this review failed to report outcome data. Although substantial changes in staff behaviour frequently were reported, one should never assume that such changes necessarily produced desirable changes in resident behaviour. One study has shown that increasing the number of training sessions conducted by staff had no significant effect on the performance of residents within those sessions (Martin et al., 1973).

In a few studies, outcome data were presented and process data were omitted (Jones and Eimers, 1975; Moore and Bailey, 1973; Quilitch, 1975; Pomerleau et al., 1973). If the treatment successfully modifies resident behaviour and experimental control is demonstrated, then obtaining only outcome data seems unproblematic. However, if the programme produced less than desirable levels of performance, then an erroneous conclusion may be made that the programme was ineffective when in fact it was not implemented correctly. This possibility emphasises the need to obtain process data at least periodically.

Experimental Design

The common designs used to evaluate staff-management techniques have been time-series designs (multiple baseline and reversal) comparing levels of staff performance or resident behaviour in the presence and the absence of the management technique (Risley and Wolf, 1972).

ABA or ABAB reversal designs were used to demonstrate experimental control of the effects of various forms of feedback and feedback plus incentives: praise (Dowrick and Johns, 1976; Montegar et al., 1977), monetary incentives (Hollander and Plutchik, 1972; Hollander et al., 1973), and work schedule incentives (Watson, 1976).

In some instances, experimental designs were weakened by trends that were not allowed to stablise (Patterson et al., 1976; Pommer and Streedbeck, 1974). In other cases, only condition means were presented, making it impossible to evaluate trends (Pomerleau et al., 1973). Some experimenters returned to different conditions than were present in the initial baseline (Pommerleau et al., 1973; Wallace et al., 1973). In all such studies, the contention that behaviour may have changed independently of the experimental intervention could not be rejected confidently.

Many of the studies reviewed employed multiple-baseline designs, across subjects, settings or behaviours. These studies demonstrated the effects of cueing (Moore and Bailey, 1973; Van Houten and Sullivan, 1975); modelling (Panyan and Patterson, 1974; Ringer, 1973); role-playing (Jones and Eimers, 1975); self-recording (Burg et al., 1979; Burgio et al., 1983; Anderson, Note 2); performance feedback (Cooper et al., 1970; Green et al., 1978; Panyan et al., 1970; Parsonson et al., 1974; Quilitch, 1975; Welsch et al., 1973); praise (Cossairt et al., 1973; Rule, 1972; Stokes et al., 1978); monetary incentives (Iwata et al., 1976); and a package of training techniques (Gladstone and Sherman, 1975; Ivancic et al., 1981, Kessel et al., 1983). Welsch et al. (1973) did not discuss issues of design. However, their study seems to represent a multiple-baseline-across-wards design, i.e., behaviour was measured simultaneously on two wards and experimental procedures were applied to each ward at different times.

Two studies (Gardner, 1972; Paul et al., 1973) employed a group design in which two groups of subjects were taught behaviour modification skills by one of two methods, i.e., role-playing or lecture. These two groups were compared statistically for any significant mean difference in treatment effects. Neither study included a non-treatment control group.

Frequently, different staff-management techniques (e.g., Bricker et al., 1972; Cossairt et al., 1973; Patterson et al., 1976), different levels of the same technique (Wallace et al., 1973; Pommer and Streedbeck, 1974), or a combination of both (Andrasik and McNamara, 1977) were introduced sequentially until a desirable effect was obtained (e.g., ABC, $AB_1B_2B_3A$, or $ABC_1C_2C_3A$). Although these designs were adequate to demonstrate experimental control, it usually was impossible to conclude the precise nature of control exhibited by each of the various techniques. Replication with additional subjects, in which the sucessful treatment technique was introduced without the preceding conditions, would complete the experimental analysis. Only three studies provided such an analysis (Patterson et al., 1976; Rule, 1972; Van Houten and Sullivan, 1975).

In general, the quality of experimental designs in the studies reviewed is good. However, exceptions have been noted. Unfortunately, in many instances it is impossible to specify a single technique as the source of behaviour change, or to see the relative significance of each technique relative to the effects of the treatment package. In some instances, an analysis of individual components may not be cost-effective, particularly when a technique appears to be a logical prerequisite or accompaniment to more complex training techniques as in the case of instructions or staff-assignments.

Single-subject designs with repeated measures seem better designs for evaluating the effects of staff-training techniques. They allow nearly immediate inspection of any effects or trends, generally require fewer subjects and circumvent variability due to intersubject differences (Kazdin, 1973). Because a reversal of experimental effects sometimes may be unexpected or undesirable e.g., administrators ardently object or undesirable effects on resident behaviour may occur, a multiple-baseline design across subjects, settings or behaviour seems most desirable. One must consider, however, whether an alteration in one subject, setting or behaviour may influence respectively, the behaviour of other subjects, behaviour in other settings, or other responses.

Reliability

Reliability was assessed in slightly more than 80 per cent of the studies reviewed excluding those by, Andrasik and McNamara, (1977); Gardner, (1972); Hollander and Plutchik, (1972); Hollander et al., (1973); Panyan et al., (1970); Watson, (1976); Welsch et al., (1973). The method of assessing reliability, when it was assessed, depended on the variables chosen for modification. When the unit of measurement was a narrowly defined target behaviour, a total score method of calculating reliability was used. In this method, two observers independently scored the occurrences of one or more target behaviours over the same period of time. The smaller observed frequency was divided by the larger and multiplied by 100. A total-score method was used to measure the number of praise statements delivered (Gladstone and Spencer, 1977); percentage of sessions conducted (Patterson et al., 1976); percentage of residents and staff present at an activity hour (Wallace et al., 1973); the number of jobs completed and new procedures implemented (Pommer and Streedbeck, 1974); the percentage of contingent reinforcers delivered (Panyan and Patterson, 1974); and the number of residents participating in a toileting programme (Green et al., 1978, Experiment 1). Kessel et al., (1983) employed a total score method across both the occurrence and nonoccurrence of the target behaviours.

Two studies used a variation of the total-score method (Ivancic et al., (1981); Parsonson et al., 1974; Anderson, Note 2). An agreement was scored only when both observers recorded that the same category of behaviour occurred, in a situation in which there were several possible ways to categorise behaviour. Reliability was calculated by dividing the number of agreements by the number of agreements plus disagreements and multiplied by 100. Reliability by individual categories as well as overall reliability scores were reported.

When the dependent variable was a composite of many responses e.g., appropriate child behaviour, then observed frequencies of the target behaviour were compared interval by interval (Cooper et al., 1970; Cossairt et al., 1973; Dowrick and Johns, 1976; Green et al., 1978; Experiment 2; Jones and Eimers, 1975; Katz et al., 1972; Moore and Bailey, 1974; Ringer, 1973; Rule, 1972; Stokes et al., 1978; Van Houten and Sullivan, 1975).

A few studies obtained momentary time-samples of behaviour (Burg et al., 1979; Burgio et al., 1983; Iwata et al., 1976; Montegar et al., 1977). At a designated signal by one observer, both observers scored the first distinguishable behaviour observed, subject by subject. An agreement was scored if both observers scored the same category during the same momentary observation.

No one method of obtaining reliability scores seems significantly more acceptable than another. The methods of assessing reliability were consistent with and appropriate for the behaviour chosen for analysis. Generally, reliabilities in all of the studies reviewed, regardless of the method of sampling, were in the 80-100 per cent range of agreement. In the few instances when reliability scores dropped below 80 per cent, the authors provided a cogent argument for why the data should be believed or they presented other reliably observed measures of behaviour (Burg et al., 1979). In general, changes in the target behaviours appeared to be real changes and not the result of possible observer error.

Future Research

There are several issues that should be considered when designing future research:

1. A detailed description of past and present training histories of experimental subjects should be reported. As noted previously, it is sometimes difficult to determine whether the purpose of a particular study was to investigate procedures designed to develop a new skill, retrain a previously learned, then lost skill, programme the generalisation of newly trained skills, or maintain skill performance. Some management techniques may be well suited for one or more of these purposes but not all of them. A detailed description would allow the reader to evaluate more accurately the nature of the experimental treatment.

2. The techniques used to train staff should be clearly specified, component by component. In several studies a technique has been identified by the authors as the single source of behaviour change. However, their description of training alluded to other training variables, e.g., instructions, staff-assignments, feedback. A careful delineation of all training techniques would allow accurate replication.

3. A sound experimental design should be employed. In some instances the scientific rigour that frequently characterises operant research has been absent in staff-management studies. In such instances, the contention that behaviour would have changed independently of the experimental intervention cannot be rejected.

4. When several training techniques are used, component analyses should occur when it is considered economical. Such an analysis would identify those variables that contribute significantly to the effects of the treatment package.

5. An estimate should be made of the staff's satisfaction with the treatment programme, because an unpopular programme is unlikely to be maintained and, if enforced, may produce unfavourable side effects such as absenteeism.

6. Other relevant behaviours should be measured before, during and following experimental treatment. Changes in staff behaviour may extend beyond the behaviour or class of behaviours treated. Obviously, not all relevant behaviour can be measured economically. However, the investigator might make assumptions based on previous research, or what might contribute to the field of knowledge, or what might be of interest to institutional administrators including possible deleterious effects.

7. Both outcome and process data should be obtained. One should never assume that changes in staff behaviour will necessarily produce desirable changes in resident behaviour.

8. Relevant behaviour changes should be assessed to extra-experimental conditions. A management technique, to be effective, generally must produce behaviour that will be displayed across a variety of nonexperimental conditions. It is important to document which techniques do and do not produce such generalised effects.

9. Unobtrusive measures of staff performance should be obtained. This paper has identified several instances in which an obtrusive observer may have set the occasion for desired staff behaviour not demonstrated in the observer's absence.

10. Relevant behaviour changes should be assessed periodically following the completion of the study to determine the durability of the treatment effects. As in the case of generalisation, it is important to document which techniques produced effects that were maintained and which required specific maintenance strategies.

11. There should occur direct and systematic replications of experimental findings. Replications would confirm what appears to be known about the management of staff behaviour and extend the generality of these findings over a

wide range of subjects and conditions (Sidman, 1960). The fact that many studies presented here involved nonstaff populations emphasises the need for replication.

Several techniques should be subjected to additional experimental analysis, since the exact source of their effectiveness is not clear. The effects of cueing staff behaviour have been confounded with the effects of the instructions that precede a cueing condition. It is unclear whether implied contingencies are necessary to produce and maintain the effects of modelling. Finally, the efficacy of self-recording may be determined in part by the presence or absence of several reactive variables described previously. Additional research is needed to determine as precisely as possible which components are necessary and must be included for the technique to be maximally effective.

Several techniques should be subjected to additional analysis because they have been demonstrated to be effective with nonstaff populations but rarely have been employed with or on direct-care staff: cueing, modelling, self-recording, and training children to alter staff behaviour.

Additional research is needed to determine whether training techniques, once behaviour has been developed, can be changed gradually in topography, provided intermittently, or removed entirely without a drop in staff performance. Modelling, self-recording and various forms of feedback have all been shown to maintain behaviour as long as they remain in effect. However, it is not clear whether these behaviours will be maintained when the amount of training input is reduced.

CONCLUSIONS

1. The literature on staff-training demonstrated that management of staff behaviour is a function of providing both discriminative stimuli and consequences for desired responses.

2. Instructional methods may be used to indicate the direction or magnitude of desired staff responses. However, they are generally ineffective unless supported by favourable

consequences. When instructional training is supplemented with training in the actual conditions in which the desired behaviour is to be displayed, it may be effective.

3. Modelling may be an effective staff-management technique in the absence of explicit consequences. However, it remains unclear whether implied contingencies are necessary as in the case of a supervisor modelling behaviour.

4. Although role-playing has not been investigated systematically, it seems a reasonably practical approach for rehearsing newly learned skills. When used in combination with other techniques such as modelling, feedback or praise, role-playing permits the trainer to programme situations common to both the training and generalisation settings, thus increasing the probability that behaviour will generalise.

5. Performance feedback has been demonstrated repeatedly to be an effective management procedure. It is unclear whether one form of feedback, written, verbal, etc., is most effective. All have been effective sometimes.

6. Feedback in combination with praise has produced changes in staff performance when feedback alone was ineffective.

7. Although there are some questions about the source of self-recording's effectiveness, it has been shown to produce desired changes in staff performance at relatively little cost. It seems particularly practical for programming generalisation and maintenance of behaviour change.

8. Monetary incentives, rearranging work schedules and allowing time-off from work all have been successful in motivating staff to increase their rate of demonstrating desirable responses already in their repertoire. However, because of practical problems e.g., money, major administrative changes, etc., their use is limited.

9. It is clear that all of the techniques described herein work sometimes but it is not clear which

ones work most often. The fact that different subjects may profit by different training procedures argues that a training package must be general enough, i.e., include a diversity of training techniques, to effect a broad range of individual differences.

10. Many of the studies described herein were concerned with increasing the **rate** of particular staff responses rather than teaching staff a new skill or shifting stimulus control. In such instances, staff were demonstrating desired behaviours but at a rate too low to effectively manage resident behaviour. One may suppose that this deficiency was a result of staff failing to generalise or maintain relevant behaviours, though it may also be supposed that training did not include **rate** as a critical element of training. For example, teaching staff the principles of positive reinforcement may not ensure that staff reinforce desirable resident behaviour at an effective level. Therefore, trainers should be sensitive to the need to train **rate** of performance rather than assume that appropriate levels of responding will occur automatically.

11. It would be most efficient to train for the generalisation of relevant staff behaviour changes rather than assume that it will occur automatically. Several programming strategies identified by Stokes and Baer (1977) could be, and in a few cases have been, used to train for generalisation. One of the most obvious training strategies is to introduce in every condition in which generalisation is desired, the same techniques used to develop behaviour. In some instances it might be possible to reduce the schedule of training, e.g., immediate feedback could be changed to delayed feedback and provided intermittently, reducing the cost of programming for generalisation. Other generalisation strategies are also possible and some have been identified in this paper: **1)** use indiscriminable contingencies (Wallace et al., 1973, in the case of supervisors modelling appropriate staff behaviour); **2)** programme common stimuli; (Gardner, 1972; in the case of role-playing), **3)** train to generalise; (Parsonson et al., 1974, in the case of performance feedback); and **4)**

introduce to natural maintaining contingencies, e.g., Stokes et al., (1978) study where residents were used to alter staff behaviour.

12. As a general rule, as soon as extrinsic consequences for staff behaviour are withdrawn, behaviour reverts to pretraining levels (Cooper et al., 1970; Dorwick and Johns, 1976; Hollander and Plutchik, 1972; Hollander et al., 1973; Katz et al., 1972; Patterson et al., 1976; Pommer and Streedbeck, 1974), although exceptions have been noted (Cossairt et al., 1973; Moore and Bailey, 1973; Parsonson et al., 1974; Van Houten and Sullivan, 1975 - all involving non-staff populations). Maintenance of staff performance when the management system remains permanently in effect is likely (Bricker et al., 1972; Bunck et al., 1979; Green et al., 1978; Panyan et al., 1970; Quilitch, 1975; Wallace et al., 1973; Wallace et al., 1973). Restructuring the management system so that consequences are scheduled intermittently may reduce the cost of training and produce behaviour more resistant to extinction. In any event, it appears that specific maintenance strategies need to be invoked as soon as training has stopped.

13. Staff who work with severely and profoundly handicapped residents may require maintenance strategies different than staff working with higher functioning residents. Loeber and Weisman (1975) describe several studies suggesting that staff performance tends to deteriorate when the probabilities of residents' responses are low. They argue that the most powerful reinforcing event for staff is a desirable change in resident responding. When the probability of desirable resident responses is low, extinction of staff responses is likely.

14. Although there exists a fairly extensive literature on how to train, an investigation is needed of what skills are critical for effective staff performance. Teaching specific responses to be demonstrated at specific times rather than teaching a general concept of behaviour modification may prove most efficient for effecting behaviour change in both staff and residents.

15. Staff performance may deteriorate or extinguish if the programmes there required to implement with residents are ineffective. Frequent evaluations of residents' progress should be undertaken and ineffective programmes should be altered as needed.

16. In many studies, it is impossible to specify a single technique as the source of behaviour change or draw a conclusion on the relative contribution of each technique to the treatment package. The exact source of effectiveness for cueing, modelling, role-playing, self-recording and various forms of feedback is unclear. In many instances the confounding variables appear to be logical prerequisites or accompaniments, i.e., instructions and staff-assignments, to more complex training techniques. In these cases, a component analysis might not be cost-effective. In other instances, a component analysis would help to either eliminate costly, insignificant variables or help to identify the package of variables most likely to be effective. Unfortunately, many researchers may not have the personnel or financial resources needed to make such extensive experimental analyses. Approximately 30 per cent of the staff-management studies reviewed in this paper were supported by grant money. Thus this paper may be making recommendations to a field constrained by financial limitations. Nevertheless, the need still exists and researchers should be encouraged to conduct component analyses whenever possible.

17. The literature on staff-training indicates that the techniques necessary to manage staff-behaviour are available. However, the field has yet to identify the ideal combination of training techniques. It would not be surprising to find that there are several different but equally effective training packages.

18. Although the question of whether it is cost-effective to train staff at all has not been addressed in this paper, it may be a pointless issue. The development of national accreditation standards for the operation of residential facilities (Accreditation Council for Facilities for the Mentally Retarded, 1971) along with the growth of legal actions concerning the right to

treatment for institutionalised persons, make it imperative that staff be trained to manage resident behaviour effectively.

REFERENCES

Accreditation Council for Facilities for the Mentally Retarded (1971) Standards for Residential Facilities for the Mentally Retarded, Joint Commission on Accreditation of Hospitals, Chicago

Andrasik, F. and McNamara, J. R. (1977) 'Optimizing Staff Performance in an Institutional Behavior Change System', Behavior Modification, 1, 235-248

Ayllon, T. and Azrin, N. H. (1964) 'Reinforcement and Instructions with Mental Patients', Journal of the Experimental Analysis of Behavior, 7, 327-331

Azrin, N.H. and Foxx, R.M. (1971) 'A Rapid Method of Toilet Training the Institutionalized Retarded', Journal of Applied Behavior Analysis, 4, 89-99

Azrin, N.H. and Wesolowski, M.D. (1974) 'Theft Reversal: An Overcorrection Procedure for Eliminating Stealing by Retarded Persons', Journal of Applied Behavior Analysis, 7, 577-581

Barton, E.S., Guess, D., Garcia, E. and Baer, D.M. (1970) 'Improvement of Retardates' Mealtime Behaviors by Timeout Procedures using Multiple Baseline Techniques', Journal of Applied Behavior Analysis, 3, 77-84

Bensberg, G.J. (1974) 'Administration and Staff Development in Residential Facilities', Mental Retardation, 12, 29-32

Blindert, H.D. (1975) 'Interactions between Residents and Staff: A Qualitative Investigation of an Institutional Setting for Retarded Children', Mental Retardation, 13, 38-40

Bricker, W.A., Morgan, D.G. and Grabowski, J.G. (1972) 'Development and Maintenance of a Behavior Modification Repertoire of Cottage Attendants through T.V. Feedback', American Journal of Mental Deficiency, 77, 128-136

Burdock, E.I., Hakerem, G., Hardesty, A.S. and Zubin, J. (1968) 'A Ward Behavior Scale for Mental Hospital Patients', Journal of Clinical Psychology, 16, 246-247

Burdock, E.I. and Hardesty, A.S. (1968). Ward Behavior Inventory Manual, Springer, New York

Burg, M.M., Reid, D.H. and Lattimore, J. (1979) 'Use of a Self-Recording and Supervision Program to Change Institutional Staff Behavior', Journal of Applied Behavior Analysis, 12, 363-375

Burgio, L.D., Whitman, T.L. and Reid, D.H. (1983) 'A Participative Management Approach for Improving Direct-care Staff Performance in an Institutional Setting', Journal of Applied Behavior Analysis, 16, 37-53

Butterfield, E. (1967) 'The Characteristics, Selection and Training of Institution Personnel', in A. Baumeister (ed.), Mental Retardation, Aldine, Chicago

Cooper, M.L., Thomson, C.L. and Baer, D.M. (1970) 'The Experimental Modification of Teacher Attending Behavior', Journal of Applied Behavior Analysis, 3, 153-157

Cossairt, A., Hall, R.V. and Hopkins, B.L. (1973) 'The Effects of Experimenter's Instructions, Feedback, and Praise on Teacher Praise and Student Attending Behavior', Journal of Applied Behavior Analysis, 6, 89-100

Daily, W.F., Allen, G.J., Chinski, J.M. and Veit, S.W. (1974) 'Attendant Behavior and Attitudes toward Institutionalized Retarded Children', American Journal of Mental Deficiency, 78, 586-591

Dowrick, P.W. and Dove, C. (1980) 'The Use of Self-Modeling to Improve the Swimming Performance of Spina Bifida Children', Journal of Applied Behavior Analysis, 13, 51-56

Dowrick, P.W. and Johns, E.M. (1976) 'Video Feedback Effects on Therapist Attention to On-task Behaviors of Disturbed Children', Journal of Behavior Therapy and Experimental Psychiatry, 7, 255-257

Favell, J.E., McGimsey, J.F. and Jones, M.L. (1978) 'The Use of Physical Restraint in the Treatment of Self-injury and as Positive Reinforcement', Journal of Applied Behavior Analysis, 11, 225-241

Ferster, C.B. and Skinner, B.F. (1957) Schedules of Reinforcement, Appleton-Century-Crofts, New York

Foxx, R.M. and Azrin, N.H. (1973) 'The Elimination of Autistic Self-stimulatory Behavior by Overcorrection', Journal of Applied Behavior Analysis, 6, 1-14

Foxx, R.M. and Brown, R.A. (1979) 'Nicotine Fading and Self-monitoring for Cigarette Abstinence or Controlled Smoking', Journal of Applied Behavior Analysis, 12, 111-125

Gardner, J.M. (1972) 'Teaching Behavior Modification to Non-professionals', Journal of Applied Behavior Analysis, 5, 517-521

Gardner, J.M. (1973) 'Training the Trainers: A Review of Research on Teaching Behavior Modification', in R.D. Rubin, J.P. Brady and J.D. Henderson (eds.), Advances in Behavior Therapy, Academic Press, New York

Gelfand, D.M., Elton, R.H. and Harman, R.E. (1972) 'A Videotape-feedback Training Method to Teach Behavior Modification Skills to Nonprofessionals', Research in Education, 7, 15

Gladstone, B.W. and Sherman, J.A. (1975) 'Developing Generalized Behavior Modification Skills in High School Students Working with Retarded Children', Journal of Applied Behavior Analysis, 8, 169-180

Gladstone, B.W. and Spencer, C.J. (1977) 'The Effects of Modelling on the Contingent Praise of Mental Retardation Counsellors', Journal of Applied Behavior Analysis, 10, 75-84

Grant, G.W.B. and Moores, B. (1977) 'Resident Characteristics and Staff Behavior in Two Hospitals for Mentally Retarded Adults', American Journal of Mental Deficiency, 82, 259-265.

Graubard, P.S., Rosenberg, H. and Miller, M.B. (1971) 'Student Applications of Behavior Modification to Teachers and Environments or Ecological Approaches to Social Deviancy' in E.A. Ramp and B.L. Hopkins (eds.), A New Direction For Education: Behavior Analysis, Support and Development Center for Follow Through, Lawrence, Kansas

Green, B.F., Willis, B. S., Levy, R. and Bailey, J.S. (1978) 'Measuring Client Gains from Staff-implemented Programs', Journal of Applied Behavior Analysis, 1, 395-412

Harmatz, M.G. (1973) 'Observational Study of Ward Staff Behavior', Exceptional Children, 39, 554-558

Hollander, M.A. and Plutchik, R. (1972) 'A Reinforcement Program for Psychiatric Attendants', Journal of Behavior Therapy and Experimental Psychiatry, 3, 297-300

Hollander, M.A., Plutchik, R. and Horner, V. (1973) 'Interaction of Patient and Attendant Reinforcement Programs: The "Piggy-back" Effect', Journal of Consulting and Clinical Psychology, 41, 43-47

Horner, R.D. (1980) 'The Effects of an Environmental "Enrichment" Program on the Behavior of Institutionalized Profoundly Retarded Children', Journal of Applied Behavior Analysis, 13, 473-492

Horner, R.D. and Keilutz, (1975) 'Training Mentally Retarded Adults to Brush their Teeth', Journal of Applied Behavior Analysis, 8, 301-309

Ivancic, M.T., Reid, D.H., Iwata, B.A., Faw, G.D. and Page, T.J. (1981) 'Evaluating a Supervision Program for Developing and Maintaining Therapeutic Staff-resident Interactions During Institutional Care Routines', Journal of Applied Behavior Analysis, 14, 95-107

Iwata, B.A., Bailey, J.S., Brown, K.M., Foshee, T.J. and Alpern, M. (1976) 'A Performance-based Lottery to Improve Residential Care and Training by Institutional Staff', Journal of Applied Behavior Analysis, 9, 417-431

Johnson, S.M. and White, G. (1971) 'Self-observation

as an Agent of Behavioral Change', Behavior Therapy, 2, 488-497

Jones, F. and Eimers, R.C. (1975) 'Role Playing to Train Elementary Teachers to Use a Classroom Management "Skill Package"', Journal of Applied Behavior Analysis, 8, 421-433

Jones, R.T., Nelson, R.E. and Kazdin, A.E. (1977) 'The Role of External Variables in Self-reinforcement: A Review', Behavior Modification, 1, 147-178

Katz, R.C., Johnson, C.A. and Gelfand, S. (1972) 'Modifying the Dispensing of Reinforcers: Some Implications for Behavior Modification with Hospitalized Patients', Behavior Therapy, 3, 579-588

Kazdin, A.E. (1973) 'Issues in Behavior Modification with Mentally Retarded Persons', American Journal of Mental Deficiency, 78, 134-140

Kazdin, A.E. (1977) 'Methodological and Assessment Considerations in Evaluating Reinforcement Programs in Applied Settings', Journal of Applied Behavior Analysis, 6, 517-531

Kazdin, A.E. (1974a) 'Reactive Self-monitoring: The Effects of Desirability, Goal Setting, and Feedback', Journal of Consulting and Clinical Psychology, 42, 704-716

Kazdin, A.E. (1974b) 'Self-monitoring and Behavior Change' in M.J. Mahoney and C.E. Thoresen (eds.), Self-control: Power to the Person, Brooks/Cole, Monterey, California

Kazdin, A.E. (1977) The Token Economy: A Review and Evaluation, Plenum, New York

Kessell, R.C., Whitman, T.L. and Reid, D.H. (1983) 'An Institutional Staff Training and Self-Management Program for Developing Multiple Self-Care Skills in Severely/Profoundly Retarded Individuals', Journal of Applied Behavior Analysis, 16, 395-415

Klaber, M. (1969) 'The Retarded and Institutions for the Retarded: A Preliminary Report' in S. Sarason and J. Doris (eds.), Psychological Problems in Mental Deficiency, Harper and Row, New York

Loeber, R. and Weisman, R.G. (1975) 'Contingencies of Therapist and Trainer Performance: A Review', Psychological Bulletin, 82, 660-688

McInnis, T. (1976) 'Training and Maintaining Staff Behavior in Residential Treatment Programs' in R.L. Patterson (ed.), Maintaining Effective Token Economies, Thomas, Springfield, Illinois

McInnes, T. (1978) 'Training and Motivating Staff Members' in D. Marholin (ed.), Child Behavior Therapy, Gardner Press, New York

McInnis, T. and Kitson, L. (1977) 'Process and Outcome Evaluation in Mental Health Systems', International Journal of Mental Health, 5, 58-72

Miklich, D.R., Chida, T.L. and Danker-Brown, P. (1977) 'Behavior Modification via Self-Modeling Without Subject Awareness', Journal of Behavior Therapy and Experimental Psychiatry, 8, 125-130

Montegar, C.A., Reid, D.H., Madsen, C.H. and Ewell, M.D. (1977) 'Increasing Institutional Staff to Resident Interactions through Inservice Training and Supervisor Approval', Behavior Therapy, 8, 533-540

Moore, B.L. and Bailey, J.S. (1973) 'Social Punishment in the Modification of a Preschool Child's "Autistic-like" Behavior with a Mother as Therapist', Journal of Applied Behavior Analysis, 6, 497-507

Nay, W.R. (1975) 'A Systematic Comparison of Instructional Techniques for Parents', Behavior Therapy, 6, 14-21

Nelson, R.O. (1977) 'Methodological Issues in Assessment Self-Monitoring' in J.D. Cone and R.P. Hawkins (eds.), Behavioral Assessment, New Directions in Clinical Psychology, Bruner/Mazel, New York

Nelson, R.O., Lipinski, D.P. and Black, J.L. (1976) 'The Reactivity of Adult Retardates' Self-Monitoring: A Comparison Among Bahaviors of

Different Valances, and a Comparison with Token Reinforcement', Psychological Record, 26, 189-201

Panyan, M., Boozer, H. and Morris, M. (1970) 'Feedback to Attendants as a Reinforcer for Applying Operant Techniques, Journal of Applied Behavior Analysis, 3, 1-4

Panyan, M.C. and Patterson, E.T. (1974) 'Teaching Attendants the Applied Aspects of Behavior Modification: An Empirical Approach', Mental Retardation, 12, 30-32

Parsonson, B.S., Baer, A.M. and Baer, D.M. (1974) 'The Application of Generalized Correct Social Contingencies: An Evaluation or a Training Program', Journal of Applied Behavior Analysis, 7, 427-437

Patterson, E.T., Griffin, J.C. and Panyan, M.C. (1976) 'Incentive Maintenance of Self-help Skill Training Programs for Non-professional Personnel', Journal of Behavior Therapy and Experimental Psychiatry, 7, 249-253

Paul, G.L. and McInnis, T.L. (1974) 'Attitudinal Changes Associated with Two Approaches to Training Mental Health Technicians in Milieu and Social-learning Programs', Journal of Consulting and Clinical Psychology, 42, 21-33

Paul, G.L., McInnis, T.L. and Mariotto, M.J. (1973) 'Objective Performance Outcomes with Two Approaches to Training Mental Health Technicians in Milieu and Social-learning Programs', Journal of Abnormal Psychology, 82, 523-532

Pomerleau, O.F., Bobrove, P.H. and Smith, R.H. (1973) 'Rewarding Psychiatric Aides for the Behavioral Improvement of Assigned Patients', Journal of Applied Behavior Analysis, 6, 383-390

Pommer, D.A. and Steedbeck, D. (1974) 'Motivating Staff Performance in an Operant Learning Program for Children', Journal of Applied Behavior Analysis, 7, 217-221

Quilitch, H.R. (1975) 'A Comparison of Three Staff-Management Procedures', Journal of Applied

Behavior Analysis, 8, 59-66

Repp, A.A. and Barton, L.E. (1980) 'Naturalistic Observations of Institutionalized Retarded Persons: A Comparison of Licensure Decisions and Behavioral Observations', Journal of Applied Behavior Analysis, 13, 333-342

Ringer, V.M.J. (1973) 'The Use of a "Token Helper" in the Management of Classroom Behavior Problems and in Teacher Training', Journal of Applied Behavior Analysis, 6, 671-677

Risley, T.R. and Wolf, M.M. (1972) 'Strategies for Analyzing Behavioral Change Over Time' in J. Nesselroade and H. Reese (eds.), Life-Span Developmental Psychology: Methodological Issues, Academic Press, New York

Romanczyk, R.G., Tracey, D.A., Wilson, G.T. and Thorpe, G.L. (1973) 'Behavioural Techniques in the Treatment of Obesity', Behaviour Research and Therapy, 11, 629-640

Rule, S. (1972) 'A Comparison of Three Different Types of Feedback on Teachers' Performance' in G. Semb (ed.), Behavior Analysis in Education, The University of Kansas, Lawrence, Kansas

Seymour, F.W. and Stokes, T.F. (1976) 'Self-Recording in Training Girls to Increase Work and Evoke Staff Praise in an Institution for Offenders', Journal of Applied Behavior Analysis, 9, 41-54

Sidman, M. (1960) Tactics of Scientific Research: Evaluating Experimental Data in Psychology, Basic Books, New York

Stokes, T.F. and Baer, D.M. (1977) 'An Implicit Technology of Generalization', Journal of Applied Behavior Analysis, 10, 349-367

Stokes, T.F., Fowler, S.A. and Baer, D.M. (1978) 'Training Pre-school Children to Recruit Natural Communities of Reinforcement', Journal of Applied Behavior Analysis, 11, 285-303

Van Houten, R. and Sullivan, K. (1975) 'Effects of an Audio Cueing System on the Rate of Teacher

Praise', *Journal of Applied Behavior Analysis*, *8*, 197-201

Wallace, C.J., Davis, J.R., Liberman, R.P. and Baker, V. (1973) 'Modeling and Staff Behavior,' *Journal of Consulting and Clinical Psychology*, *41*, 422-425

Warren, S.A. and Mondy, L.W. (1971) 'To What Behaviors do Attending Adults Respond?', *American Journal of Mental Deficiency*, *75*, 449-455

Watson, L.S. (1976) 'Shaping and Maintaining Behavior Modification Skills in Staff Using Contingent Reinforcement Techniques' in R.L. Patterson (ed.), *Effective Token Economies*, Thomas, Springfield, Illinois

Watson, L., Gardner, J.M. and Sanders, C. (1971) 'Shaping and Maintaining Behavior Modification Skills in Staff Members in an MR Institution', *Mental Retardation*, *9*, 39-42

Weissman-Frisch, N., Crowell, F.A. and Inman, D.P. (1980) 'In-servicing Vocational Trainers; A Multiple Perspective Evaluation Approach', *Journal of the Association for the Severely Handicapped*, *5*, 158-173

Welsch, W.V., Ludwig, C., Radiker, J.E. and Krapfl, J.E. (1973) 'Effects of Feedback on Daily Completion of Behavior Modification Projects', *Mental Retardation*, *11*, 24-27

Reference Notes

1. Meseke, J., and Anderson, S. R. (May, 1980) *The effects of a play program on the behavior of institution children and staff*. Paper presented at the meeting of the Association for Behavior Analysis, Detroit

2. Anderson, S. (1981) *Programming incidental language training opportunities*: *An analysis of teacher and child behavior*. Unpublished doctoral dissertation, University of Kansas

PART II: TRAINING IN SPECIFIC TECHNIQUES

Chapter 4

DELAYED PROMPTING: A METHOD FOR INSTRUCTING CHILDREN WITH SEVERE LANGUAGE HANDICAPS

J.H. Halle and P. Touchette

The difficulty of teaching persons with severe handicaps to generalise newly trained language to natural settings is well documented (Guess, Keogh and Sailor, 1978; Harris, 1975; Warren, Rogers-Warren, Baer and Guess, 1980). From a stimulus control perspective, the same problem would be stated differently: how to broaden the stimuli controlling particular responses to those that are both appropriate and available in natural settings. Generalisation or broadening of stimulus control is not a phenomenon that occurs automatically (Marholin and Touchette, 1979; Stokes and Baer, 1977); it must be actively and carefully programmed. Delayed prompting represents a procedure that has been used in natural settings to promote generalisation or the transfer of control from contrived prompts to stimuli that exist naturally in ordinary everyday environments.

In the pages that follow, applications of delayed prompting in both artificial, highly constrained therapeutic settings and in naturally occurring settings will be discussed. First an historical perspective of the evolution of operant language training is offered. A rationale is constructed for moving the context of language training from the highly constrained therapy setting to the natural environment. The focus then shifts specifically to the use of delayed prompting in the natural environment. Functions that it may serve and historical studies that used delay without formalising it as a procedure are described. Two specific examples of teaching delayed prompting to teachers and parents are detailed with special emphasis on the training procedures, child behaviour change resulting from caregiver delay use, generalisation of caregiver delay use, maintenance of caregiver delay use, and social validation of delayed prompting as a procedure. The final section of the paper delineates strategies for arranging the environment to set the occasion for delayed prompting by caregivers and language use by target individuals.

Students may be handicapped as much by handicapping environments as by their primary disability. Institutional, classroom, and home settings may not offer sufficient and appropriate opportunities for acquiring skills. Consider language as a case in point. Particular conditions within institutions for handicapped people fail to encourage language use. For example, high staff-resident ratios, ability grouping, poorly trained staff, inflexible programme schedules, and low levels of social and physical stimulation greatly limit available language opportunities and thereby reduce the probability of its acquisition and use.

Classroom and home environments available to handicapped individuals are superior in some respects to that of the institution. Adult-child ratios are improved, schedules tend to be more flexible (especially at home), and the physical setting usually is rich with varied materials and activities. However, other factors in these potentially superior environments may discourage language display. As in institutions, classrooms often are arranged by student abilities, thus severely handicapped students have few competent language users with whom to interact. In institutions, classrooms, and homes, caregivers either have been excluded from language training or have relinquished the responsibility. Unintentionally, current language training programmes may be contributing to a lack of generalised use of language by handicapped students because those who are most often in contact with these individuals have abdicated their role as language teacher and facilitator - perhaps because they were told that this training was someone else's province.

In all three environments - institutions, classrooms, and homes - well intentioned caregivers have been overly responsive to the needs and wishes of their severely handicapped charges. Mittler and Berry (1977) discussed this issue in the context of under functioning by retarded individuals. They hypothesised that retarded people may achieve less than their capabilities warrant because adults working closely with them fail to provide appropriate settings of demand, expectation, and opportunity for language use in ordinary everyday situations. By anticipating what students want, caregivers remove functional reasons for language use such as obtaining assistance or exercising control over the environment. For example, if a student were struggling to tie a shoe and a teacher provides the assistance without waiting for a request, the teacher has eliminated the motivation to ask for assistance.

Although non-handicapped children acquire language at a young age simply by interacting with their natural environment, these same conditions often are insufficient for establishing a language repertoire in severely handicapped students. Operant language researchers responded to these less-than-optimal natural settings by developing ideal conditions for training language in a special environment - the training setting. Operant language training programmes developed in the 1960s and 1970s were conducted in these special environments. The special environments were created to bring the language of handicapped students under very narrow stimulus control i.e., the stimuli to which the student responds are highly restrictive. This objective was accomplished by (a) conducting training in isolated settings where distrations are minimised; (b) maintaining one-to-one trainer-to-student ratios with the same trainer working with the same student; (c) training directly attention to the trainer and the task at hand; (d) controlling how and when relevant and distracting stimuli are introduced; (e) applying prompting hierarchies when required; (f) and programming and scheduling reinforcement contingencies as determined by the accuracy of the response and the level of response mastery. Massing carefully orchestrated trials together provided numerous opportunities to practise highly discriminated responses.

The optimal conditions operating in the training setting produced relatively rapid results; students successfully were taught language forms e.g., noun and verb labels, pluralisation, question-asking. However, these responses were learned under highly discriminative conditions and therefore were not displayed in natural settings - they were not under appropriate stimulus control (Guess, Keogh and Sailor, 1978; Harris, 1975; Rincover and Koegel, 1975; Warren, Rogers-Warren, Baer and Guess, 1980). This discussion is not meant to be an indictment of highly structured training settings; the systematisation and structure may be necessary to teach particular individuals. Indeed, a major section of this chapter has been dedicated to the use of delay procedures in controlled environments. The narrowing of the stimuli controlling language succeeded at making acquisition not only possible, but efficient. However, it was at the cost of generalised use. Students learned language under a narrow range of stimuli, and unless these stimuli were present, a response was not forthcoming. The students discriminated when the training conditions were and were not operating. The stage was set for tackling an applied problem - how to teach severely handicapped students to use their newly trained language functionally in their natural environment or alternatively how to bring their new responses under the control of stimuli available in their ordinary everyday settings.

Probably the most influential work on generalisation in the applied behavioural literature was written by Stokes and Baer (1977). Drawing from the previous 10 years of literature, these authors summarised the generalisation literature and its "implicit embryonic technology". They induced nine categories of generalisation-promotion strategies from the existing literature. Most of their strategies assume that the training environment requires modification to simulate the natural environment (e.g, introduce the natural maintaining contingencies, train loosely, use indiscriminable contingencies, and programme common stimuli). Although this has been the predominant assumption in the generalisation literature (and one worthy of investigation), another assumption is gaining popularity. It is the converse of the former: the natural environment requires modification to simulate, at least in some respect, the training environment.

Halle (1982) offered several reasons for adopting the natural environment as a setting for language facilitation and training: (a) The problem of transferring stimulus control of trained responses from the training setting to the natural environment is eliminated. (b) Persons (parents, staff, teachers) who are typically a part of the students' natural environment are exposed to, and perhaps involved in, language training, thus increasing the likelihood of facilitative interactions even when formal training is not in effect. (c) When training and facilitation occur in natural settings, the consequences for resulting responses are relevant to and functional in the setting. If language displayed in everyday settings results in consequences natural to the settings, the transfer from artificial, unrelated reinforcers used in training settings to natural consequences would be unnecessary.

The idea of training and facilitating language use directly in the natural environment was proposed by Hart and Risley (1968, 1974, 1975), Hart and Rogers-Warren (1978) and Mittler and Berry (1977). In recent years at least three different, but overlapping, training procedures have been developed and demonstrated experimentally to produce language in the natural environment. They are mand-model, delay, and incidental teaching. Although the procedures differ, they all refer to language training strategies that are (a) brief and positive; (b) conducted in everyday settings where opportunities for teaching functional language naturally occur, and (c) occasioned by student interest in a topic that will become the focus of training (Halle, Alpert and Anderson, 1984). Taken together, these procedures comprise an integrative model of natural environment language training (Alpert, 1984; Halle, 1982; Halle et al., 1984; Hart, 1985; Nordquist and Raab, in press). This chapter is devoted to issues related to training caregivers to implement the delay procedure. For further information on the integrative mode, the reader is referred to the references above.

FUNCTIONS OF THE DELAY PROCEDURE

Delays may serve a number of functions in natural settings. By delaying at critical moments in an interactive exchange, an adult may set the occasion for language that otherwise would not have occurred (e.g., a teacher simply delays the giving of a preferred toy until the student makes a request). Thus, one function of delay is to provide an opportunity or a reason for a language response. A second function of delay is related to assessment. Stimulus control exercised by local conditions can be assessed when a student's repertoire is known.

Delayed Prompting

For example, if a student requests a toy when the teacher holds it in front of her, will she request the same toy if it appears on a shelf and the teacher delays (i.e., teacher focuses attention on the student and waits for a response)? Delays programmed in applied settings may also function to transfer stimulus control from one stimulus to another. Halle, Marshall and Spradlin (1979), for example, used models immediately following 15-second delays to teach meal requesting. These researchers found that three of the subjects participating began to anticipate, that is, they requested their meals before the model was provided. When these anticipated requests occurred, control had been transferred from the model to other stimuli (e.g., withheld food tray or a waiting adult).

Teaching by transferring stimulus control

Students, parents and teaching staff find the process of language acquisition aversive when progress is minimal and errors proliferate. It is to everyone's advantage to minimise errors especially during the early stages of language learning. Skinner (1968) first suggested the virtues of reducing or eliminating errors during learning. Later, Sidman and Stoddard (1966, 1967) and Touchette (1968) demonstrated empirically that instructional programmes based on stimulus control transfer both eliminated errors and improved the functional quality of what was learned. Learning can progress more rapidly when there are few or no errors. The approach is clearly appropriate for those with serious learning handicaps. Acquisition of new skills is accelerated, retention is improved (Touchette, 1968) and most importantly, skills which might be unattainable by trial-and-error are readily learned by stimulus control transfer.

The term transfer, though broadly accepted, is somewhat misleading. What we are really interested in is **establishing** stimulus control. The language-delayed child may fail to name people, objects, activities, relations (expressive language) and also may fail to identify these stimuli when a teacher speaks corresponding words to the child (receptive language). At the outset, environmental stimuli are not sufficient to produce relevant language behaviour. The problem is how to **establish** control by the target stimuli without producing errors and confusion. One solution is to transfer control of the desired behaviour from a prompt to the currently ineffective environmental stimuli. The point in time at which a prompt is delivered can be manipulated in order to encourage the transfer of stimulus control. When the prompt is no longer employed and the child continues to respond appropriately, stimulus control is said to have transferred.

Prompts are stimuli which the teacher employs because they control or produce the target behaviour. But when a teacher employs a prompt, the correct behaviour is produced by the wrong stimulus. If the target is to select the picture of a shoe when the teacher says "Show me what you put on after your socks", then the teacher might prompt the response by touching the correct picture. A student can then touch the correct picture simply by imitating the teacher. At this point the student is emitting the correct response (selecting the shoe) for the wrong reason (because the teacher touched it). The teacher's mission is to arrange things in such a way that the student will select the correct picture from among others in response to the request rather than solely when the teacher touches it.

Some technique must be employed to transfer control from teacher supplied imitative prompts to the request for information which approximates an ordinary verbal interaction. Later, the task will be to establish the child's verbal repertoire by transferring control from adult imitative verbal prompts to specific objects. Finally, we will attempt to get stimulus control by the natural environment. The child who learned to identify a shoe in response to a request, and later learned to name a shoe in a teaching setting, will now learn to say "shoe" when he has finished putting on his or her socks and cannot find the next item of apparel he or she needs before going outside. At each juncture, the correct response will be prompted and the teaching technique will **transfer** control exerted by the prompt to naturally occurring, environmental stimuli.

Unfortunately, no one knows how to guarantee transfer of stimulus control from a prompt to appropriate environmental stimuli. Teachers whose students have severe language handicaps must be prepared to set up conditions which make the transfer of stimulus control likely. If necessary, they succeed, because prompting is the only way for them to **establish** rudimentary communicative behaviour in these students.

Delayed Prompting

Early studies of learning without errors employed procedures which accomplished the desired result by making a series of very minor alterations in the prompt stimuli. In each case a prompt was gradually eliminated in steps so small that each was unlikely to disrupt the ongoing performance. The sequences of graduated stimulus changes had little in common except that each was composed of many small steps. All gradual change procedures are typically lumped under the heading of **fading.** An empirically derived programme of prompt-fading can work very well, producing rapid errorless learning. There is, however, a good reason why this approach has not been universally adopted. The development of an effective fading programme can be very costly in terms of time, effort and material. Moreover, there is no guarantee that the programme which emerges will be relevant to the next instructional problem. Equally unfortunate, the programme may work well with only a few clients who have similar prior training histories. What is a teacher to do when faced with an instructional problem for which no fading programme currently exists?

Delaying a prompt is a way to eliminate it.

Delayed prompting offers an alternative to fading. Something about inserting a delay prior to the presentation of a prompt encourages transfer of stimulus control. The procedure is far simpler than fading. It requires no special preparation of material. Delaying the onset of a controlling stimulus (prompt) following the presentation of the target stimuli can and usually does result in errorless transfer of stimulus control (Touchette, 1971; Touchette and Howard, 1984). In fading, controlling and target stimuli are paired, then the controlling stimuli are gradually eliminated. In delayed prompting, controlling and target stimuli are paired, then the controlling stimuli are delayed so that they follow the presentation of the task-intrinsic stimuli. The delay provides an opportunity on every trial for the student to respond appropriately prior to the presentation of the prompt. When correct responses occur consistently prior to the delivery of the prompt, stimulus control has transferred and the prompt is no longer necessary. This may happen almost immediately, or it may take an extended period of time; student performance determines the time required for training. In either case, when a response occurs before the prompt (anticipation) and it is correct, the teacher has an easily observable indication of the transfer of stimulus control. Current evidence suggests that not just a few, but many language instruction goals can be achieved by inserting a delay prior to the delivery of a stimulus (a prompt) which controls the behaviour of interest. The objective of delaying the prompt is to shift control from stimuli supplied by the instructor to stimuli inherent in the task or setting.

The essence of delayed prompting is that a stimulus which controls the response of interest (a prompt) is presented concurrently with the task related stimuli. A delay is then interposed between the presentation of the task and the onset of the prompt. Stimulus materials do not appear to be critical and there is no need to develop elaborate, subtle, and sometimes unique, graduated changes necessary for effective fading (Etzel, LeBlanc, Schilmoeller and Stella, 1981). A number of studies have shown that this approach can teach useful discriminations to handicapped and young unimpaired children (Johnson, 1978; Smeets and Striefel, 1976; Stremel-Campbell, Cantrell and Halle, 1977; Striefel, Bryan and Aikins, 1974; Striefel, Wetherby and Karlan, 1976).

Delayed prompting is a technique that teachers can easily add to their repertoire. The approach can then be applied in a broad variety of tasks and settings. The only prerequisites are a prompt that works and a way of presenting it in an orderly manner in company with the stimuli which are the target for transfer.

Stepping and fixed delays.

Initial laboratory research into the impact of delays on stimulus control transfer was done with an adjusting delay value (Touchette, 1971). At first, the stimuli to be associated were presented simultaneously. If the subject responded correctly, the controlling element (prompt) was delayed one-half second. With every correct response, the delay increased another one-half second.

Following Touchette's (1971) paradigm, a number of researchers have used delayed prompting to teach receptive language skills. Striefel, Bryan and Aikins (1974) taught their students to follow verbal instructions using a delay to promote transfer of stimulus control. All of their students were able to imitate motor behaviour modelled by the teacher. The instructional target was to bring the motor behaviour under the control of the teacher's verbal instructions. The verbal instruction and a physical model were initially presented simultaneously. A delay was then inserted and following each correct response the delay between instruction and model was increased. All of their students learned to follow simple verb-noun instructions, responding correctly before the teacher modelled the behaviour. A review of several receptive language studies of this sort can be found in Striefel, Wetherby and Karlan (1976).

Smeets and Striefel (1976) first taught a student with a severe learning handicap to select pictures that corresponded to manual signs. They then extended the procedure to include an expressive language component by teaching signs which corresponded to the pictures. Both receptive and expressive signing were taught by inserting a delay between the initial stimuli and the teacher-supplied prompt. In the expressive-signing component of this study the teacher presented a picture, waited the specified delay interval, then modelled the appropriate manual sign. The delay was once again increased after every correct trial. Instruction was complete when the student produced the correct signs in the presence of the pictures without waiting for the teacher's model (prompt). Stremel-Campbell, Cantrell and Halle (1977) used a similar approach to teach retarded students first to imitate a manual sign, then to respond with the correct sign when the teacher presented an object and asked "What is this?". This study dealt more comprehensively with problems of establishing initial communication skills in seriously learning-handicapped students. Delayed prompting was used in two stages of instruction. First, the students were taught to imitate manual signs by manipulating the child's hand so that it closely approximated the desired configuration (prompt). Then the students were taught to make the appropriate sign when an object was presented. The delayed prompt was the teacher's model of the sign.

Recently Touchette and Howard (1984) taught retarded students to choose letters and written words "named" by an instructor. As in the studies above, the instructor supplied a model of the correct response as a prompt. The prompt was delayed longer each time a correct response was made and the prompt delay was reduced if errors occurred. The flow chart (Figure 1, after Touchette and Howard, 1984) demonstrates how this approach works. In addition to the delay increment, this procedure includes a delay decrement should errors occur.

The sequence described by the flow chart in Fig. 1 could be as follows. The teacher places before the student an array of cards with letters printed on them. Usually there are between 3 and 6 cards, a manageable number of all which can be seen and reached easily. The teacher then says "please touch the letter B" while simultaneously placing a finger on the printed letter. The letter named is the S+ (the correct stimulus); all other choices (distractors) are S-'s. On every trial the teacher will name a different letter, in an unpredictable sequence. After a few familiarisation trials, a delay is interposed after the teacher speaks and before the correct card is touched. As the student continues to respond correctly (following the prompt), the delay is increased in half-second or one-second increments. Thus, the first few delayed presentations are so short that they are below the time taken for most students to respond. This guarantees that students will experience the delay but respond following the prompt. They literally cannot anticipate at the outset. As the length of the delay increases, students will begin to respond before the prompt is delivered. If some of these responses are errors, the delay can be reduced to one short enough to eliminate the errors. Once an error-free performance is recaptured, the delay can once again be increased to encourage anticipatory responses.

The procedure could be exactly the same if the teacher were training expressive rather than receptive naming. The difference in the expressive paradigm is only in the stimuli presented and the response required, not in the delay procedure. Let us assume a teacher presents a student with a picture of a horse and simultaneously asks "What is this?". Following the prescribed delay, the teacher will name the picture if the student has not already done so. If the student does not imitate verbally, then manual signs would be used as in the Stremel-Campbell, Cantrell and Halle (1977) study.

Fig. 1. The events and decisions occurring with a stepping-delay procedure.
(Source: Touchette & Howard, 1984)

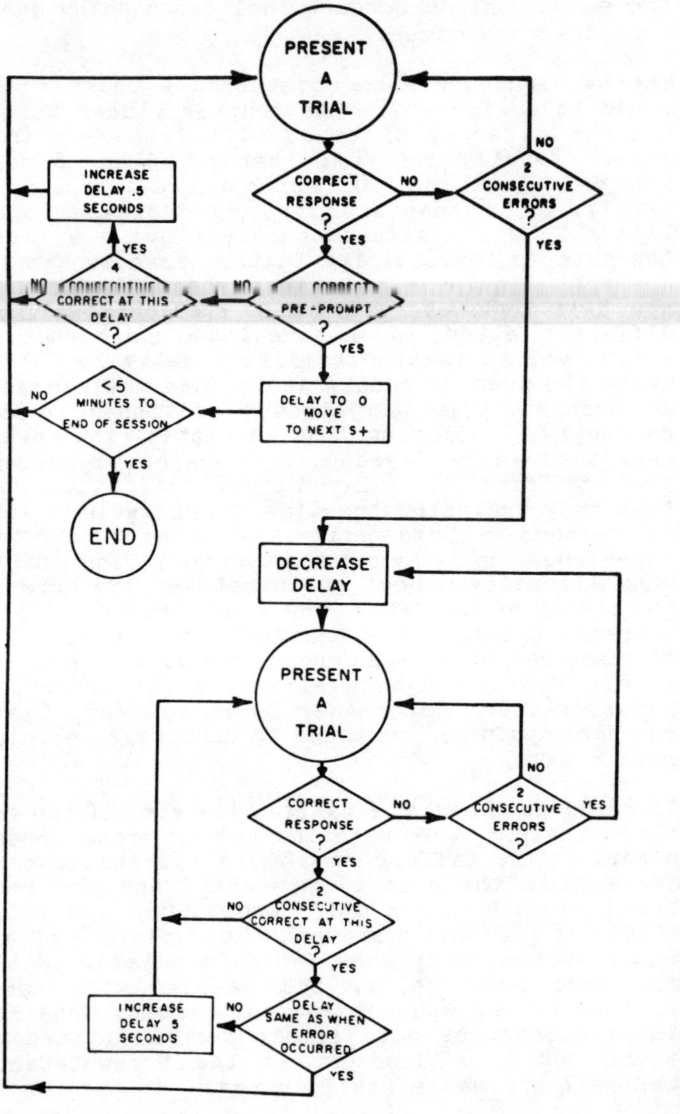

The basic receptive and expressive paradigms can be simply diagrammed as follows:-

RECEPTIVE (Designating)

Prompted

Teacher	Teacher		Teacher	Student	
Presents	Names	DELAY	Touches	Touches	:Reinforcement
Stimuli	S+		S+	S+	

Final Performance

Teacher	Teacher	Student	
Presents	Names	Touches	: Reinforcement
Stimuli	S+	S+	

EXPRESSIVE (Naming)

Prompted

Teacher		Teacher	Student	
Presents	DELAY	Names	Names	: Reinforcement
S+		S+	S+	

Final Performance

Teacher	Student	
Presents	Names	: Reinforcement
S+	S+	

There are advantages to starting with no delay and gradually extending the time between the presentation of the task and the prompt. As we pointed out above, errors are minimised in this way, especially with the student who has little or no experience with the procedure. On the other hand, increasing and decreasing delays can be a difficult process. If the task is not acquired in a single session, then difficult decisions result such as what the appropriate, initial delay interval ought to be. An alternative is to use a fixed, rather than an adjusting, delay interval. A much simpler process occurs then a fixed delay is used. For example, a 4-second delay is interposed between presentation of the task and the prompt. Errors have no impact on the procedure. There is a clear advantage here in terms of teaching the instructor how to use the procedure. Fixed delay procedures are easily implemented. The missing elements from the procedure, however, mean that more discipline and attentional prerequisites are demanded of the student. If these are not gratuitously present, they must be taught or the student should be excluded from the procedure until such time that its demands can be handled.

Johnson (1978) demonstrated that a fixed, 4-second delay was effective in teaching a series of visual discriminations to an adolescent with multiple handicaps. The student learned the discriminations virtually errorlessly with an overall accuracy of 99.3 per cent for all of the problems presented. If a teacher is to use a fixed rather than an adjusting delay, how will he select the duration to be employed? Touchette has suggested a 4-second delay for simple discrimination, naming and matching tasks. This selection was based on informal laboratory and field studies and it has proven suitable in many circumstances. Some tasks will take the naive student four seconds or more to execute e.g., find the "H" in this scrambled alphabet. Some multiply handicapped students may take longer to execute a choice, sign or verbal response. Those with cerebral palsy cannot be expected to respond at the same rate as their motorically nonimpaired peers. In these cases, the teacher must begin by determining the minimal time necessary for this student to execute a task of this type. The fixed delay can then be set at approximately twice the minimal latency. That turns out to be about four to five seconds for most table-top tasks. Direct observation of the student to-be-taught is always an excellent idea. Touchette and Howard (1984) found that a 13-year-old girl diagnosed as having severe cerbral palsy anticipated at or below a 4-second delay value in every one of 19 discrimination tasks. We had expected her responding to be slower than her motorically nonimpaired peers. She was faster than one and slower than another.

Contingencies of Reinforcement

A disparity in reinforcement density is inherent in delayed prompting. Unprompted responses are closer to the trial initiation, and prompted responses can occur only after the delay has timed out. This means that when the schedule of reinforcement is the same for prompted and unprompted responses, the actual density of reinforcement over time is higher when a response preceded the prompt. Instead of waiting for the prompt, the student can respond right after a trial has been initiated, and get reinforced sooner. The disparity can be very large when long delays are used. Delay values have ranged as high as 30 seconds in laboratory studies (Touchette, 1971) but shorter delays are typically used in clinical applications.

The decision of whether to apply disparate or uniform consequences of pre and post prompt responses is a practical one. Providing high reinforcement probability for anticipatory responses can produce more rapid transfer of stimulus control. The drawback in application is that the procedure is more complex when different schedules of reinforcement apply to responses before and after the prompt. The alternative of using uniform consequences for all correct responses does not prevent or seriously retard transfer of stimulus control, although more trials and longer delays will result in some cases.

FADING vs. DELAY:

The essence of delayed prompting is that a stimulus which controls the response of interest (a prompt) is presented concurrently with the task related stimuli. A delay is then interposed between the presentation of the task and the onset of the prompt. Stimulus materials do not appear to be critical and there is no need to develop elaborate, subtle and sometimes unique graduated changes necessary to effective fading (Etzel, LeBlanc, Schilmoeller and Stella, 1981). A number of studies have shown that this approach can teach useful discriminations to handicapped and young unimpaired children (Johnson, 1978; Smeets and Stiefel, 1976; Stremel-Campbell, Cantrell and Halle, 1977; Striefel, Bryan and Aikins, 1974; Striefel, Wetherby and Karlan, 1976).

WHAT WILL BE LEARNED?

The specific stimulus-response relations which have been programmed will be learned in the context in which they are taught. The criterion phase in which anticipations occur demonstrates this phenomenon. No assumption beyond this is warranted without a test to determine its validity. Stimulus generalisation (to another setting, trainer, time of day), response generalisation (to other members of the stimulus class taught e.g., (similar words or objects), and maintenace of responding (attributable to naturally occurring contingencies of reinforcement) may or may not occur.

Few assumptions of incidental learning are reliably validated among the severely learning handicapped. Each individual must be tested to determine what, if any, learning has occurred beyond that which was programmed (Marholin and Touchette, 1979; Rincover and Koegel, 1975). Desirable controlling relations can emerge spontaneously following training of related discriminations (Sidman, 1971; Spradlin, Cotter and Baxley, 1973) but most must be directly taught (Stokes and Baer, 1977).

HISTORICAL STUDIES

The first operant approaches to teaching language to handicapped children in their natural environments occurred in the mid 1960s. Without labelling it as such or studying it in its own right, these applied operant pioneers used delays to transfer control from prompt stimuli to "naturally occurring stimuli". They used structured training, as described above, to teach the rudiments of speech (e.g., imitation and labelling). After establishing a small labelling vocabulary, control was shifted from verbal models to the circumstance itself. For example, Lovaas (1966) taught autistic children to make demands by prompting the desired response, then fading the prompt, and finally "waiting the child out". Once children could label "milk", they would receive milk only after requesting "milk". Or, if they wanted to go outside, they could do so only after verbalising "out".

Risley and Wolf (1967) used an "anticipation procedure" with an autistic child who did not attend closely to picture stimuli that he was expected to label. He did not have to look at the pictures to make a correct response and receive reinforcement; he needed only to imitate the modelled label. To discourage waiting, the anticipation procedure was introduced. The trainer presented a picture and waited for several seconds before giving the prompt. By anticipating the correct response, the child could receive the reinforcer sooner than if he waited for the prompt. After teaching object and action labels using edible reinforcement, the trainer shifted to natural consequences as a means of maintaining labelling. "Out" (or in) the door", was maintained by opening the doors to and from the training room. The trainer would model, "Out the door" and when the child imitated, the door would be opened. Over trials, the trainer faded to partial verbal prompting and later to no verbal prompting - the trainer put his hand on the door knob and looked at the child, who responded by saying, "Out of door". As in the Lovaas procedure, the trainer transferred stimulus control of the label from a verbal prompt to the circumstance itself by pausing in a naturally occurring situation where the expectations for the child were clear.

Hartung (1970) provides a further example of waiting for a response and then programming natural consequences to maintain it, once it is emitted. This researcher discovered that particular idiosyncracies could be exploited to generate motivation for speech. For example, an autistic boy immediately would squirm away when a hand was placed on top of his head; thus it was inferred that he did not like anyone's hand on his head. The trainer capitalised on this idiosyncracy by placing a hand on the child's head and simultaneously modelling, "Stop it". If the child imitated these words, the trainer placed his hand on the child's head and delayed the model, thus allowing the child to anticipate the response. Within 30 minutes, the child no longer required any prompt to respond correctly with "Stop it" each time a hand was placed on his head.

The investigators involved in this pioneering research employed this two-pronged approach - "waiting the child out" and programming natural consequences - in a very restricted manner. Studying delay procedures was not their intent. They used delays in natural settings to transfer control from prompted stimuli to naturally occurring stimuli. They did not investigate experimentally the efficacy of using delays.

In contrast to the use of delay to transfer stimulus control, Hall and Broden (1977) employed delays to provide more salient opportunities for responding. The students participating in the study had been reluctant to volunteer to answer teacher questions. Therefore, the teacher increased the latency (i.e., delayed) between the time she asked a question and called on students to respond. This very simple procedure more than doubled the number of students volunteering to answer questions.

EXPERIMENTAL CASE EXAMPLES OF TRAINING CAREGIVERS TO USE DELAYS IN NATURAL SETTINGS.

A multitude of experimental investigations have included delay use in natural settings (e.g., McGee, Krantz, Mason and McClannahan, 1983; Oliver and Halle, 1982; Schepis, Reid, Fitzgerald, Faw, van den Pol, and Welty, 1982; Woods, 1982). Very few, however, have measured the effect of delay training on caregivers' use of delay. More often, caregiver delay training is assumed and child behaviour is measured. Due to these circumstances, the discussion of caregiver training of delay use will encompass two experimental case examples: delay training with teachers (Halle et al., 1981) and delay training with parents (Alpert, 1984).

Before reviewing these studies, it seems appropriate to suggest a format that can be used as an organisational tool that will guide the discussion and lend continuity across case presentations. Each study will be discussed in terms of the following issues: (1) What procedures were used to train caregivers and how effective were they? (2) Did student behaviour change as a function of caregiver behaviour change, since "...the behaviour of the client remains the most relevant unit of analysis for determining the effectiveness of programme implementation and hence, techniques intended to encourage it" (Greene, Willis, Levy and Bailey, 1978)? It could be argued that teaching caregivers to engage in new behaviour is itself unimportant unless newly acquired skills result in child behaviour change. In other words, the true test of the relevance and importance of caregiver behaviour change is its correlated (or preferably casual) effect on child behaviour. (3) How did the researchers define delay? Enumerating the specific observable behaviours that comprise a delay is needed to assess the similarity of the procedure across studies. (4) Was the environment arranged to set the occasion for delay use? Once teachers and parents are taught to use delays, the next training objective is to bring their use under appropriate stimulus control. The question of **WHEN** to use delays becomes germane. (5) Did **NEW** stimuli begin to set the occasion for caregiver delay use? Once teachers have been trained **WHEN** delays are to be employed, will they generalise their delay use to appropriate novel situation? (6) Will caregivers maintain their use of delay when they are no longer undergoing training and if so, for how long? (7) Were social validation measures used? Wolf (1978) defined three levels on which a researcher's work could be validated by society. (a) Do the **GOALS** selected coincide with what society really wants? (b) Do the consumers of the treatment (e.g., participants, caregivers) find the **PROCEDURES** acceptable? (c) Are the consumers satisfied with the **RESULTS**? For any applied training endeavour these three questions could, and should, be asked. Using the seven criteria outlined above, the two studies will be reviewed and critiqued.

HALLE, BAER, and SPRADLIN'S (1981) STUDY

Halle et al. taught classroom teachers to delay their assistance and their provision of materials in naturally occurring situations and thereby to provide additional opportunities for language by 12 moderately retarded language-delayed students. Additional objectives of the investigation included the transfer of stimulus control from prompt to naturally available stimuli and the assessment of teachers' generalised use of delay to occasion language use.

Criterion 1. Teacher training was accomplished in a one-hour meeting of the trainer and the teachers. The trainer identified and described verbally a number of pre-established naturally occurring opportunities for language requests (see Criterion 3 below). The teachers were given a list of these opportunities with accompanying descriptions to study at their leisure. The trainer then described the eight steps of the delay procedure and modelled its proper use with role play using simulated opportunities from the list. The trainer also modelled and role played how teachers were to respond to the different ways that the children might make requests. If children responded correctly, teachers were instructed to model an appropriate request and wait for an imitative response before praising and fulfilling requests. The trainer encouraged the teachers to generalise their use of delay by telling them that the delay opportunities identified were only examples of a much larger set of delayable opportunities and that teachers should feel free to apply the procedure whenever it seemed appropriate. In addition to the training that occurred in the one-hour meeting, the trainer provided immediate feedback to the teachers about their implementation of delays during the first week of intervention.

Criterion 2. Halle et al. collected data on teachers' use of delay and on children's vocal initiations (see Figure 2). By collecting data on both teacher and child behaviour, two studies were ongoing simultaneously. In one, the effect of delay training on teacher use of delay was assessed; in the second, the effect of teacher delay use on children's vocal initiations was assessed. A multiple-baseline design across children was used to demonstrate experimental control in the second study. Each time the teachers increased their delay use with untreated children, the children's vocal initiations increased. This finding was replicated six times as may be seen in Figure 2. The effectiveness of the delay training is difficult to determine because the teachers were trained together in one session. Only a baseline phase (prior to treatment) and an intervention phase occurred. Thus, an AB design characterised this study from which functional relations cannot be determined. Note, in Figure 2 that although the teachers introduced delays on different days for different children, they were trained to use delays only once and were asked to apply the procedure to additional children only when instructed to do so.

Criterion 3. In the Halle et al. study, delays were defined by five required conditions and four optional conditions. They are : REQUIRED 1. Teacher does not vocalise. 2. Teacher is in close proximity to the child (i.e. within 3 feet). 3. Teacher's head is orientated toward the child. 4. The orientation of the child's head is directed toward the teacher at least intermittently to ensure that the child has noted the teacher's attention. 5. Conditions 1-4 are in effect for at least 5 seconds or until a child vocal initiation occurs. OPTIONAL 1. Teacher uses some form of visual prompt (e.g. holding juice). 2. Teacher assumes a questioning or expectant look (e.g. pursed lips, raised eyebrows, eye contact). 3. Teacher's body is orientated toward the child. 4. Teacher kneels down to be at eye level with the child.

Criterion 4. Prior to the beginning of the study,

Fig. 2 Daily percentages of training opportunities (those identified by the experimenter and used to teach the teachers to recognise delayable opportunities) used by teachers to delay and by children to initiate vocally. Points connected by solid lines represent percentages of teacher delays; shaded areas represent percentages of child vocal initiations. Spaces between points and shaded areas represent teacher delays during which children either did not vocalise or did not make an appropriate vocal initiation. Numbers along abscissa represent number of daily opportunities or denominators used to calculate the daily percentages. (Source: Halle Baer & Spradlin, 1981)

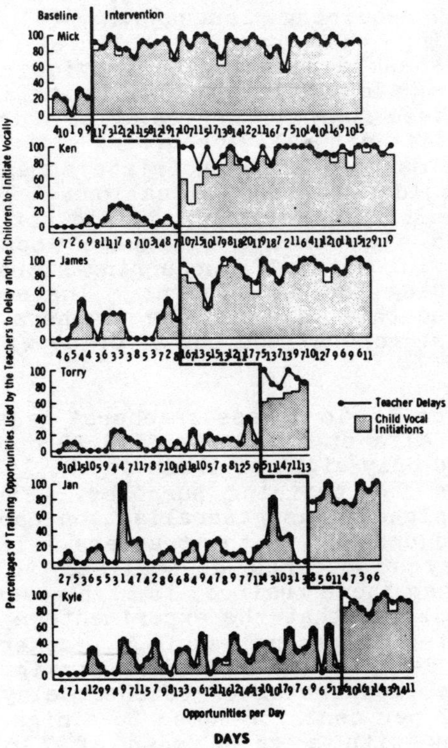

an experimenter observed the classroom routine for two months to identify naturally occurring situations that could be used or rearranged slightly to create language opportunities for the handicapped participants, simply by teachers' delaying at critical moments. From the observations the experimenter induced four strategies for recognising language opportunities: (1) Observe routines, i.e., the daily schedule of activities and the steps required to complete each activity offer many potential opportunities, especially when the beginning and ending of each is considered. (2) Note environmental preempting where highly preferred materials are readily accessible to the students, negating teacher assistance and thus opportunities for language interactions. (3) Note nonverbal preempting that includes those occasions when materials or activities are not readily accessible to students, but teachers provide access to them without requiring language. (4) Note verbal preempting that occurs on those occasions when teachers ask a question or provide a prompt before students have sufficient time to initiate a response. Using these four strategies allowed the experimenter to identify naturally occurring situations, however, delays inserted at appropriate moments were needed to mould these situations into language opportunities. Halle et al. did not directly train teachers to create language opportunities by identifying naturally occurring situations and then rearranging the environment. Instead, the trainer performed this task for the teachers. However, the teachers' generalised use of delay was assessed (see below).

Criterion 5. To assess teachers' generalised use of delay, Halle et al. identified 20 opportunities and included only eight of these on the list given to the teachers for training purposes. The remaining 12 were designated as generalisation opportunities and remained unknown to the teachers. If teachers' use of delay procedures generalised to opportunities other than those trained, it might overlap with those opportunities that the experimenters identified and designated as generalisable. Teachers' generalised use of delay is illustrated in Figure 3. During baseline, mean rates of teacher delay varied from a low of 2 per cent for James to a high of 10 per cent for Mick with a group mean of 7 per cent. The introduction of the delay procedure with training

Fig. 3 Daily percentages of generalisation opportunities (those identified by the experimenter, but unknown to the teachers) used by teachers to delay and by children to initiate vocally. Points connected by solid lines represent percentages of teacher delays; shaded areas represent percentages of child vocal initiations. Dashed vertical lines indicate point at which teacher delays were begun during training opportunities with individual children. Spaces between points and shaded areas represent teacher delays during which children either did not vocalise or did not make an appropriate vocal initiation. Numbers along abscissa represent number of daily opportunities or denominators used to calculate daily percentages. (Source: Halle, Baer & Spradlin, 1981)

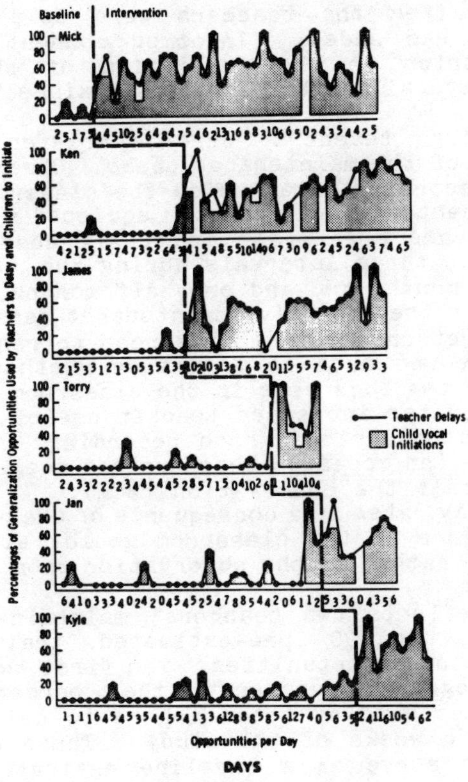

opportunities was associated with large increases in teachers' use of delays during generalisation opportunities. The mean rates of delays varied from a low of 48 per cent for James to a high of 68 per cent for Kyle with a mean of 56 per cent for the group.

Due to the manner in which the generalisation data were collected, it is likely that the extent of teachers' generalised use of delay is grossly underestimated. The percentages stated above reflect only those occasions where teachers delayed in situations that overlapped with the experimenters' pre-established list of 12 opportunities. On other occasions (those not appearing on the list) when teachers delayed, the observation system failed to record these generalised instances.

Criterion 6. To assess the maintenance of teachers' use of delay, unobtrusive data collection was continued after the teachers were told that the experiment had ended. Informed consent had been obtained prior to the initiation of the study, however, several months had elapsed since that time.

Participating teachers were debriefed at the conclusion of the maintenance phase. Observers, who had been recording data inside the classroom, moved to an adjacent observation room equipped with a one-way mirror and speakers. Fifty-six sessions were conducted at three intervals during the maintenance phase: one month, two and one-half months, and five months. For the last five maintenance sessions, the observers returned to the classroom to record data. This change was made to determine whether (a) the presence of the observers in the classroom would set the occasion for increased teacher use of the delay and (b) the observation room recordings were truly unobtrusive (on occasion teachers had seen observers enter and exit the observation room). A change in teacher delay rates as a consequence of the observers' clear presence in the classroom would validate the unobtrusive nature of the observation room measures.

Figure 4 reflects two teachers' maintained use of delays in the 20 pre-estimated training and generalisation opportunities. The first two bars in both histograms represent the percentage of opportunities used by the teachers to delay during the last two weeks of the study. These data were included to serve as a baseline against which to

Fig. 4 Percentages of opportunities used by each teacher to delay during maintenance. Open bars designate training opportunities; shaded bars designate generalisation opportunities. Teacher 1's data appear in upper graph and Teacher 2's in lower graph. Not shown, but pertinent to data displayed is average percentage of opportunities (both training and generalisation) used by each teacher during baseline of study, 10% for Teacher 1 and 5% for Teacher 2. (Source: Halle, Baer & Spradlin, 1981)

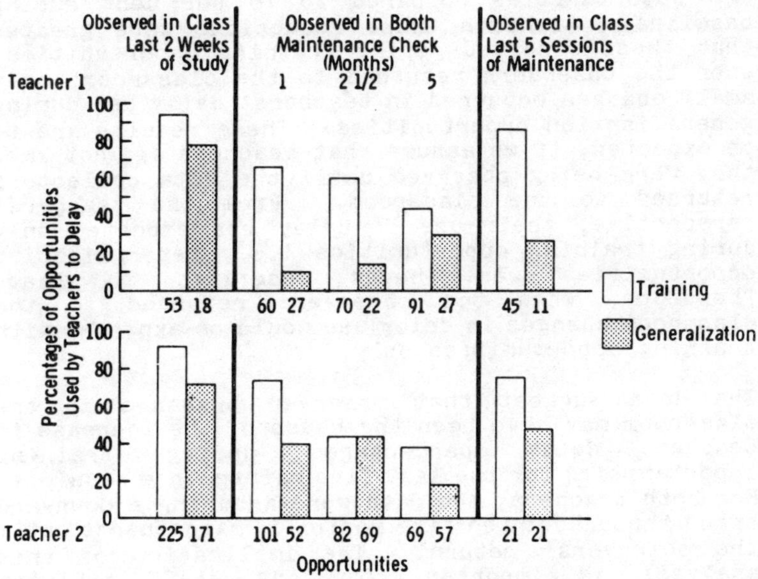

measure delay use during the maintenance phase. For training opportunities both teachers' delay use decreased throughout the five-month maintenance period to a level about half as frequent as that established during the last two weeks of the study. When the observers returned to the classroom, the teachers' delay data increased to levels slightly lower than baseline comparison.

The teacher's percentage of delay use during generalisation opportunities assumed a different pattern. When the observers moved from the classroom to the observation room, the delay data decreased sharply. Teacher 1's data dropped from 80 to 10 per cent; Teacher 2 delayed during only 40 per cent of the opportunities compared to 75 per cent during baseline. Although these reductions were greater than those observed during training opportunities, when the observers returned to the classroom, only small changes occurred in teachers' delay use during generalisation opportunities. These results are to be expected, if we assume that teachers did not know they were being observed until the data collectors returned to the classroom. From the teachers' perspective, their use of delay was expected only during training opportunities i.e., generalisation opportunities were never described to them. Therefore, when the observers returned to the classroom changes in delay use would be expected with training opportunities only.

The data suggest that observer presence in the classroom may have been the cause of the increase in teacher delay percentages during training opportunities for the last five maintenance sessions. For both teachers, the data were assuming a downward trend throughout the five months of maintenance until the observers' return. The implication of this analysis is important for any staff training endeavour: the stimulus control exercised by the trainer may be an influential variable in maintaining trained skills. Maintenance should be evaluated in the absence of the teacher unless the trainer is indigenous to the natural setting.

Criterion 7. Halle et al. attempted to answer Wolf's (1978) three questions related to social validity by asking the participating teachers to respond to a short questionnaire. Questions about the usefulness and the effectiveness of the delay procedure were included. Teachers commented that their major goals were socialisation and language and that using delays furthered both. Related to usefulness and effectiveness, teachers mentioned that delays were "extremely easy to implement" and "...(they) worked well with all the subjects". Although the questionnaire produced positive results, this method of social validation is incomplete. Kazdin (1982) refers to this type of social validation as subjective evaluation and it does provide social validation (a) of the treatment GOALS by asking a group of experts (teachers) if the goals are appropriate; (b) of the delay PROCEDURE by asking those who used the procedure about their satisfaction and concerns with its use; and (c) of the EFFECTS of treatment by questioning those who are in a position to judge its success.

However, the subjective evaluation method by itself does not allow for an anchoring of the validation procedure. That is, teachers may observe changes in their students' behaviour and thus evaluate positively the effect of the procedure even though the effect has fallen short of bringing the behaviour within the normative level when compared to the students' peer group. Similarly when treatment goals are evaluated, teachers provide only their subjective opinions of the appropriateness of these goals. Also needed is an evaluation that includes an assessment of the behavioural repertoires of peers to determine whether the target behaviours selected appear in the normative repertoires.

ALPERT (1984) STUDY

Alpert (1984) trained six mothers to be language interventionists with their own language-delayed preschool children. She used the natural environment as the context for training. Her objectives were twofold: (a) to train parents to teach their children language responses that would produce functional control of the environment and (b) to obtain children's functional use of language in environmental and conversational contexts in which communication naturally occurs. Alpert taught the participating mothers a series of four "Milieu" intervention procedures: model, mand-model, time delay, and incidental teaching (Hart and Rogers-Warren, 1978). She used a multiple baseline design across dyads as well as a multiple baseline across procedures. My discussion here will be confined to the training of time delays and the results of this training on mother and child behaviour.

Criterion 1. Mothers individually attended a clinic-based training session that began with a lecture on the delay procedure. Lectures included: (a) experimental applications of delay and its effect on child language; (b) anticipated goals of delay use; (c) rules for using delays; and (d) steps required for using delay correctly. To facilitate consistency across mothers, the trainer lectured from a written outline. Mothers were encouraged to ask questions at any time to clarify presented material. The lectures varied in length from 30 minutes to one hour, depending on the amount and complexity of material covered and the number of questions and comments by mothers.

Following the lecture, three 10-minute video training tapes were shown of the trainer using delays with three different language-delayed preschoolers, one of whom was the mother's own child. As the tapes were played, the experimenter identified when she was delaying and noted each step of the procedure. Specific language objectives that might be accomplished with delays were discussed and mothers were encouraged to use delays incidentally throughout the day as opportunities naturally arose. At the conclusion of the clinic-based session, the trainer gave the mothers notebooks containing handouts highlighting the information that had just been presented. The trainer asked the mothers to read the handouts before the first home-based training session that was always scheduled within two days of the clinic-based session.

Home-based training included the following elements: (a) the trainer provided descriptive and graphic feedback on the mother's rate and accuracy of using delays during the previous home-based session; (b) the trainer played pre-selected audiotape examples from the previous session of the mother's correct and incorrect use of delay and accompanied these with explanations of how delays were used correctly or incorrectly; (c) the trainer modelled use of delays with the child; (d) the trainer gave verbal feedback after the mother practised delaying with her child; (e) the trainer asked the mother to use delays during a 10-minute audiotaped play interaction with the child; (f) the trainer provided feedback about the mother's use of delay during the immediately preceding 10-minute interaction (audiotape feedback also was provided); (g) the mother practiced using delays in an additional 5-minute audiotaped play interaction with the child; and (h) the trainer gave feedback on the mother's delay performance during the preceding five minutes. Although Alpert used all of these elements in the home-based training, she noted that some (e.g. audiotape feedback, trainer modelling, and practice accompanied by feedback) were excluded or faded as their need diminished.

If a mother had particular difficulty mastering delay use, reflected in the accuracy of application data, an "Intensive Training" session was scheduled. Intensive training was conducted at the clinic and consisted of: (a) a thorough description of the steps involved in delaying; (b) a videotape demonstration of the trainer using delays with the mother's child; (c) a discussion of the specific problems that the mother was experiencing in delivery delays; (d) role-playing with the trainer acting as the child, accompanied by trainer feedback; (e) the mother practising delays with a language-delayed child other than her own, accompanied by trainer feedback; and (f) the mother's use of delay with her own child, accompanied by trainer feedback.

Alpert used a multiple-baseline design across dyads and therefore introduced delay training to one dyad at a time while the remaining dyads were maintained in baseline. Later delay training was introduced sequentially to each untreated dyad until all six mothers had received training. The results of training mothers to delay with their language-handicapped children appear in Figure 5. It is clear that both the frequency and percentage of mothers' correct use of delay increased when training was introduced with each mother.

This figure, however, does not reflect changes in children's linguistic skills. The results of this study are reported, but the data are collapsed across the package of four milieu procedures. The findings demonstrate that mothers' use of the package was associated with improvement in a variety of linguistic skills by the children. However, the effect of mothers' use of delay alone on their children's linguistic skills cannot be isolated. In contrast to Halle et al. (1981), Alpert could not determine

Fig. 5 **Frequency and percentage of correct use of time delay in training sessions and in maintenance sessions. (Adapted from Alpert, 1984)**

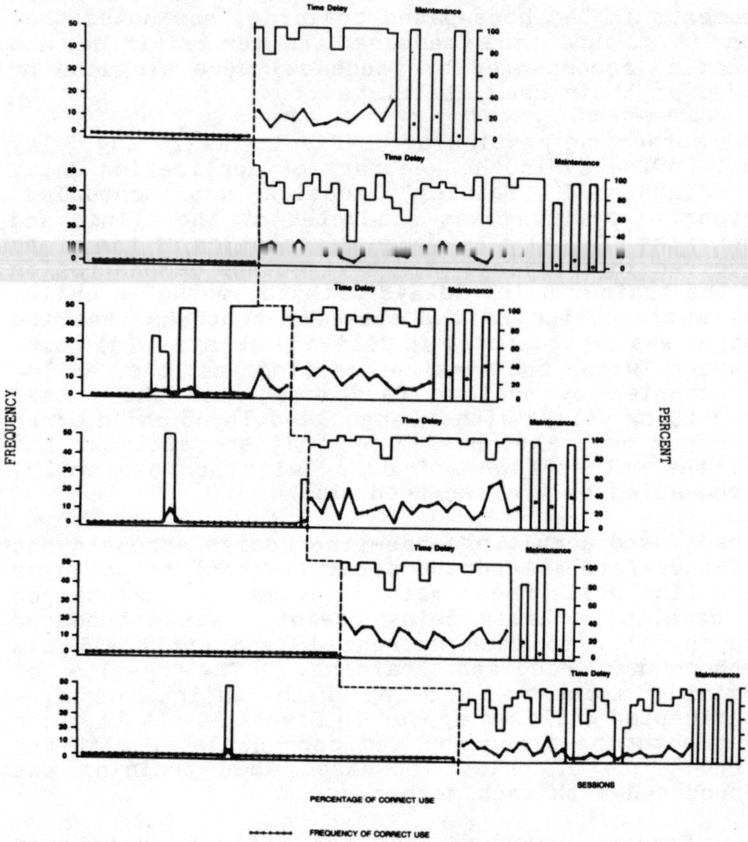

the effect of delay on child behaviour. However she did demonstrate the effect of delay training on mothers' delay use with the multiple-baseline design; Halle et al. used a less powerful design (an A-B) to demonstrate the effect of delay training on teachers' delay use.

Criterion 2. Alpert reported data on both mothers' use of the four milieu language teaching procedures, including delay, and correlated changes in children's linguistic skills. Delay was measured in terms of its frequency of correct use and the percentage of correct use. The children's linguistic skills measured included responsiveness, rate of vocalisation, upperbound (longest utterance), mean length of utterance (MLU), novel and total number of words produced, and intelligibility. As in the Halle et al. study, the effect of the delay training on mothers' use of delay was assessed. Also the effect of mothers' delay use, in combination with the other three milieu procedures, on their children's linguistic repertoire was assessed.

Criterion 3. The definition of delay in the Alpert (1984) study was essentially the same as that used by Halle et al. (1981).

Criterion 4. According to Alpert, effective use of each of the four milieu language training procedures is predicated on adults' skills in selecting materials of potential interest to children and on their efforts to control access to assistance and materials. These should be provided contingent on acceptable child responses when possible. Due to the significance of the selection, arrangement and control of materials, a training lecture on these topics preceded the training of milieu procedures.

Alpert identified three conditions under which children are most likely to talk to adults: when they NEED ASSISTANCE or INFORMATION or when they HAVE INFORMATION to share. She suggested ways that adults might arrange the environment to produce these three conditions: (a) To create a need for the child to request adult assistance, make available a variety of toys or materials with which the child can play. Select novel materials that you think the child would enjoy, as well as those known to be enjoyed. Arrange the materials so that they are in view of, but not accessible to, the child without requesting assistance or permission from the adult. Finally, occasions can be arranged such that once the child obtains an object that another request is required because the adult withheld other objects that the child needed, e.g., dry paint, water, paper, paint brush. (b) To increase the likelihood that the child will request information from the adult, make unfamiliar objects available. The child is more likely to communicate about novel things than familiar things. (c) To increase the likelihood that the child will have information to share with the adult, make available materials that are novel and have demonstrated interest for the child. Also objects that can be manipulated and thereby changed, e.g., tinker toys, should be made available. Materials and objects such as these provide opportunities for the child to share information with a nearby adult.

Criterion 5. Alpert assessed generalisation of mother's delay use by collecting data in two situations, Domestic Chore (DC) and Television On (TO), that differed from the training situation. DC was a time when the mother washed dishes or dusted and the child played with nearby toys; TO meant the mother and child sat in front of the television and the child had access to toys. These two generalisation probes were conducted at the end of baseline and after each milieu procedure was trained to criterion. At no time was graphic or descriptive feedback provided for mothers' teaching efforts during the generalisation sessions. The frequency and percentage of mothers' correct use of delay during generalisation sessions constitute the relevant data for our analysis. All six mothers increased their delay use during generalisation sessions relative to baseline. In baseline generalisation sessions they rarely used delays; in generalisation sessions that followed delay training, the six mothers averaged 6 delays per session during DC and 4 per session during TO. Their percentage of accurate use was near 0 during baseline and increased to an average of 77.5 per cent during DC and 91 per cent during TO.

Criterion 6. Following the completion of formal training on all four milieu procedures and generalisation probes, the trainer discussed with each mother the importance of the continued use of the four language-training procedures. The content of the discussion included (a) the improvement in the child's language correlated with mother's use of the procedures; (b) the need for continued use of procedures to ensure continued progress; (c) encouragement to use the procedures incidentally throughout the day whenever opportunities arose; (d) request continued use of the procedures for at least 10 minutes each week to maintain mastery; and (e) the need to conduct three monthly maintenance checks.

Maintenance sessions differed from training sessions in two ways: no feedback about the mother's use of the procedures was provided and, during the first half of the session, the mother applied the procedures while playing with the child as in training sessions and during the second half, the mother applied the procedures while engaged in a domestic chore or while watching television as in generalisation sessions.

Figure 5 also reveals the results of mothers' maintained use of delay during maintenance sessions for each of the six participants. Mother E delayed most frequently (46 times) in the three maintenance sessions; Mother C delayed least frequently (eight times). The average number of delays by mothers for each session was seven. For all six mothers, the percentage of correct delay use within any maintenance session fell below 75 per cent only twice i.e., 50 per cent for Mother C and 68 per cent for Mother E.

Criterion 7. Following the trainer's discussion of maintenance, a consumer satisfaction survey was given to each mother with the request that she complete and return it to the trainer during the following week. Twenty questions were include. Most questions centred on mothers' opinions of and satisfaction with training; one asked for their ratings of improvement in the language skills of their children as a function of training and others queried mothers about the relevance and frequency of use of procedures outside of training. The results of the survey revealed that all mothers believe that training made them more effective language teachers; that the milieu procedures could be used in most situations when they were with their child and that they did use the procedures frequently at times other than training. Furthermore, four mothers thought that their children's skills improved as a result of training. Modelling was rated as the most effective training method with lectures and videotape playback of correct and incorrect procedural applications as next most preferred.

Delayed Prompting

Although mothers answered many other questions and their responses were informative and provided one type of social validation, subjective evaluation, social comparisons are lacking. As in the Halle et al. (1981) study, Alpert's investigation may have been strengthened by the inclusion of social comparison data - data that reflect the language skills of an appropriate comparison group of same-aged children who are functioning adequately with regard to language. Social comparisons provide a baseline measure against which the levels of the treated behaviour can be compared.

ARRANGING THE ENVIRONMENT: STRATEGIES FOR RECOGNISING AND CREATING LANGUAGE OPPORTUNITIES

Although a number of these strategies were discussed in relation to Criterion 4 of the above reviews, they are such an integral part of delay use in natural settings that more extensive coverage is appropriate.

RECOGNISING PREEMPTING. Throughout the day countless occasions arise in which caregivers preempt opportunities for language. In a free play activity, children are allowed ready access to reinforcing materials or events without having to request them (environmental preempting). During a fine motor task, students are given crayons and paper and thus have no reason to ask for them (nonverbal preempting). When a teacher spies a child struggling with her coat zipper and asks "What do you need?", the opportunity for the child to initiate "Help" is lost (verbal preempting). In every one of these episodes if the caregivers had modified the setting in very small ways (e.g. placed the materials in sight, but out of reach; held back the crayons and paper; approached the child and waited silently) and had implemented delays, they would have created new opportunities for language.

ARRANGE FOR CONTINGENT ACCESS TO REINFORCERS. For severely handicapped students with very limited language, we must concentrate on the motivation for language use. We need to give them reasons to use the language they currently possess and to learn new language forms. We must be able to show them that language has a function for them. In order to accomplish these lofty objectives, materials, events and activities that are established reinforcers for an individual may be provided contingently. That is, a rule is established: you may have access to these things that you enjoy, but only when you request them or describe them or make a sentence about them. The rule will depend upon students' current skill levels.

During a free time period, for example, Halle et al. (1981) observed teachers pulling a wagon full of students or spinning a big plastic ball in which a student had crawled. In both cases the students smiled and laughed while in motion and they seemed to communicate that they wanted more when the teacher stopped the activity. A new rule was established for students participating in the study: No wagon pulls or ball spins until students said either "Spin", "Pull", "Ball", "Wagon", or some acceptable combination. To provoke opportunities for the rule to be implemented, teachers were instructed to give the students a very short ride or spin (reinforcer sampling, see Allyon and Azrin, 1968) and then stop and wait (delay a prompt) for a request.

A variation of the above strategy is CREATE SITUATIONS TO PROVOKE LANGUAGE. By prohibiting access to materials or activities that are accessible to other students, provocation is established (Klein et al., 1981) and a reason for language is thereby created. For example, if going for a ride in the school van is a potent reinforcer and every student in the class except one is given a ticket redeemable for a van ride, the remaining students' probability of language use may increase greatly. If a request is not forthcoming, delayed prompting could be invoked to assure a correct response and thus a ride.

CREATE ROUTINES. If chains of behaviour or routines are established, then they can be interrupted by withholding the next step or omitting a step altogether. Chain interruption may set the occasion for language and thus constitutes a strategy for creating language opportunities. When students day-after-day put on their coats, line up at the door and then proceed outside to recess, a routine has been created. If the first two steps of the routine are completed and then the teacher waits at the door, students have a reason to communicate. The teacher has wisely withheld access to the last step of a routine that leads to a potentially potent reinforcer.

Delayed Prompting

Motivation is highest just prior to reinforcement delivery.

Hall (1980) investigated the effect of chain interruption on requesting behaviour of two retarded, language-delayed students. Rather than surveying the environment for naturally occurring routines, Hall trained short, functional, and reinforcing motor routines. Each required particular objects and sequences of behaviour. For example to make soup, students needed to find a packet of soup, a bowl, and a spoon; they also needed to pour water into a kettle, boil the water, and pour the water into the bowl with the dry soup mixture. In addition to training the motor routines, the labels of the objects needed to complete the routine were taught. With these prerequisites mastered, Hall made all the necessary objects available, except one, and waited for a request for the newly trained object label. Interrupting the short, motor routines created language opportunities for these language-delayed students to practise their newly acquired language.

RECOGNISE ALTERNATIVE FORMS OF COMMUNICATION. Clear opportunities for language exist on those occasions when currently other forms of communication are occurring. Although some of these forms are developmental precursors of spoken or sign language and as such are appropriate. Over time, their use can become counterproductive. Extended eye gaze, pointing, gesturing, and tapping adults are examples. Consider a language-delayed child who takes his mother by the hand and leads her to the refrigerator and points to the freezer section where the ice cream is located. This form of communication is often reinforced by obtaining access to the ice cream. Thus a rudimentary form of communication becomes functional. Why learn new, maybe more difficult to produce, forms of communicating if you are able to influence your environment sufficiently with current forms? By delaying at critical moments, new opportunities for language use are created.

In addition to the prominent alternative forms of communication already mentioned, various topographies of aberrant behaviour have recently been characterised as communicative. Carr (1983) and Schuler and Goetz (1981) hypothesised that particular forms of aberrant behaviour such as self-injury, aggression, and tantrums may serve a communicative function and therefore their presence may signal an opportunity for socially appropriate language. Experimental demonstrations have been conducted by Carr, Newsom, and Binkoff (1980) and Durand and Carr (in press). If precursors of the aberrant behaviour can be identified, then delayed prompting may be used to set the occasion for socially appropriate alternative language forms. Although the recommendation awaits experimental validation, using graduated (stepping) delayed prompting on these occasions in the natural environment may increase the probability of success. During the acquisition of a new communicative form, it may be unwise to wait for the new form to occur when the old form (e.g., aggression) has a higher probability of occurrence. The use of an immediate model of the socially appropriate alternative with graduated delays makes sense intuitively.

This chapter deals with teaching a procedure that encourages the acquisition and use of language by those children who do not spontaneously acquire these skills. We have discussed the training of delayed prompting in artificial, highly constrained therapeutic settings (e.g., language therapy rooms) and in "natural" less constrained settings (e.g., classrooms, lunchrooms, and homes). Different training procedures have evolved for teaching delayed prompting in these two diverse contexts. A research-validated, integrated continuum of staff-training procedures to teach delayed prompting does not currently exist. Therefore, this technology must await some future date when opinion and dogma have given way to more comprehensive research findings. We look forward to that day and report here the state of the art.

ACKNOWLEDGEMENT

The authors wish to thank Cathy Alpert for generously providing a copy of her dissertation. Her procedures for teaching parents provide an elegant model for teaching staff to use any instructional technique. Furthermore, the authors acknowledge the time and efforts of Sally Brown for her patience and tenacity in the preparation of this manuscript.

REFERENCES

Alpert, C. (1984) Training Parents to Use Incidental Teaching as a Means of Improving the Communication Skills of their Language-delayed Children, Unpublished doctoral dissertation, University of Kansas, Lawrence

Ayllon, T. and Azrin, N.H. (1968) 'Reinforcer Sampling: A Technique for Increasing the Behavior of Mental Patients', Journal of Applied Behavior Analysis, 1, 13-20

Carr, E.G. (1983) Application of Pragmatics to the Conceptualization and Treatment of Severe Behavior Problems in Children, presented at the Annual Convention of the American Psychological Association, Anaheim, Calif.

Carr, E.G., Newsom, C. D. and Blinkoff, J. A. (1980) 'Escape as a Factor in the Aggressive Behavior of Two Retarded Children', Journal of Applied Behavior Analysis, 13, 101-117

Durand, V.M. and Carr, E.G. (in press) 'Self-injurious Behavior: Motivating Conditions and Guidelines for Treatment', School Psychology Review

Elzel, B., LeBlanc, J., Schilmoeller, K. and Stello, M. (1981) Stimulus Control Procedures in the Education of Young Children' in S. W. Bijou and R. Ruiz (eds.), Contributions of Behavior Modification to Education, Lawrence Erlbaum, Hillsdale, N. J.

Greene, B.F., Willis, B.S., Levy, R. and Bailey, J.S. (1978) 'Measuring Client Gains from Staff-implemented Programs', Journal of Applied Behavior Analysis, 11, 395-412

Guess, D., Keogh, W. and Sailor, W. (1978) 'Generalization of Speech and Language Behavior: Measurement and Training Tactics', In R. L. Schiefelbusch (ed.), Bases of Language Intervention, University Park Press, Baltimore

Hall, G. (1980) Establishing Mands with Language-delayed Children using Chain Interruption and Imitative Prompt Procedures, Unpublished master's thesis, Western Michigan University, Kalamazoo, Mich.

Hall, R.V. and Broden, M. (1977) 'Helping Teachers and Parents to Modify Behavior of their Retarded and Behavior-disordered Children' in P. Mittler (ed.), Research to Practice in Mental Retardation: Education and Training, Vol II, International Association for Scientific Study in Mental Deficiency.

Halle, J.W. (1982) 'Teaching Functional Language to the Handicapped: An Integrative Model of Natural Environment Teaching Techniques', Journal of the Association for the Severely Handicapped, 7, 29-37

Halle, J.W. (1984) 'Arranging the Natural Environment to Occasion Language: Giving Severely Language-delayed Children Reasons to Communicate', Seminars in Speech and Language, 5, 185-197

Halle, J.W., Alpert, C.L. and Anderson, S. R. (1984) 'Natural Environment Language Assessment and Intervention with Severely Impaired Preschoolers', Topics in Early Childhood Special Education, 4, 36-56

Halle, J.W., Baer, D.M. and Spradlin, J.B. (1981) 'Teachers' Generalized Use of Delay as a Stimulus Control Procedure to Increase Language Use in Handicapped Children', Journal of Applied Behavior Analysis, 14, 389-409

Halle, J.W., Marshall, A.M. and Spradlin, J.E. (1979) 'Time Delay: A Technique to Increase Language use and Facilitate Generalization in Retarded Children', Journal of Applied Behavior Analysis, 12, 431-439

Harris, S. (1975) 'Teaching Language to Non-verbal Children: With Emphasis on Problems of Generalization', Psychological bulletin, 82, 565-580

Hart, B, (1985) 'Environmental Techniques that may Facilitate Generalization and Acquisition' in S.F. Warren and A.K. Rogers-Warren (eds.), Teaching Functional Language, University Park

Press, Baltimore

Hart, B. and Risley, T.R. (1968) 'Establishing Use of Descriptive Adjectives in the Spontaneous Speech of Disadvantaged Preschool Children', Journal of Applied Behavior Analysis, 1, 109-120

Hart, B. and Risley, T.R. (1974) 'Using Preschool Materials to Modify the Language of Disadvantaged Children', Journal of Applied Behavior Analysis, 7, 243-256

Hart, B. and Risley, T.R. (1975) 'Incidental Teaching of Language in the Preschool', Journal of Applied Behavior Analysis, 8, 411-420

Hart, B. and Rogers-Warren, A.K. (1978) 'A Milieu Approach to Teaching Language' in R.L. Schiefelbusch (ed.), Language Intervention Strategies, University Park Press, Baltimore

Hartung, J.R. (1970) 'A Review of Procedures to Increase Verbal Imitation Skills and Functional Speech in Autistic Children', Journal of Speech and Hearing Disorders, 35, 204-217

Johnson, C.M. (1978) 'Errorless Learning in a Multihandicapped Adolescent', Education and Treatment of Children, 1, 25-33

Kazdin, A.E. (1982) Single-case Research-Designs: Methods for Clinical and Applied Settings, Oxford University Press, Oxford

Klein, M.D., Wulz, S.N., Hall, M.K., Waldo, I.K., Carpenter, S.A., Rathan, D.A., Myers, S.P. Fox, F. and Marshall, A.M. (1981) Comprehensive Curriculum Communication Guide, Early Childhood Institute, University of Kansas, Lawrence

Lovaas, I. (1966) 'A Program for the Establishment of Speech in Psychotic Children' in J.K. Wing (ed.), Childhood Autism, Pergamon Press, Oxford

Marholin, D. and Touchette, P. (1979) 'The Role of Stimulus Control and Response Consequences' in A. Goldstein and F. Kanfer (eds.), Maximizing Treatment Gains, Academic Press, New York

McGee, G.G., Krantz, P.J., Mason, D. and McClannahan,

L.E. (1983) 'A Modified Incidental-teaching Procedure for Autistic Youth: Acquisition and Generalization of Receptive Object Labels', Journal of Applied Behavior Analysis, 16, 329-338

Mittler, P. and Berry, P. (1977) 'Demanding Language' in P. Mittler (ed.), Research to Practice in Mental Retardation: Education and Training, Vol.II, International Association for Scientific Study in Mental Deficiency.

Nordquist, V.M. and Raab, M.M. (in press). 'A Naturalistic Approach to the Problem of Establishing Functional Language in Home and Community Settings' in S. Adler (ed.), A Multidisciplinary Treatment Program for the Preschool Aged Exceptional Child, C.C. Thomas, Springfield, Illinois

Oliver, C. and Halle, J. (1982) 'Language Training in the Everyday Environment: Teaching Functional Sign Use to a Retarded Child', Journal of the Association for the Severely Handicapped, 7, 50-62

Rincover, A. and Koegel, R. (1975) 'Setting Generality and Stimulus Control in Autistic Children', Journal of Applied Behavior Analysis, 8, 235-246

Risely, T. and Wolf, M. (1967) 'Establishing Functional Speech in Echolalic Children', Behaviour Research and Therapy, 5, 73-88

Schepis, M.M., Reid, D.H., Fitzgerald, J.R., Faw, G.D., van den Pol, R.A. and Welty, P.A. (1982) 'A Program for Increasing Manual Signing by Autistic and Profoundly Retarded Youth within the Daily Living Environment', Journal of Applied Behavior Analysis, 15, 369-379

Schuler, A.L. and Goetz, C. (1981) 'The Assessment of Severe Language Disabilities: Communicative and Cognitive Considerations', Analysis and Intervention in Development Disabilities, 1, 333-346

Sidman, M. (1971) 'Reading and Auditory-visual Equivalences', Journal of Speech and Hearing Research, 14, 5-13

Sidman, M. and Stoddard, L. (1966) 'Programming Perception and Learning for Retarded Children' in N.R. Ellis (ed.), International Review of Research in Mental Retardation (Vol. 2), Academic Press, New York

Sidman, M. and Stoddard, L.T. (1967) 'The Effectiveness of Fading in Programming a Simultaneous Form Discrimination for Retarded Children', Journal of the Experimental Analysis of Behavior, 10, 3-15

Skinner, B.F. (1968) The Technology of Teaching, Meredith Corporation, New York

Smeets, P.M. and Striefel, S. (1976) 'Acquisition and Cross-modal Generalization of Receptive and Expressive Signing Skills in a Retarded Deaf Girl', Journal of Mental Deficiency Research, 20, 251-260

Spradlin, J., Cotter, V. and Baxley, N. (1973) 'Establishing a Conditional Discrimination without Direct Training: A Study of Transfer with Retarded Adolescents', American Journal of Mental Deficiency, 77, 556-566

Stokes, T. and Baer, D. (1977) 'An Implicit Technology of Generalization', Journal of Applied Behavior Analysis, 10, 349-367

Striefel, S., Bryan, K.S. and Aikins, S.A. (1974) 'Transfer of Stimulus Control from Motor to Verbal Stimuli', Journal of Applied Behavior Analysis, 7, 123-135

Striefel, S., Wetherby, G. and Karlan, G. (1976) 'Establishing Generalized Verb-noun Instruction-following Skills in Retarded Children', Journal of Experimental Child Psychology, 22, 247-260

Stremel-Campbell, K., Cantrell, D. and Halle, J. (1977) 'Manual Signing as a Language System and as a Speech Initiator for the Nonverbal Severely Handicapped Student' in E. Sontag (ed.), Educational Programming for the Severely and Profoundly Handicapped, Council for Exceptional Children, Reston, Virginia

Touchette, P. (1968) 'The Effects of Graduated

Stimulus Change on the Acquisition of a Simple Discrimination in Severely Retarded Boys', Journal of the Experimental Analysis of Behavior, 11, 39-48

Touchette, P.E. (1971) 'Transfer of Stimulus Control: Measuring the Moment of Transfer', Journal of the Experimental Analysis of Behavior, 15, 347-354

Touchette, P.E. and Howard, J.S. (1984) 'Errorless Learning: Reinforcement Contingencies and Stimulus Control Transfer in Delayed Promoting', Journal of Applied Behavior Analysis, 17, 175-188

Warren, S.F., Rogers-Warren, A., Baer, D.M. and Guess, D. (1980) 'The Assessment and Facilitation of Language Generalization' in W. Sailor, B. Wilcox and L. Brown (eds.), Methods of Instruction for Severely Handicapped Students, Pan H Brooks, Baltimore

Wolf, M.M. (1978) 'Social Validity: The Case for Subjective Measurement or how Applied Behavior Analysis is Finding its Heart', Journal of Applied Behavior Analysis, 11, 203-214

Woods, T.S. (1982) 'Generality in the Verbal Tacting of Autistic Children as a Function of 'Naturalness' in Antecedent Control', Presented at the Conference on Behavior Analysis in Education, Ohio State University, Columbus

Chapter Five

EVALUATION OF A SELF-INSTRUCTIONAL TEACHING PACKAGE

Colin Robson

A. Project TASS

This chapter focuses on the effects on teachers' behaviour of their involvement with a self-instructional training package which aims to give them the skills of running short, effective structured teaching sessions with severely mentally handicapped pupils. This training package was an outcome of the work of Project TASS (Teaching and the Severely Subnormal) carried out at Huddersfield Polytechnic in association with the Hester Adrian Research Centre, University of Manchester, over the period 1976-1982.

The central rationale for the Project was to seek ways in which the already existing research evidence on learning processes in people with severe mental handicap could be made accessible to teachers, with concentration on various projects which had been carried out at the Hester Adrian Research Centre.

Existing reviews of the evidence (e.g. Clarke and Clarke, 1974; Clarke and Clarke, 1975) and a further review carried out by the Project team (Jones and Robson, 1979a) provided strong support for the view that the learning and development of people with severe mental handicap can be enhanced by the use of structured teaching with regular, short sessions and a specific teaching objective closely geared to the child's present level of attainment. Hence the primary aim of Project TASS became the production, development and evaluation of materials which would assist the teacher to acquire the skills needed to do this.

To fulfil the aim, the Project Team produced a

'Minicourse' (cf Borg, Kelly, Langer and Gall, 1970). This is a self-instructional multi-media package consisting of written material (a teacher's handbook and workbook and a co-ordinator's handbook), instructional video-tapes and self-evaluated practical sessions (Robson, Jones and Storey, 1982). The focus of the material is on language, specifically the child's expressive language. This does not so much reflect the view that the structured approach is specifically appropriate to language, but more the need to concentrate on a particular aspect of the curriculum in order to give coherence to the material presented. By focusing on language, it also becomes possible for this project to assist in the dissemination of materials, findings and techniques from several completed projects (e.g. Jeffree and McConkey, 1976; Leeming, Swann, Coupe and Mittler, 1979; Thomas, Gaskin and Herriot, 1973).

In Phase One of the project, pilot trials of the material were carried out with a group of 20 teachers from one local authority area in the North of England and modifications made in the light of feedback from the participants and the experience gained. Field trials of the revised material have been held in successive terms in three other areas involving 19 teachers and 38 children. Modifications to the material of a minor nature were made after the first field trial, taking into account the additional feedback from the teachers involved. The main evaluation of the effectiveness of the Project material has been directed toward these field trials.

A follow-up project evaluated a series of four trials of the material in different schools in successive terms where more generalised effects of the intervention on the school and in the classroom were assessed. It also mounted a series of trials run by local personnel with no involvement by this project team. Data from a total of 24 further teachers and 48 children were analysed.

The training course

Table 1 shows the suggested organisation of the course, although this was varied in minor respects to suit local conditions. Typically, the course would have two or three teachers from each of up to four schools in an area. It is seen as important to have

SUMMARY OF COURSE ORGANISATION AND ACTIVITIES

	Length of Time	At 'centre' or in school	In school
Phase One PREPARATORY	Flexible - but two weeks minimum.	Preliminary group meeting (to give out 'Teacher's Workbook - go through it and confirm arrangements). Teacher's handbook given out at this meeting or, at the latest, one week before group meeting.	Teachers select 2 children; obtain, transcribe and analyse language samples using Workbook. Tape Recorder needed. Video-taping at least one 10 minute session with each child. VTR monitor, microphone and camera needed.
Phase Two MAIN PART OF COURSE	Five Weeks	Weekly group meeting to view Instructional and Modelling tapes (3/4 hr.) VTR and monitor needed. Teachers to have read handbook chapter before meeting.	Two ten-minute video sessions per week each followed by self-evaluation using workbook (approximately 30 minutes each). VTR, microphone and camera needed.
Phase Three PRACTICE	Flexible	Post-course group meeting (party?) - feedback from course members and suggestions for future activitives.	10 minutes sessions with each child, or with groups of children (number and frequency of sessions are flexible). Video-taping preferable but not essential (If video-taped) VTR, monitor, microphone and camera needed.

more than one teacher involved in each school, mainly so that they can provide mutual support during the course. It is also possible for the course to be totally based on one school.

An important and integral part of the course consists of practical sessions in school where the teacher tries out the techniques for him/herself with children he/she is already teaching. To get the most out of the course teachers are advised to work with two children who are beyond the 'one word' stage. The 'Teacher's Workbook' gives advice on selection based upon sections of the PIP Language Development Charts (Jeffree and McConkey, 1976) as a screening device.

Table 2 gives chapter headings from the Teacher's Handbook. Chapters one to five indicate the course content for weeks one to five respectively. Thus week one is mainly concerned with teaching objectives but also gives some attention to the amount and complexity of teacher language in relation to child language. In week two the 'Basic Structuring Techniques' referred to are essentially the behaviour modification techniques including the appropriate use of verbal reinforcement, provision of verbal models, eliciting imitation, providing verbal prompts and requesting a non-imitative utterance from the child following a successful imitation. For this session the teachers are asked to work to a single word language objective which permits them to concentrate on the structuring skills themselves, with the language aspect kept to the simplest possible.

In week three the teachers switch to a language objective based on the child's present level of language use - as assessed by them from the pre-course exercises. Particular attention is given here to the type of question asked by the teacher and the teacher's treatment of answers from the child (Jones and Robson, 1979a). A systematic approach based on 'targeting the missing element' in a child's utterance derived from the Schools Council project 'questioning technique' (Leeming et al, 1979) is advocated. The practical sessions also provide the opportunity for further practice of the basic structuring techniques, but in the context of a more complex language objective. In week four the techniques involved are substantially identical, but now addressed to a language objective which represents a 'next step' in language development. Information is given to the

Table 2. CHAPTER HEADINGS FROM TEACHER'S HANDBOOK

Chaper One	:	Introducing the Course Using Objectives and Watching Your Language
Chapter Two	:	Basic Techniques of Structuring
Chapter Three	:	Using Structuring Techniques to Encourage Full Use of the Child's Present Language
Chapter Four	:	Using Structuring Techniques to Extend the Child's Use of Language
Chapter Five	:	Using Structuring Techniques in a Group Setting
Chapter Six	:	Conclusion - Where Do We Go From Here?

teachers about sequences of language development to assist in their choice of an appropriate objective.

Whereas the first four weeks are concerned with one-to-one work, the fifth week shifts to the use of structuring techniques in a small group setting. Again the practical sessions provide further practice in the use of structuring techniques but there is also the need to distribute time and attention between individual children in the group and to check on the achievement of individual objectives. The final chapter is mainly concerned with ways in which structured sessions can be incorporated into the teaching day and with various aspects of generalisation. Extensive appendix material is provided partly for use during the course, but mainly for reference following the course.

B. Evaluation of the Minicourse: Phase One

The central task was taken to be an assessment of the extent to which teachers taking the course can develop the skills and techniques of structured teaching covered in the course so that they can run effective structured sessions themselves. To that end, in all field trials, there has been a short series of pre-course teaching sessions at weekly intervals and a corresponding series of post-course teaching sessions. Various aspects of teacher's and child's behaviour, primarily language, were analysed and pre- and post-course performance compared.

The strategy adopted has been to analyse and interpret the key or central aspects of the data for teachers on all field trials. Six dependent variables have been selected for analysis in this fashion - four of them being essentially measures of teacher behaviour ("Total sequences", "Modal target proportion", "Teacher-Initiating Structuring" and "Encouragement"), one of teacher behaviour relative to child behaviour (Mean Length of Response for teacher compared to Mean Length of Response for child), and one of child behaviour ("Length Complexity Index" for child language). Details are given below. For the nine teachers and eighteen children on the first field trial a more detailed analysis was carried out, covering a series of five pre-course sessions and five post-course sessions and a retention session three months after the last post-course session. In this way it is possible to provide illumination and further interpretation of the findings established with the full sample.

For teachers in both Phase One and follow-up trials there was a series of three to five pre-course sessions. In this main analysis, the second and the third sessions are used, an average figure being computed for the 'pre-course' and 'post-course' sessions. In a more detailed analysis of the first field trial, each of the five pre-course and five post-course sessions were used, together with the retention sessions.

In this presentation, analysis of the Phase One trials will be presented separately and comparison subsequently made between the two sets of trials.

Inter-Observer Agreement

The sessions from field trials constituting the data base were transcribed by two transcribers. The 'pre'- 'post'- and 'retention' transcripts and associated video-tapes were coded 'blind' in randomised sequence by two coders. It was so arranged that the coders (Robson, 1980a Appendix 7) did not code any sessions for which they had been responsible for making the transcript. The coding and analysis were carried out, using a detailed set of 'Rules for Coders'. The rules were originally developed using transcripts and tapes from the pilot trials; development and coder training continuing until acceptable initial levels of inter-observer agreement were achieved. During coding and analysis of the Phase One field trial transcripts and tapes, a series of 21 reliability trials was carried out with independent coding of the same transcript/tape and subsequent consensual coding of categories to minimise inter-observer drift. Table 3 shows inter-observer agreement statistics for the various aspects of coding of the data (P_0 = proportion of agreement, K = Cohen's Kappa, which corrects for chance agreement). The meaning of the various types of coding is developed below, but it appears that the agreement values are at an acceptably high level, with the more subjective "child utterances which 'should' or 'should not' be encouraged" predictably having the lowest K.

Analysis of Transcripts and Video-Tapes

A brief description of each of the central measures

is presented, followed by a summary of the findings of the analysis on these measures. Each measure is then considered in turn and a more detailed analysis and interpretation attempted, drawing upon the findings of the full analysis of the first field trial. If the teacher is using the structured method as developed on the course, this should be discernible in various ways from the tapes and transcripts of the sessions. Apart from the specific structuring techniques (e.g. use of verbal reinforcement, models etc.), which will be considered below, some rather more global aspects should be detectable.

a) Sequences. A characteristic of 'non-structured' interactions between teacher and child noted in pilot work and amongst others, by the Schools Council Project Team (Leeming et al, 1979) is the way in which the teacher 'hops' rapidly from one topic, or question or point of attention, to another in an unconnected and apparently random way. If order is present, it appears to be much more constrained by the material used (often picture cards) and not order in the sense of concentration on a particular language form or aspect of language.

In the course, considerable stress is placed on the value of specifying a language objective and focusing the situation, the questions, demands etc., so that there is a concentration on the language form(s) indicated by the objective. It is predicted that the teacher who does this will be likely to stay on any particular topic for a longer period of time. To assess this, the transcript is divided into sequences - (by which is meant a set of utterances, usually consecutive, which appear to relate to same topic or target).

It should be noted that it is not necessary to specify the particular target for each sequence - the requirement is simply that the point where one sequence ends and another starts should be found. As can be seen from Table 3, this can be specified with adequate reliability.

b) Modal Target. Following the division into sequences as discussed above, the resulting sequences were labelled according to their apparent target. The basic categories used were:-

Table 3. INTER-OBSERVER AGREEMENT - PHASE ONE TRIALS

	P_O	K
SEQUENCE BOUNDARY	0.80	0.94
SEQUENCE LABELLING	0.84	0.78
TEACHER UTTERANCE LABELLING	0.76	0.85
CHILD LCI	0.89	0.93
UTTERANCES	0.99	0.98
CHILD UTTERANCES WHICH "SHOULD" OR "SHOULD NOT" BE ENCOURAGED	0.87	0.70

i) 'Single word', subdivided into 'single noun' (a sequence where the apparent target is a single noun, e.g. teacher asks "what's this?", child replies "dog" and teacher accepts the reply); 'single verb'; 'single other' (most commonly adjective).

ii) 'Multi-word' subdivided according to the language form of the multi-word target, (e.g. Preposition, Noun; Noun-Verb-Noun, etc.).

iii) 'Non-Verbal' (e.g. where the teacher is checking comprehension by getting the child to do something).

iv) 'Child-Initiated' where the child spontaneously introduces a new topic. Sequences where the child is making the first utterance as response to material presented by the teacher are considered as teacher-initiated rather than child-initiated.

If it was not possible to assign one of the above labels to the sequence it was labelled 'uncertain'. The 'Rules for Coders' (Robson, 1980a, Appendix 7 gives detailed category definitions). Inter-observer agreement in respect of sequence labelling was again adequate.

While several aspects of sequence labelling and the relative occurrence of different categories are of interest, the concentration here is on the Modal Target. That is, given that the teachers are working with children above the single word level of language development and that they are also working to a specific language objective, we would expect that they would tend to concentrate on a specific language form (or possibly, in the case of multiple objectives, on two or three specific language forms). Considered in terms of sequences and targets, this is equivalent to hypothesising that a particular language form multi-word target will predominate. So we would expect that the modal multi-word target (i.e. the most frequently occurring multi-word target) will occur in a large proportion of the sequences.

Conversely if a teacher is not working to a

specific objective, no one language form will predominate and the modal multi-word target will have a low relative frequency of occurrence.

c) Mean Length of Response. The course seeks to sensitise teachers to the length and complexity of their utterances as related to the length and complexity of the child's utterances. While no specific rules or guidelines are laid down, it is hypothesised that, in particular, the complexity of teacher utterances will be more closely matched to that of the children, following the course. The measure used is that of mean length of response (MLR) which is simply the average number of words per utterance. Hence we are concerned with the ratio of Mean Length of Response for Teacher (MLR_T) to Mean Length of Response for Child (MLR_C).

d) Structuring Skills. The basic structuring skills are introduced at week two of the course, and their use is further practised in weeks three to five with addition of further 'targeting' skills in week three. Clearly these skills form a central part of the course and it is of importance to determine the extent to which the course assists teachers to acquire and use them. The initial pre-course level is also of considerable interest in view of the claim sometimes made (e.g. by teachers at initial meetings giving information about the course) that "I do all this already". It is convenient to partition these skills into two sub-categories - covering those which are primarily either 'teacher-initiating' or 'teacher-reacting' to a child utterance.

'Teacher-initiating' structuring skills are taken as:

i) provision of verbal models
ii) provision of verbal prompts
iii) request for imitation
iv) request for non-imitative utterance (following a successful imitation by the child)
v) targeting a missing element.

'Teacher-reacting' structuring skills are essentially concerned with the use of verbal reinforcement. An important element of the structured method resides in the teacher's response to and treatment of utterances which are produced by the child. In analysis such responses were sub-categorised as 'encouragement', 'discouragement' or 'neutral'. The term 'encouragement was used throughout the course as a synonym for the more usual 'verbal reinforcement' (although there are precedents for the usage adopted here). This step was taken as a matter of policy following pilot work where it appeared that a sizeable minority of teachers reacted unfavourably to the term 'reinforcement'. A further subcategory of 'enthusiastic encouragement' was also created.

While it is by no means straightforward to supply a complete algorithm specifying the appropriate teacher treatment of each child utterance, the basic position is that child utterances which fulfil the objective, or are steps along the road to doing so, should be encouraged. Inappropriate responses should be treated neutrally. Discouragement (e.g. 'Don't be silly', or 'No' in a harsh or angry tone) should not be used. It was found that in both pre- and post- sessions there was a vanishingly small incidence of 'discouragement'. This may be an instance of certain aspects of the somewhat artificial pre- and post-sessions causing the teachers to behave in an atypical fashion - perhaps in the knowledge that the tapes would be seen and analysed by the research team. However, informal observation in the classroom gave further support for the view that 'discouragement' occurred very infrequently.

e) Analysis of Child Language. While the research evidence indicates strongly that the use of structured teaching techniques with teaching objectives keyed to the child's present level of ability will enhance the severely mentally handicapped child's development and attainment, it is valuable to demonstrate that there are actual changes in child behaviour and language. The child utterances in teaching sessions were analysed using the Length-Complexity Index. Table 4 summarises the scoring procedures - full details are given as Robson, 1980a, Appendix 8. It should be noted that imitations by the child are excluded from the LCI computation.

Results of Analysis of Key Dependent Variables

These results are summarised in Table 5. While it is necessary to qualify to some extent the simple picture presented here, in the more detailed discussion given in the following sections, it can be seen that there is a significant change in the hypothesised direction in relation to each of the six variables.

Specifically the teacher:

i) drops from over 6 sequences per minute pre-course to just over 2 post-course. That is, whereas before the course she was switching from one "topic" to another at 10 second intervals, she is subsequently staying on the same topic for nearly 30 seconds;

ii) increasingly concentrates on a specific aspect of language following the course, (changing from fewer than 1 in 10 being concerned with any one 'multi-word' language form to more than a half);

iii) triples the number of 'initiating' structuring utterances;

iv) increases the number of times she encourages the child's utterances by 50%;

v) decreases the complexity of her language in relation to the child's language from over 3½ to 2½;

and

vi) the length and complexity of the child's language is increased noticeably from an LCI value of 1.63 to 2.33.

The results provide a striking confirmation that, following the course, the teachers are going about these video-taped sessions in a markedly different way from that in which they did prior to the course.

Both the importance and the limitations of these findings is taken up in the concluding section of this chapter.

Detailed Analysis of First Field Trial

Graphs 1 to 2 show the pre-post and retention measures

TABLE 4. SUMMARY OF SCORING PROCEDURES FOR LENGTH COMPLEXITY INDEX

(For greater detail see Robson, 1980a Appendix 8. "The LCI - A Revision of Scoring Procedures for Project TASS").

i) Eliminate (ie. mark as -----)

unintelligible utterances
imitations (unless there is change of intonation or child's utterance includes elements not present in teacher's).
repetition (unless intervening teacher utterance, or 'no response' from teacher. Exact repetitions and cases where one child utterance is contained within the one following or preceding).
stereotypes
starters (including Yes, No, except primitive negative)
incomplete single words and imitations of prompts (not the completion of a prompt).

ii) Score
1 point for each word (treat compounds as one word)
1 point for each -ing ending
1 point for each past tense ending
1 point for each plural inflection
1 point for each possessive inflection
1 point for each combination of modifiers

iii) Score
1 point for each negative with negative at start or end of utterance.
2 points for each negative (no, not, can't, don't) when included within the utterance.

iv) Score 1 point for each conjunction.

vi) Non-grammatical word combinations score 0 (minor non-grammaticality being ignored).

Table 5. ANALYSIS OF KEY DEPENDENT VARIABLES

	Mean Pre-Course Value	Mean Post-Course Value	F[1]	Significance
Sequence Totals (normalised to 10 minutes session)	67.6	22.9	179.13	****
Proportion of Sequences having Modal Target	0.097	0.578	37.28	****
Teacher Initiating Structuring	11.5	33.8	36.34	****
Teachers' Use of Encouragement	12.68	18.69	6.27	*
MLR_T/MLR_C	3.59	2.34	11.96	***
Child's LCI	1.63	2.33	8.82	**

[1] from ANOVA (Hierarchical design).

KEY * $p < 0.05$; ** $p < 0.01$; *** $p < 0.005$; **** $p < 0.001$

for the first trial. For sequence totals Graph 1 shows a significant pre-course trend[1] which casts some doubt on the attribution of the pre-post difference on this variable as being related to the experiences provided by the course. A comparison of pre- and post-course scores with the retention scores three months later shows a significant difference between pre-course and retention but no difference between post-course and retention. A somewhat similar picture is presented by the modal target variable in Graph 2.

It should be noted that the definition of 'modal target' is couched in terms of multi-word targets so that a teacher who was, say, working to a single word objective would not score on the modal target measure. It is, of course, appropriate to work toward a single word language objective for children at a low level of language development and hence it may be that the picture presented is distorted. The dashed line in Graph 2 excludes children with a relatively low level of language development. The exclusion criterion is an average pre-post child LCI score below 1.5 which leads to the dropping of seven children. This is a generous exclusion criterion as, in fact, only one child is indubitably at the single-word level. The picture is not greatly changed by this exclusion although there is somewhat higher pre-course level and a more marked increase in proportion in the final pre-course session.

Analysis of the mean proportions of sequences where the target is the 'modal target' pre-course, post-course and at the retention trial indicates a significant difference between pre-course and retention and no difference between post-course and retention.

For teaching initiating structuring skills as shown in Graph 3 'a straight forward picture of lack of trend both pre- and post-course emerges. The pre-

---

1 *Analysis of variance shows both a significant pre-course linear trend and a marginally significant deviation from linearity using the Greenhouse & Geisser technique recommended by Winer (1971, p.523). Details of this and other analyses are presented in Robson (1980a)*

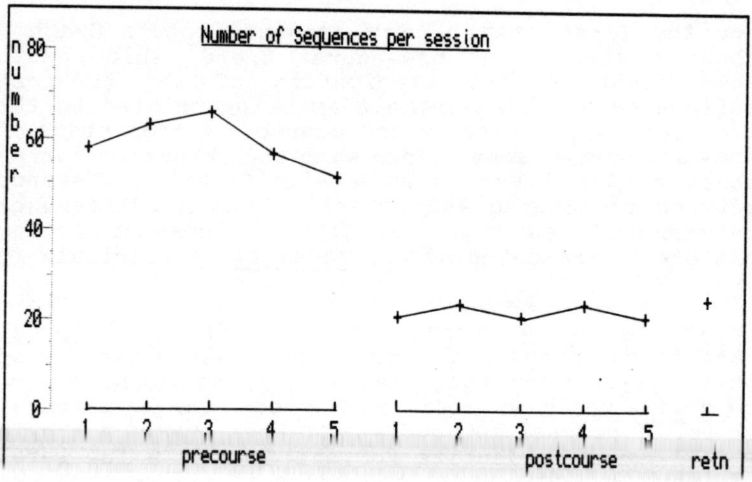

GRAPH 1 Total number of sequences per session : Field trial 1.

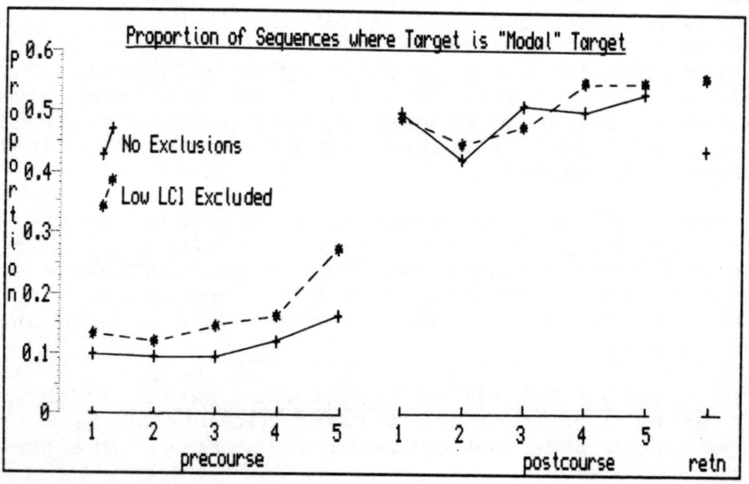

GRAPH 2 Proportion of sequences where the target is the 'modal' target.

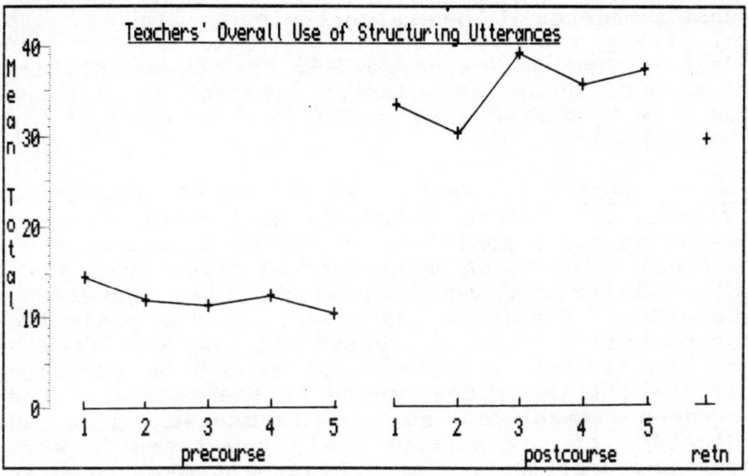

GRAPH 3 Teachers' overall use of 'structuring' utterances, i.e. models, prompts, imitation requests, requests for non-imitative child utterance and targeting missing element. (Mean totals per ten minute sample.)

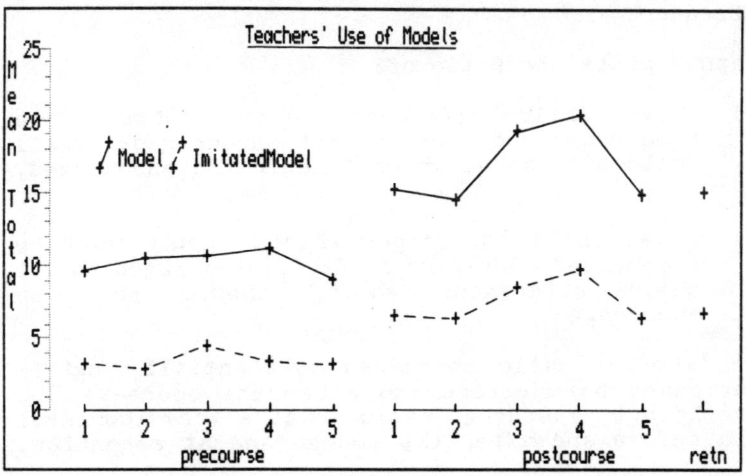

GRAPH 4 Teachers' use of models. (Mean total per five minute samples.)

course incidence of these structuring skills is almost exclusively attributable to the teachers' use of models as shown in Graphs 4 and 5. The general picture for each of these variables is substantial increase from pre- to post-course, which is maintained at the retention stage.

<u>Encouragement</u> (i.e. verbal reinforcement) also shows a very clear picture (Graph 6) with lack of trend pre-course and a positive linear trend post-course, the final value being maintained at retention, three months later, although not further increased. Separate consideration of 'Enthusiastic Encouragement' shows a substantial increase from a very low pre-course value. It should be stressed that the counts of occurrence of the teachers' use of encouragement do not in themselves give an indication of how appropriately the teachers were using encouragement. As this aspect was strongly stressed in the course, it is important to attempt some assessment of appropriateness of use. This was done in two ways, first, by categorising separately those child utterances which the teacher 'should' and 'should not' encourage according to the structuring approach; second, by relating the use of encouragement to the syntactical complexity of the child's utterance.

Graph 7 plots the ratio of:

i) those child utterances which 'should' be encouraged and were in fact encouraged, to all child utterances which 'should' be encouraged,

and

ii) those child utterances which 'should not' be encouraged, but were in fact, encouraged to all child utterances which 'should not' be encouraged.

The 'should' ratio increases substantially and is stationary both before and after the course. The 'should not' encourage ratio is at a very low level both before and after the course and at retention.

These 'should not' ratios are not considered to be particularly meaningful as the heavily restricted set of categories used as indicators for 'should not' be encouraged meant that few instances were in fact coded. It should perhaps also be noted that inter-

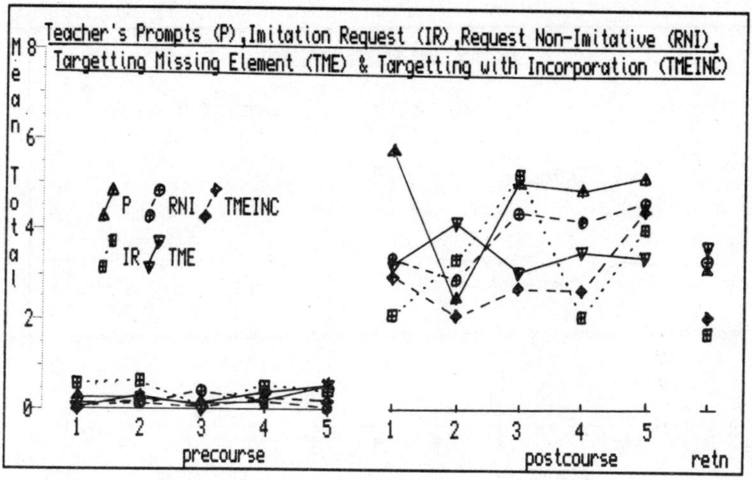

GRAPH 5 Teachers' use of prompts (P), imitation requests (IR), request non-imitative (RNI), targeting missing elements (TME) and targeting with incorporation (TME-INC).

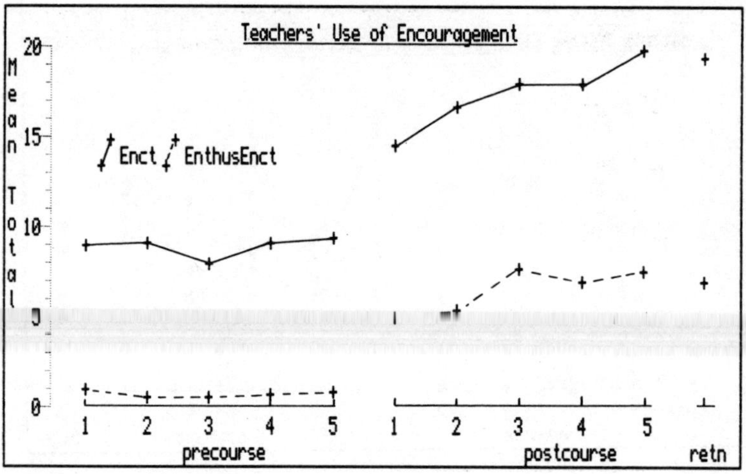

GRAPH 6 Teachers' use of encouragement. (Mean totals for 5 minute samples.)

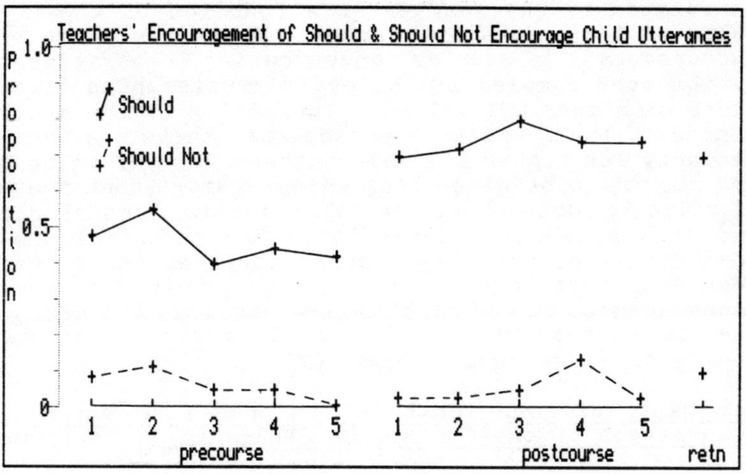

GRAPH 7 Teachers' encouragement of 'should encourage' and 'should not encourage' child utterances. (Overall ratio, i.e. total number encouraged to totall occurring for 5 minute sample.)

observer agreements was lowest for this measure (see Table 3).

Graph 8 shows the proportion of child utterances encouraged by the teacher as a function of the LCI value of the child's utterance. Appropriate use of encouragement is seen as concentrating encouragement on the more complex of the child's utterances (i.e. those of higher LCI value). Inspection of the graph suggests that whereas pre-course there is some tendency for higher LCI value utterances (of value 4 and above) to be given less encouragement than those of value 3, post-course the relationship is monotonic and in the expected direction. The essential pre-post difference in this respect appeared to be that teachers post-course were more likely to give encouragement to the child's more complex utterances, whereas pre-course their encouragement was not consistantly related to complexity.

The ratio of mean length of teacher's response to mean length of child response (MLR_T/MLR_C), is shown as Graph 9. There is some indication of a pre-course trend downwards in this ratio which casts doubt on the interpretation that the lower mean level post-course is due to the intervention. The post-course value shows no evidence of trend. Similarly there is no difference between the post-course mean and that at retention. The ratio MLR_T/MLR_C is clearly a highly derived one as both numerator and denominator are themselves ratios (mean length of response = number of words/number of utterances). In an attempt to throw further light on the drop in the ratio of MLR_T/MLR_C, separate consideration was given to each of the constituents (viz. teacher words, teacher utterances, child words, child utterances). Graph 10 shows these variables for pre-course, post-course and retention sessions. An interesting and relatively complex picture emerges from analyses of these data. Teachers use significantly fewer words post-course than they did pre-course, while their number of utterances does not change. Hence the teacher's MLR (Mean Length of Response) drops following the course. However, any interpretation is complicated by the significant linear trend downwards for both teacher words and teacher utterances and hence, interpretation of the pre-post difference as related to the teachers' experience during the central five weeks of the course is vitiated. It appears likely, as confirmed by comments from several teachers, that

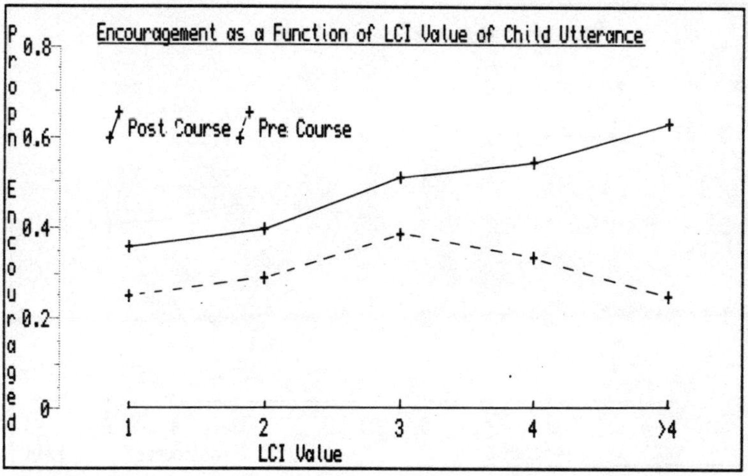

GRAPH 8 Teachers' encouragement of child utterances as a function of LCI value of utterance.

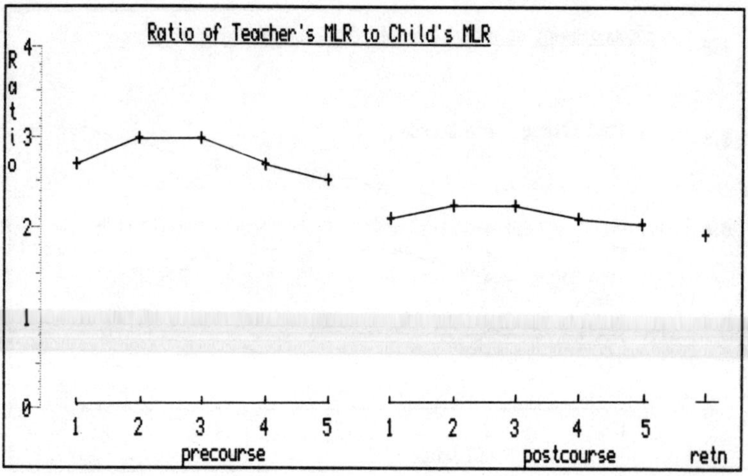

GRAPH 9 Ratio of teachers' mean length of response to child's mean length of response.

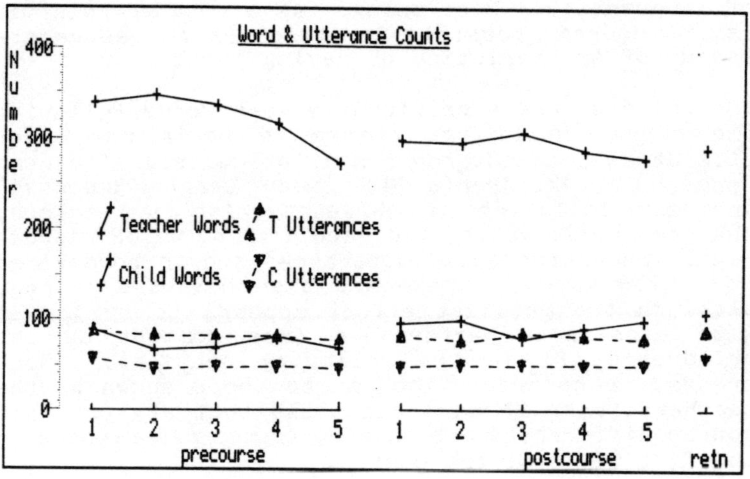

GRAPH 10 Word and utterance counts. (Mean totals for 5 minute samples.)

an effect of the teachers being asked to make transcripts of their pre-course sessions (for the purpose of analysing the child's use of language), had the function of sensitising them to the amount of language they were using. As a related point it is, of course, possible for teachers to reduce the labour of transcription by saying less.

The children use significantly more words following the course while the change in their number of utterances does not reach statistical significance. Hence, the children's MLR (Mean Length Response) increases following the course. As with the teachers, the pre-course values indicate a trend which reaches significance for child utterances and is borderline for child words. These are also downward trends, although the greatest effect appears to be linked with session 1 performance (see comment on the children's LCI in the following section). Such trends, in contradistinction to those shown by the teachers, make it more plausible that any pre-post course differences are related to the experiences in the five weeks of the course.

The Length-complexity Index (LCI) for the children's speech is shown as Graph 11. While statistical analysis provides no evidence for either pre- or post-course trends in LCI value, the high value of the pre-course session 1 is notable. The undoubted absence of any indication of a positive trend in LCI value prior to the course lends support to the attribution of the post-course increase in LCI as related to aspects of what occurs either in the five weeks of the course itself or subsequently. Analysis of pre-course mean LCI compared with post-course and at retention shows a highly significant pre-course to retention increase and no difference between the post-course and retention values.

Discussion of Findings in Phase 1 Trials

Inspection of the findings as listed above gives strong support to the view that the minicourse package does assist the teachers involved to acquire the skills and techniques identified as involved in structured teaching. It has also been possible to show that the children targeted by the teachers working on the course have a marked increase in the complexity of their utterances. The course material is also very well received by participating teachers

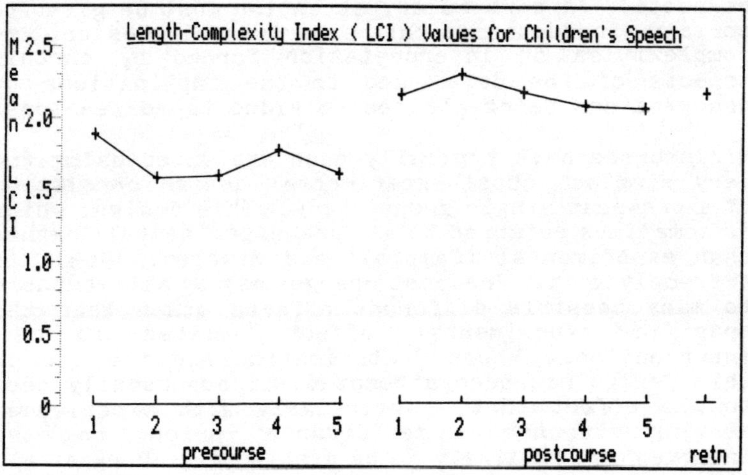

GRAPH 11 Length complexity index values for children's speech.

(Robson, 1980a). However, these results must be set in an appropriate context. In particular it must be stressed that confidence in the results and in the utility of the findings has to be qualified in certain respects. In particular, attention must be given to certain inadequacies of experimental design, to complexities of interpretation forced by certain aspects of the data, and to the implications of observations being limited to video taped sessions.

Minicourses have typically been evaluated using the very simplest quasi-experimental design consisting of a pre-post single group study. This design, which is sometimes referred to as 'pre-experimental' rather than experimental (Campbell and Stanley, 1963), is extremely weak. Pre-post changes may be attributable to many possible different effects other than the specific experimental effect related to the intervention. Where justification for the use of this design has been attempted, it has usually been to the effect that, particularly with experienced serving teachers, performance prior to the intervention is likely to be stable (e.g. Borg et al, 1970; Perrott, Applebee, Heap and Watson, 1975). This argument might have been employed with the present project and could perhaps be justified to an even greater extent in connection with measures of child behaviour and development in that several studies have produced data indicating little or no change or development on several language indices over short periods in the absence of structured intervention (e.g. Fenn, 1976; Leeming et al, 1979). However, it appeared highly desirable to attempt some strengthening of the design and sufficient data were collected to analyse the first field trial using what has been termed a 'Cross-sectional Time-Series Design', (Simonton, 1977). This approach which, inter alia, seeks to establish the stationarity or otherwise of performance on the various measures of teacher and child behaviour, provides the potential for making much stronger statements about associations between pre-post differences and the intervention. It should be noted that after exploratory modelling attempts, the autoregressive model put foward by Simonton was judged inappropriate and recourse was made to the more usual Greenhouse and Geisser approach to the problems posed in repeated measures designs (cf. Cook and Campbell, 1979, e.g. p.235).

The analyses and interpretation presented above

provide several examples of pre- and post-course trends in the data. The discussion here will be limited to trends in the values of the six key dependent variables - Sequence Totals, Proportion of Sequences having Modal Target, Teaching-initiating Structuring, Teachers' Use of Encouragement, Ratio of Teacher to Child Mean Length of Response and Child LCI. In only one case (Sequence Total) is there a clear indication of a pre-course trend in the data. Inspection of this trend shows it is associated largely with a decrease in the number of sequences for the fourth and fifth weeks pre-course. There is no ready explanation for this apart from the possibility that teachers having received the course handbook at about this time, appreciate from their reading the need to concentrate for a longer time on some specific aspect of language. Whatever the explanation, this trend casts doubt on the interpretation of the massive pre-post difference in sequence totals as being solely related to the teacher's experiences during the five cycles of the course. No other result is brought into question in this way. The only other strong trend is that of 'Use of Encouragement' post-course. This positive trend does not so much cast doubt on the effectiveness of the course in this regard as suggest that the effect continues to strengthen in the weeks following the course. This is supported by comments from several teachers during the post-course sessions to the effect that they felt less inhibited about giving strong encouragement to the child as they gained increasing confidence.

The analysis presented here has been restricted to video-taped sessions before and after the main part of the course. This restriction arose from a conscious evaluation of priorities by the project team. It was felt that the first priority was to establish whether or not participation in the course assisted the teachers to acquire the skills of structured teaching and, given this, whether there was any detectable increase in the complexity of the children's language. It is necessary for the purposes of the course to have a short series of video-taped preparatory sessions where the teacher is working with an individual child, both before and after the course. Hence, the setting for an evaluation of pre- and post-course performance arises naturally from the teachers' involvement with the course.

While every attempt was made to present the pre- and post-course sessions to teachers and children in an identical manner with identical instructions it is, of course, possible that they are viewed differently by the teachers and hence, that pre-post differences relate to what they think is required of them rather than to techniques and skills acquired on the course. Instructions were couched in a deliberately general form, inviting teachers to teach a short, 10 minute maximum, lesson concentrating on the child's use of language. They were similarly invited to write down an objective for the lesson. It is possible to argue that a more constrained set of instructions, effectively inviting teachers to perform in a structured manner would have been more appropriate. However, pilot work indicated problems in framing generally understandable instructions along these lines and, on balance, it appeared advisable to retain the general instructions.

The restriction of analysis to the video-taped sessions does raise serious questions as to the generalisability of the teachers' and children's behaviour. It is freely admitted that simply because teachers can use the techniques for ten minutes when they are videotaped there is no guarantee that they will use them outside these sessions. Similarly, just because the child can use more complex language when interacting with the teacher in this somewhat artificial one-to-one situation, there is no guarantee that this more complex language will transfer to other settings or with other people. An extension to the project enabled some purchase to be gained on these issues through the follow-up trials discussed below.

C. The Follow-up Studies

The follow-up studies concentrated on two main areas.

i) Evaluation of the effectiveness of the 'Minicourse' material in its 'operational revision' form when used with minimal involvement by the Project team (the 'Distance' trials).

ii) Evaluation of the effectiveness of the course in modifying the teachers' approach and the child's use of language outside the specific test sessions (the 'Near' trials).

The 'Minicourse' model envisages the course package, when developed, as used in a self-instructional form and run by a 'co-ordinator' who has a primarily organisational role. The trials in the first phase which were fully evaluated were run directly by the research team. In the follow-up study, a set of 'distance trials' were run using the final 'operational revision' of the material. These trials were run by local personnel with the minimum of involvement of the research team.

The first priority in Phase One of the project was to attempt to demonstrate changes in the way in which teachers dealt with short structured sessions with individual children. These were usually specially timetabled and took place in any convenient small room in the school, e.g. where the video equipment is located. This was not usually the room where the teacher did most of her teaching, although schools are asked wherever possible to use rooms where the children are used to having teaching sessions. Following the microteaching model, it was seen as necessary for a teacher to gain practice in the use of the structured skills and techniques in the somewhat simplified situation if she is to incorporate them into her teaching repertoire.

However, there is no guarantee that this incorporation will happen, even though the coure stresses the importance of this and other forms of transfer or generalisation. In the follow-up study, some general aspects of the pre- and post-course teaching and other activities of a sub-group of those teachers were monitored. Particular attention was given to the extent to which the teacher made use of individual and small group structured sessions. Such observation also permitted the collection of samples of children's language pre- and post-course in the classroom and hence an assessment of the extent to which the increases in complexity of the children's language which have been demonstrated in the video-taped sessions generalise to other situations. For these purposes, it was clearly necessary for the project team to have a much greater degree of involvement with the schools and teachers taking part in the trials, than that minimal involvement for the 'distance' trials described above. These trials are referred to subsequently as the 'near' trials (indicating their geographical accessibility to the Project team. A member of the Project team acted as 'co-ordinator' for the minicourse and spent a minimum of three full days per week in the field trial school for effectively the whole of one term.

A detailed account of these trials is presented in Robson (1981c). The present account is limited to an analysis of tapes and transcripts of video-taped sessions to provide comparative data to that obtained in Phase 1. Data on classroom behaviour of teachers and children outside the video-taped sessions are presented in Storey (1982).

Inter-Observer Agreement

The same procedure as that used in Phase 1 was employed to obtain and assess inter-observer agreement. Table 6 shows the agreement obtained.

TABLE 6. INTER-OBSERVER AGREEMENT

	P_0	K
Sequence Boundary	0.945	0.820
Sequence Labelling	0.778	0.686
Teacher Utterance Labelling	0.867	0.726
Child LCI	0.953	0.927

P_0 = proportion of agreement

K = Cohen's Kappa Coefficient

Scores are means of 10 sessions

The figures compare reasonably well with those obtained in the first phase of the project and suggest that the categories continue to be used in an acceptably consistent manner. It should be noted that the coding of "Child Utterances which 'should' or 'should not' be Encouraged", which had the lowest degree of inter-observer agreement on the original project, has now been dropped - partly for this reason and partly as a component of a general attempt to simplify the coding procedure. Conversely 'utterance' coding was not carried out formally as this had appeared to be non-problematic with essentially perfect agreement.

Analysis of Transcripts and Video-Tapes

The analysis constituted a replication of that carried out in Phase 1. Table 7 compares the result obtained with the Phase 1 trials. They are based on 12 teachers (and 24 children) from 'Near' trials and 12 teachers (and 24 children) from 'Distance' trials.

The results of the analysis of pre- and post-course video-tapes and associated transcripts arising from the follow-up project replicate and hence corroborate the findings of Phase One of the project. In each of the trials, i.e., the Phase One trails, the 'near' trials and the 'distance' trials of the follow-up project, the changes are significant statistically and in the expected direction.

A comparison of the performance on these variables for the 'near' and 'distance' trials shows that there is little difference between the trials, either in relation to the teachers' performance overall (i.e. their pre/post average) or in the gains they make from pre-course to post-course. In only one of the five variables is there an overall difference between 'near' and 'distance' trials. This occurs with 'encouragement' and is in the direction that teachers on the 'distance' trials make more use of encouragement than those on 'near' trials. This significant effect is associated with the average of pre- to post-course figures. The greater increase in encouragement from pre- to post-course by teachers on the 'distance' trials is not significant, although that for 'enthusiastic encouragement' taken separately does reach significance.

Similarly there is only one of the five variables in which the pre- to post-course gains differ between 'near' and 'distance' trials. This occurs in 'sequence total' where the slightly higher pre-course mean for teachers on the 'near' trials is changed to a noticeably lower post-course mean, the comparison being with the 'distance' trial in each case. There is a somewhat similar effect for structuring skills but this does not reach significance.

Table 7. **ANALYSIS OF KEY DEPENDENT VARIABLES - 'NEAR' AND 'DISTANCE' TRIALS COMPARED WITH 'PHASE ONE' TRIALS**

	'Near' Trials		'Distance' Trials		Phase One Trials	
	Mean Pre-Course Value	Mean Post-Course Value	Mean Pre-Course Value	Mean Post-Course Value	Mean Pre-Course Value	Mean Post-Course Value
Sequence Totals	66.9	19.3	63.2	28.[illegible]	67.6	22.9
Proportion of Sequences having Modal Target	0.120	0.550	0.150	0.522	0.097	0.578
Teachers' Initiating Structuring	14.6	38.9	13.9	29.[illegible]	11.5	33.8
Teachers' Use of Encouragement	9.55	17.14	10.22	22.60	12.68	18.69
MLR_T/MLR_C	2.73	1.75	3.38	2.[illegible]0	3.59	2.34
Child LCI	1.79	2.81	1.73	2.58	1.63	2.33

Taken overall, there is then little indication in the follow-up trials of a pattern of superiority for one type of trial over another in the teachers' use of structuring. There is a similar lack of consistent difference when comparisons are made between these trials and the Phase One trials.

There is a consistent increase in the length and complexity of child utterances (as indexed by the LCI score) from pre-course to post-course in each of the sets of trials. There is some suggestion that post-course the children on the 'near' trials achieve higher LCIs than those in the Phase One trials. These results refer to the child's language in the video-taped sessions; results from the classroom are presented in Storey (1982).

It should perhaps be added at this point that in contradistinction to the findings on the teachers' use of structuring and on the children's use of language, the teachers' evaluation of the course does show a quite consistent pattern of difference between the types of trial. Simply expressed, the finding is that the 'near' trials are given the highest ratings on a variey of indices, the 'Phase One' trials are given intermediate ratings, and the 'distance' trials are given the lowest ratings on the three.

The ratings in the case of the 'distance' trials can still be regarded as being acceptably high. In only one single case out of a multiplicity of ratings does the mean value fall below the '3' which is the centre-point of the scale. However, the differential between 'near' and 'distance' trials is in many cases considerable, e.g. for 'overall value' of course, the respective means are 4.92 and 3.94 on a 1-5 scale, and is particularly noteworthy when one bears in mind the fact that identical handbooks, manuals, instructional video-tapes and practical exercises were involved in each case.

D. Discussion of Findings

The results of the 'distance' trials, where local personnel carry out the minicourse for themselves in the absence of the research team, show that the material is effective in assisting teachers to develop the skills needed to run effective, short structured sessions. This is demonstrated by the analysis of the series of pre-course and post-course video-taped sessions. The results in this respect do not differ for these trials from the 'near' trials of the follow-up projects, where a member of the research team acted as coordinator and was present in the school for a large proportion of the time that the course was running. Hence one can conclude that the direct involvement of a member of the research team is not essential for the effectiveness of the material.

Similarly, there do not appear to be differences of substance between the teachers' use of the structuring techniques in these 'near' and 'distance' trials from the trials which made up Phase One of the project. These 'Phase One' trials were closer to the 'near' trials than to the 'distance' trials in that the project team fulfilled the coordinator's role but there was a considerably smaller amount of involvement with the teachers than took place in the 'near' trials. The 'Phase One' and 'follow-up' trials also employed slightly different versions of the mini-course materials. The differences in these two versions are minimal (see Robson 1981c: Appendix One). Their main thrust can be seen as towards maximising the acceptability of the materials, e.g. by cutting down on what was viewed by some teachers as unnecessary repetition. Obviously the simultaneous change in both degree of project staff involvement and nature of course material renders the separate assessment of their effects problematic but it would appear that neither of the two variables have discernible effects on the teacher's development of the structured teaching techniques.

The results of the follow-up trials also replicate the earlier trials in connection with the children's language in the video-taped pre- and post-course sessions; in all trials there is a significant increase in the length and complexity of the child utterances (as indexed by LCI). However, while there are no differences pre-course, in this case the post-course performance on the 'near' trials is significantly superior to that on the Phase One trials. In attempting to explain this, one cannot call on any differences in teacher performance of the structured skills as indexed by the video-tape pre- and post-course sessions since, as discussed above, the differences from one type of trial to another are minimal.

However there is one respect in which the trials

produce quite different results - the teachers' evaluations. 'Near' trials achieve consistently higher ratings than 'distance' trials with the Phase One trials occupying an intermediate position. It has been argued above that the most obvious dimension on which these trials differ is that of the degree of involvement of the project team - the greater the involvement the higher the rating.

Several factors may be suggested as mediating this relationship. If the project staff are closely involved with the teaching staff, it may be that the latter give an inappropriately high rating for the various aspects of the course because they do not wish to hurt the feelings of the project staff, or regard themselves as involved not only with the project but also with its successful outcome. It is difficult to disprove the possible existence of such effects but the strong impression gained, particularly in the near trials, was that the relationship in fact encouraged candour. Such candour, demonstrated for example by comments about internal workings of the school, is regarded as tending to the expression of truthful evaluations of the course.

It may be that the presence of the project team led to the teachers involved having a 'better' course, which then led to the higher ratings. Superficially this would appear unlikely as the course package is essentially a fixed entity. However there are various possible sources of difference. Variations in relation to the handbooks are unlikely. It is possible that the quality of the instructional video-tapes, as actually viewed on the different trials, could vary. Certainly some critical comments on Phase One trials had been traced to badly adjusted video-recorders and/or monitors which led to unacceptable degrees of picture break-up. As far as is known, however, this did not take place on the distance trials, no evidence for this coming from discussions with coordinators. The most likely difference concerns the video-taped practical sessions, with the further possibility of differences in the conditions under which teachers view their tapes of practical sessions in order to self-evaluate them.

Such possible differences appear to stem from the perceived greater importance of the minicourse when it is being run by a member of the project team.

Because of this greater importance, a priority could be given to minicourse activities which might otherwise have to take their chance amongst other school activities. This effect is in clearest focus for the video-taped practical sessions, as they have to take place at times when the children are available, usually involve the cooperation of another member of staff or the help of a teaching assistant, and often involve the use of a room which has different users at different times of the week. Given the establishment of priority and regular routine, the two ten-minute sessions per week need cause little problem. If the arrangements are ad hoc and need to be renegotiated each week, then this can be a source of considerable difficulty.

It could also be argued that the 'near' trial teacher has a 'better' course because of the extra input that the project team coordinator might provide by comparison with a local coordinator. Again, it is difficult to assess such possible effects. The agreed role of the project team coordinator was the normal one for a coordinator. As explained in the 'Coordinator's Handbook', the role is primarily organisational - to ensure that the various materials and equipment are available and that the activities making up the course are programmed and actually take place. The experience and close involvement by the project team coordinator in the development of the minicourse would suggest that he might be in a better position to implement this role than a coordinator who is involved for the first time.

In general terms, the project overall has achieved what it set out to do. A self-instructional package, firmly rooted in empirical research findings, has been shown to have quite marked effects on the teachers' ability to use skills and techniques featured in the package, with associated changes in the targeted children's language.

In designing and developing the package, several compromises had to be made, most noticeably between all that we would wish to include (and which others would wish us to include) and what could be reasonably included in a short course carried out over and above the teachers' normal responsibilities. Similarly there are strong tensions between the simplicity and clarity of a prescriptive approach for a self-instructional format and the need to preserve sufficient flexibility to deal appropriately with the idiosyncratic challenge provided by each individual child. The fact that the package has been well received by teachers augurs well for those teachers who have acquired new skills seeking to continue to use the structured approach. There are however clear deficiencies which are to some extent intrinsic to the format chosen for the course. Teachers would clearly like, and in some cases have obviously benefited from, the supplementation of the self-instructional course by specialist assistance and advice, particularly in relation to aspects of language.

The teachers' relative preference for the course when run by project staff (as in the 'near' trials) compared with the course run in the absence of the project staff (as in the 'distance' trials) is not mirrored by a corresponding difference in its effectiveness in developing structured teaching skills. However the highest possible evaluation of the course material is clearly desirable, if only in providing teachers with what they see as a more satisfying and useful experience. It is also reasonable to hypothesise that such high ratings would be linked to higher levels of use of structured teaching sessions.

It would appear that the key aspects of the contribution made by the project staff member as coordinator were his detailed knowledge of the minicourse and his availability and regular presence in the school. In this way, it is possible to ensure that the teachers involved are in a position to carry out the various activities making up the course and can seek reassurance about anything connected with the course. These observations suggest a model where trained coordinators work in a range of schools with this minicourse and similar packages. This type of peripatetic trainer, who would ideally be an experienced teacher with the personality and skills needed for working with adults, when armed with the appropriate training materials, would be a potent instrument for change and progress in the education of children with special needs.

The work of Project TASS, from which this chapter arises, has been funded by grants from the Department of Education and Science, London; this support is gratefully acknowledged.

Publications on the work of Project TASS

The main theme covered in this chapter is the relationship of teacher behaviour as videotaped prior to the course, to corresponding behaviours after the course. Other themes have been addressed elsewhere. Thus teachers' behaviour during the course is analysed and discussed in Jones and Robson (1983, 1985) and Jones (1981). The wider effects of the course, particularly effects in the classroom, are discussed in Storey (1982). More specifically linguistic issues are covered in Jones (1978), Jones and Robson (1979a, 1979b) and Robson (1984). General accounts of the work are available in summary form in Robson (1978, 1981a, 1981b), Robson and Barwick (1979) and in detail in two Project reports presented to DES (Robson, 1980a, 1981c). These include details about the teachers involved and about the children and the teachers' evaluation of the course. Particular research issues related to the work of the project are covered in papers on observation systems (Jones and Robson, 1977), evaluation techniques for in-service training (Tatum and Robson, 1977a), assessment of language (Tatum and Robson, 1977b) and methodology (Robson, 1984, 1985). Apart from work relating directly to the minicourse, staff and research students associated with Project TASS have been carrying out work on the curriculum for children with severe learning difficulties (Robson, 1980b; Freeman, 1983; Robson and Freeman, 1985; Carden, 1983; Carden and Robson, 1985) and on the use of the microcomputer as a curriculum and recording aid when using structured teaching and an objectives-based curriculum (Robson and Mushin, 1985). Current work being carried out by students working in related areas includes the modification of Crystal's LARSP technique (Crystal, Fletcher and Garman, 1976) for use with children with severe learning difficulties and the piloting and assessment of microcomputer-controlled interactive video systems in developing community living skills.

References

Borg, W. R., Kelly, M. L., Langer, P. and Gall, M.D. (1970) The Minicourse: A Microteaching Approach to Teacher Education, Collier Macmillan, London

Campbell, D. T. and Stanley, J. C. (1963) Experimental and Quasi-Experimental Designs for Research,

Rand McNally, Basingstoke

Carden, N. (1983) An Assessment Procedure for Use in Planning Programmes to Develop Cognitive Skills in ESN(S) Children, M. Phil. Thesis, Huddersfield Polytechnic

Carden, N. and Robson, C. (1985) 'A Survey of Curriculum Aims and Context for Children with Severe Learning Difficulties', Special Education: Forward Trends, British Journal of Special Education (in press)

Clarke, A. M. and Clarke, A. D. B. (1974) Mental Deficiency: The Changing Outlook. 3rd Edition Methuen, London

Clarke, A. M. and Clarke, A. D. B. (1975) Recent Advances in the Study of Subnormality, National Association for Mental Health, London

Cook, T. D. and Campbell, D. T. (1979) Quasi-Experimentation: Design and Analysis Issues for Field Settings, Rand McNally, Basingstoke

Crystal, D., Fletcher, P. and Garman, M. (1976) The Grammatical Analysis of Language Disability, Edward Arnold, London

Fenn, G. (1976) 'Against Verbal Enrichment' in P. B. Berry (ed.), Language and Communication in the Mentally Handicapped, Edward Arnold, London

Freeman, A. (1983) Curriculum Aims and Objectives for Use with Mentally Handicapped Children, M. Phil. Thesis, Huddersfield Polytechnic

Jeffree, D., and McConkey, R. (1976) Let Me Speak, Souvenir Press, London

Jones, A. A. (1978) 'Project TASS: Language Assessment in Three Contexts' in J. Inman (ed.), Aspects of Curriculum Development: Teaching Language to Handicapped Children, Westhill College, Birmingham

Jones, A. (1981) Teachers of Severely Subnormal Children: Their Behaviour during Microteaching Sessions in a Self-Instructional Minicourse, M. Phil. Thesis (CNAA), Huddersfield Polytechnic

Jones, A. A. and Robson, C. (1977) Observation Systems: Problems and Procedures (with Special Reference to Observation in the ESN(S) School), Project TASS Research Paper No 2

Jones, A. and Robson, C. (1979a) 'Language Training the Severely Mentally Handicapped' in N. R. Ellis (ed.), Handbook of Mental Deficiency Research : Second Edition, Laurence Erlbaum Associates, New Jersey

Jones, A. A. and Robson, C. (1979b) 'Do We Ask the Right Questions?', Special Education: Forward Trends, British Journal of Special Education, 6, 11-13

Jones, A. A. and Robson, C. (1983) 'Within-course Effects of a Training Package for Teachers of the Severely Mentally Handicapped', Special Education: Forward Trends (Research Supplement), British Journal of Special Education, 10, 17-20

Jones, A. A. and Robson, C. (1985) 'Effects of Discrimination Training and Self-Evaluative Feedback in a Minicourse for Teachers of Mentally Handicapped Children, Programmed Learning and Educational Technology, 22, 49-56

Leeming, K., Swann, W., Coupe, J. and Mittler, P. (1979) Teaching Language and Communication to the Mentally Handicapped, School's Council Project of Education of Severely Educationally Subnormal Pupils, Evans/Methuen Education, London

Perrott, E., Applebee, A. N., Heap, B. and Watson, E. P. (1975) 'Changes in Teaching Behaviour after Completing a Self-Instructional Microteaching Course', Programmed Learning and Educational Technology, 12, 348-362

Robson, C. (1978) 'A Self-Instructional Course on Language Development Through Structured Teaching' in J. Inman (ed.), Aspects of Curriculum Development: Teaching Language to Handicapped Children, Westhill College, Birmingham

Robson, C. (1980a) Project TASS - Phase One. Final Report to DES. Huddersfield Polytechnic

Robson, C. (1980b) 'Evaluation of Curriculum for the

Severely Mentally Handicapped' in B. N. Crawford (ed.), Curriculum Planning for the ESN(S) Child, BIMH, Kidderminster

Robson, C (1981a) 'A Minicourse in Structured Teaching', Special Education: Forward Trends: British Journal of Special Education, 8, 26-27

Robson, C. (1981b) 'Developing Structured Teaching Skills', Teaching and Training, 19, 23-26

Robson, C. (1981c) Project TASS - Follow-up. Final Report to DES, Huddersfield Polytechnic

Robson, C. (1984) 'Issues in the Development of Language Intervention Programmes', Journal of Mental Deficiency Research, 28, 89-100

Robson, C (1985) 'Small N: Case Studies', in P. Evans and S. Hegarty, (eds.), Evaluation Methodology in Special Education, NFER Nelson, Windsor

Robson, C. and Barwick, D. (1979) 'Developing Structured Teaching Skills', Learning, 1, 43-45

Robson, C. and Freeman, A. (1985) 'Teachers' Views on the Relative Importance of Different Curriculum Areas for Children with Severe Learning Difficulties', Research in Education, (in press)

Robson, C., Jones, A. and Storey, M. (1982) Language Development through Structured Teaching, A Minicourse for Teachers of the Mentally Handicapped, Drake Educational Associates, Cardiff

Robson, C. and Mushin, D. (1985) C.A.R.A. (The Curriculum and Recording Aid), Teachers' Handbook and Program Disks, Huddersfield Polytechnic

Simonton, D. K. (1977) 'Cross-Sectional Time-Series Experiments: Some Suggested Statistical Analyses', Psychological Bulletin, 84, 489-502

Storey, M. (1982) An Investigation of Factors Affecting the Implementation of a Structured Teaching Approach in Several ESN(S) Schools, M. Phil. Thesis, Huddersfield Polytechnic

Tatum, S. and Robson, C. (1977a) Research Methodology: An Appraisal of Evaluation Techniques for an In-Service Teacher Training Course, Project TASS - Research Paper No 3, Huddersfield Polytechnic

Tatum, S. and Robson, C. (1977b) Assessment of Language in Evaluation Studies, Project TASS - Research Paper No 4, Huddersfield Polytechnic

Thomas, B., Gaskin, S. and Herriot, P. (1973) Jim's People, Hart-Davis Educational, London

Winer, B. J. (1971) Statistical Principles in Experimental Design, 2nd Edition, McGraw Hill, New York

Chapter Six

EVALUATING THE IMPACT OF TRAINING, SUPERVISOR FEEDBACK, SELF-MONITORING AND COLLABORATIVE GOAL SETTING ON STAFF AND CLIENT BEHAVIOUR

Alan A. Jones, Roger Blunden, Enid Coles, Gerry Evans and Jan Porterfield

1. INTRODUCTION

In the late nineteen-sixties and early seventies, training for staff responsible for mentally handicapped clients underwent a revolution, first in content and then in form. Part of the impetus for these changes came from the recognition that since front line staff such as nurses, and other care staff, and families, rather than professionals such as psychologists or psychiatrists, spent most time with clients, they had the greater potential as agents for producing change in their clients (Ayllon and Wright, 1972). Added to this was an impetus from the discovery of an effective technology for producing such changes. Professionals working with mentally handicapped people demonstrated repeatedly that the use of behaviour modification techniques could produce improvements in a wide range of existing client behaviours and develop new repertoires (J. Gardner, 1971; W. Gardner, 1971). Thus the revolution in content was the introduction of behaviour modification as a topic in the training of care staff; the revolution in form was the application of behavioural techniques not only to the training of clients but to the training of staff as well.

Surprisingly, the logic of this strategy was not seen immediately. Kazdin (1973) noted that most of the problems involved in teaching new skills to handicapped clients were also encountered in training staff in new practices, yet while behavioural approaches were widely employed for changing client behaviour, staff training still relied mostly on methods such as lectures and reading assignments designed to transmit knowledge rather than to provide skills in particular techniques. He concluded "if we believe that principles and techniques of behavior modication are well suited to behavior change, this applies to staff as well as client behaviors". (Kazdin, 1973, p.135). In the decade since Kazdin's paper, a great deal of work has been carried out which demonstrates the efficacy of behavioural techniques in changing staff behaviour. Anderson (this volume) provides a comprehensive review of research findings, and so no attempt will be made to summarise them in this chapter. However, one trend which is discernible in this research is an increased emphasis on what might be termed "management" as opposed to "training" strategies.

Various writers have conceptualised this distinction in their own individual fashion, but the basic difference is that "training" consists of changing staff behaviour through describing and demonstrating particular techniques, (usually intensively and often away from the regular workplace) whereas "management" involves some modification of the working environment so as to change behaviour through cues (stimulus control) or feedback or reward (reinforcement control) or a combination of these. Miller and Lewin (1980, pp.296-297) conceptualised "training" as, in part, "...the teaching of behaviors not presently in the aide's repertoire, through modeling and instructions, rules, or guidelines...while...management is concerned with the increase and maintenance of behaviors presently in the aide's repertoire".

Kushlick (1975) distinguished between issues of staff training and staff management in a particularly striking way: "The question is... 'if the life of the person who should carry out the performance were at stake, could he or she succeed in doing it?' If the answer to this question is yes, the problem is not one of lack of skills and the answer does not lie in a training programme." Instead, he suggested the use of various types of "job aid" - a term which covers detailed job descriptions (which Miller and Lewin include, as "rules and guidelines", in their list of "training" methods), revised rotas and timetables, etc. - in other words, changes in the organisation of the service which encourage staff to use skills they already possess by reminding them to do so, by reminding them **how** to do so, and by removing constraints on them doing so. Bruininks, Kudla, Wieck and Hauber (1981, p.127) advocate such approaches on the grounds of economy and efficiency: "Training activities may be conducted...out of sheer desperation to 'do something' in response to staff needs. Such an approach can severely drain resources...and often be unresponsive to staff needs. Modifying job functions through environmental changes can often alleviate job problems at far less cost than expensive short-term training programs for staff members who typically remain in their positions for relatively short periods."

Such opinions were, in part, a response to evidence that the typical staff training programme, which was held away from the regular workplace, often had little effect on staff-client interactions back on the ward unless supplemented by some modification of the working environment of the kind suggested above. Three research studies on this issue (Panyan, Boozer and Morris, 1970; Welsch, Ludwig, Radiker and Krapfl, 1973; Fielding, Erickson and Bettin, 1971) provide typical illustrations of the types of staff behaviours tackled, methods used to control them and the results obtained.

In the study by Panyan et al. (1970), each of the staff of eleven living units in a mental handicap institution received a four-week course in operant conditioning. Upon their return to the wards, a system of feedback on their performance was introduced to the wards, in a multiple-baseline across settings. The researchers calculated, from staff records, the percentage of possible training sessions which staff had actually carried out, and in the feedback condition, gave staff a weekly summary of these percentages. This feedback appeared to be effective in maintaining a high percentage of training sessions. In one ward, where the condition was introduced immediately after training, the percentage of sessions was maintained at a high level (between 69 per cent and 100 per cent) for 34 weeks. In each of the three other wards for which Panyan et al. presented data, the percentage of sessions conducted was initially high but declined during the course of baseline (e.g. from 63 per cent - 20 per cent in a four week baseline, from 79 per cent in the fifth week of baseline to 8 per cent in the 34th week of baseline). In each case the introduction of the feedback system brought about a marked improvement in performance.

Similar procedures were adopted by Welsch et al. (1973) on two wards of a state hospital for mentally handicapped people. In each case, staff had previously been trained in the use of behaviour modification and were responsible for carrying out daily "behaviour modification projects" with the clients. In the first ward, performance decreased over the 42 days of baseline. 96 per cent of projects were completed in the first three days, but for the whole phase the average was 61.6 per cent. When the head of each shift was made responsible for recording the percentage completed on a publicly posted graph, the average increased to 97.9 per cent. On the second ward, each staff member was responsible for recording his or her completion of projects on a publicly posted chart. In baseline, 28.3 per cent of projects were completed on average when individuals were made responsible for charting completed sessions.

Fielding et al. (1971) found that, although they had trained staff to use methods of reinforcement to encourage mentally handicapped people to move around a ward independently, staff only used these techniques at the set times that "the project" was in operation. At other times they resorted to the methods of pulling and carrying clients which they had originally employed. The researchers then put up a satirical poster, with a caption, depicting a resident being towed by a breakdown truck. During the following four weeks, the use of these inappropriate methods of moving clients was completely discontinued.

These and similar experiments demonstrated the "restorative" effects of management techniques: in each case staff had acquired skills through training but their use of them was inconsistent or decreasing. However, another set of studies suggests that such manipulations of conditions of the workplace may be essential to the introduction of new work practices, because skills taught elsewhere may not be transferred to the work setting even immediately after training unless some management intervention is made. A study by Quilitch (1975) suggests that they may be a prerequisite of change. He compared the effectiveness of memoranda to staff, training workshops and feedback to staff on client's behaviour. The staff behaviour of concern was running scheduled leisure sessions for mentally handicapped residents of an institution. Unfortunately, Quilitch only measured the number of clients participating in these activities and did not take any direct measures of staff behaviour, so his results are only suggestive of changes in staff practice. However, in a multiple baseline across settings, he showed that substantial change only occurred after the introduction of feedback. Matlock and Adams (1978) studied the nature of staff-client interactions, in one "cottage" of a mental handicap institution with particular regard to the appropriateness of the assistance and reinforcement which staff gave to clients. Although all staff had been trained, in a classroom setting, to use behaviour modification techniques, in baseline they used cues and reinforcement correctly in only 12 per cent of the observation intervals. Staff were not given any further training, but "management" interventions were employed, consisting of grouping clients together according to their ability and providing feedback to staff on their level of appropriate interaction. Grouping residents alone led to an increase in appropriate interaction to 29 per cent of observations. Feedback to staff increased this effect, raising the level of appropriate interaction by about 10-15 per cent.

These studies have concerned themselves with very specific topics of management and their effect upon staff-client interactions. However, at the same time, researchers working with a very different theoretical orientation were suggesting that more general day-to-day management practices in residential settings for mentally handicapped people might have a significant impact on the development of clients (King, Raynes and Tizard, 1971; Raynes, Pratt and Roses, 1979). Descriptive studies of institutions for mentally handicapped children and adults in Britain and the USA, (Morris, 1969; Blatt, 1967) and the accounts of poor practice which emerged from government enquiries (e.g. D.H.S.S., 1969) had drawn attention to the often appalling conditions in such places. Raynes and her colleagues attempted to discover the determinants of the quality of care provided in different settings, using concepts derived from sociological accounts of the detrimental effects of psychiatric hospitals on long-stay patients (e.g. Goffman, 1961). They identified care staff behaviour and styles of speech which appeared broadly to be geared to the smooth running of institutional routines or to the acceptance of clients as individuals and valued people. They examined the relationship of these variables to others such as number of residents in each "living unit" (ward, villa, etc), quality of the physical environment, residents' skill level, care staff characteristics, and size and administrative structure of the setting. Studies took place in hospitals for mentally handicapped and physically ill children in Britain (King et al., 1971); large institutions for mentally handicapped adults in the USA (Raynes et al., 1979), "group homes" serving 8-12 mentally handicapped adults in Canada (Pratt, Luszcz and Brown, 1980) and small hospital units in Britain (Hemming, Lavender and Pill, 1981).

Naturally enough, there has been considerable variation in the results reported in the various studies and a brief account inevitably oversimplifies the issues. A particularly significant finding, however, is that the mere size of the setting (large hospital versus smaller unit) does not have the major influence on the style of staff-resident interactions which simplistic accounts of institutionalisation suggested.

Institution-oriented practices were on the whole far more prevalent in very large hospitals, less so in smaller ones, and least common in smaller units. However, within similar **types** of service (e.g. across the range of hospitals considered "very large") the actual size of the setting was not related to the approach to client care (McCormick, Balla and Zigler, 1975; Pratt et al, 1982). The variables most closely associated with positively-valued staff-client interactions were more closely related to the day-to-day running of the living unit: they were factors such as direct-care staff feeling that their role was flexible and that they played a part in decision-making in the unit (Raynes et al., 1979).

Raynes et al. singled out the role of the supervisor as a particularly important one. For example direct care staff who had responsibility for organising their workload and the activities of their clients were by and large those whose interactions with clients were positive: but these practices were also influenced by the behaviour of their immediate supervisors. Although the correlational analysis of Raynes et al. could not indicate the direction of any causal influence, it was observed that where "building heads" were more actively involved with the residents, the direct-care staff felt their role was more flexible;

in turn, this was related to a better quality of verbal interactions between staff and clients. More generally, insofar as the supervisor actually has some responsibility for organising staff and resident activities, then he or she is in a position to delegate this responsibility, thereby creating this valuable flexibility for front-line staff. However, this naturally depends on the administrative structure of the service and the amount of authority actually invested in the supervisor. Without a degree of influence by the supervisor over services provided by departments outside the living unit (e.g. meals, laundry, education), opportunities for involving direct-care staff in the management of the residents' day are considerably reduced.

At first sight, the two lines of research on the "management" of good practice in mental handicap services seem quite distinct. One considers very specific issues, suggesting that certain behaviours of direct care staff can be changed when other professionals clearly specify what is to be done, and when cues to carry out such tasks are introduced or feedback on this performance is provided (often from the care staff's immediate supervisors). The other suggests that various types of positive interaction with clients are related to, and probably result from, a sense of flexibility, responsibility and involvement by care staff and their supervisors. However, it seems possible to draw upon both lines of research to produce a strategy for developing staff practices in directions favourable to clients, which takes into account the specificity of the first approach and the more generalised effects of organisational climate. Such a strategy would require collaboration by "change agents" and the supervisors and direct care staff of the setting in defining improvements desirable in the service and designing interventions to achieve these. While the intervention might well be of the specific job-aid/feedback type, the involvement of the staff directly responsible for carrying out new practices might be expected to provide not only greater commitment to the specific intervention but also more generalised changes in the running of the service.

This chapter describes a number of studies carried out by the Mental Handicap in Wales - Applied Research Unit which have attempted to address these issues. In each one the aim of the intervention was to increase client behaviours regarded as desirable by manipulating the cues and feedback available to staff. Although some training took place, it was not of the same intensity as that often provided for staff of mental handicap services (e.g. Milne, 1982). Instead, the emphasis was on manipulating "management" conditions (in the sense used by Kushlick, 1975, and Bruininks et al., 1981, rather than by Miller and Lewin, 1980). Experimental interventions consisted of providing staff with written guidelines to new procedures and various types of feedback on their performance. In each of the studies, a collaborative approach as outlined above was adopted to some degree although it was not possible to manipulate this aspect experimentally.

The first of the studies took place in a day setting for severely handicapped adults, and attempted to increase clients' participation in activities by defining more clearly the role of staff supervising them and providing them with feedback on the extent to which they fulfilled this role. The next study consisted of a replication of this work in a hospital setting, and the third was an elaboration of this whereby a system of feedback more in keeping with the hospital management hierarchy was introduced to ensure maintenance of the procedures. The fourth study also took place in a hospital setting. It attempted to change staff practices so as to allow residents more independence in self-care and domestic routines, through training carried out by charge staff and a recording system intended to allow staff to provide themselves with feedback on their own performance. The final piece of work was concerned with improving particular aspects of a residential service selected for alteration by a meeting of clients' families, staff, and researchers. The interventions, in the form of procedural guides and supervisor feedback, were thus to a large extent determined by those responsible for carrying them out.

Although these studies have several themes in common, the interventions were geared to particular problems of the different settings. consequently, it was not possible to undertake a thorough evaluation of particular approaches to staff training and management. However, we hope, by examination of the elements common to these studies and the relative success of the various interventions, to draw an outline of a possible general strategy for staff training and management which could provide the basis for further advances in research and practice in this field.

2. ESTABLISHING ACTIVITY PERIODS IN A DAY SETTING FOR PROFOUNDLY HANDICAPPED ADULTS

2.1 Background

A repeated criticism of services for handicapped people is that both residential and day care services often provide their clients with very little stimulation or opportunity for purposeful activity (Cataldo and Risley, 1974; Quilitch, 1975; Horner, 1980). Such "impoverished" environments are damaging to clients in at least two important ways. Firstly, they deny clients the opportunity to use their existing skills, or to consolidate newly acquired behaviours through practice (Hart and Risley, 1976). Secondly, research suggests that unstimulating environments are associated with higher rates of self-injurious behaviour (Iwata, Dorsey, Slifer, Bauman and Richman, 1982).

It is frequently pointed out (e.g. Jones, Brown, Cunningham, Roberts and Williams, 1975) that low staff-client ratios contribute significantly to the poor quality of these environments, with available person-hours largely taken up with meeting the clients' basic physical needs. Educational activities may be limited further by a lack of available materials or by the practice of restricting clients' access to such materials for fear of loss or breakage of the materials or injury to the clients.

The project reported here (Porterfield, Blunden and Blewitt, 1980) was concerned with developing staff procedures for increasing clients' participation in activities, which would not require extra staff or new materials. It was also considered important that these procedures should be easy to incorporate into the daily routine of the setting concerned and that they could easily be maintained by the head of the setting.

2.2 Setting and Participants

The study was carried out at a purpose built Special Needs Day Unit in South Wales designed for the provision of day care and training for 20 adults considered too severely handicapped to attend the local Adult Training Centre. At the time of the study, the staff responsible for the care of clients comprised a Unit manager and a deputy manager, four care instructors and two care assistants, all of whom were women. Eighteen clients attended the Unit and each was allocated to one of two groups. These groups occupied separate rooms in the Unit for most of the day.

The group consisted of eight clients (five women and three men) whose ages ranged from 17 to 26 years. Their abilities were assessed using the Social and Physical Incapacity Scale and the Speech, Self Help and Literacy Scale (Kushlick, Blunden and Cox, 1973). One of the clients was non-ambulant and four presented severe behaviour problems to the staff. Five were unable to speak, read, write or count and had very few self-help skills. Two trainees were regarded as incontinent despite frequent toilet training sessions which had reduced the occurrence of such problems. Four of the clients had been assessed by the manager of the Special Needs Unit as too severely handicapped to benefit from attendance.

The staff participants in this study were the two care instructors normally responsible for this client group and the head of the Unit. One of the care instructors had no professional training, but had been a teacher in a mental handicap hospital school for 11 years prior to coming to the Special Needs Unit just before the study began. The other was a qualified Nursery Nurse and had worked with mentally handicapped children for eight years before joining the unit staff three months before the start of the study. The Unit head had been trained as an occupational therapist and had worked with mentally handicapped people for 16 years. She had been manager of the unit for 18 months when the study began.

2.3 Intervention

Preliminary observations suggested a number of aspects of the Unit's running which might be changed in order to achieve the goal of increase client participation in activities and reduced behaviour disturbances. Following work by Ayllon, Layman and Kandel (1975) and Ayllon and Roberts (1974), it was considered that distruptive behaviour might be reduced by providing positive contingencies for purposeful activity. Clients' engagement in such activities appeared to be limited by a number of factors independent of their handicap. Firstly, materials with which they might occupy themselves were not always readily available. Secondly, staff attention was frequently (although not exclusively) contingent upon disruptive behaviour, and conversely clients received little attention from staff when they were occupying themselves. Thirdly, having to attend to clients' disruptive behaviour or incontinence was not the only interruption faced by staff. They were often called to carry out duties elsewhere in the unit, or had other staff visit the room to discuss something or to join in the activities. Therefore it was decided that an appropriate intervention would be one aimed at making materials easily accessible to clients; at encouraging clients to use them; at making staff attention contingent upon appropriate rather than inappropriate behaviour; and at maintaining sufficient staff in the room to apply these procedures consistently. Also, in view of the literature on the importance of feedback to direct care staff, it seemed necessary to incorporate in the intervention some sort of constructive feedback from the Unit head to staff on their performance of new routines. Staff were therefore trained in a new routine known as the "room manager procedures"; and the Unit head was trained to use a feedback system known as "positive monitoring".

Room manager procedures

In following the room manager procedures, the two care instructors were required to alternate as "room manager" for two half-hour periods. During this time (the "activity period") seven key performances, designed to increase clients' participation, were required of the room manager:

a) giving each client a choice of recreational or educational materials to work with (e.g. jigsaws, plasticine, building bricks);

b) briefly prompting clients who did not independently begin using these materials;

c) placing other materials within each client's reach;

d) talking to clients who were using materials or

who were interacting with other people;

e) praising clients who had completed a task;

f) offering a choice of alternative materials when clients tired of the ones they were using;

g) dealing with disruptive behaviour.

The other care instructor was to work individually with three clients for about 10 minutes each, and was available in case of emergency.

Training

The room manager procedure was informally developed by researchers in collaboration with the staff during three pilot activity hours. Staff and researchers then reviewed and revised a written draft of the procedures which formed the basis of training.

The experimenter carried out five daily one-hour training sessions before the study. Training involved staff reading the written instructions, the experimenter describing the procedures and modelling them for staff, and practice with feedback. One care instructor would try the procedure with the clients while the other observed, recording her performance on a training checklist which listed important components of the procedure. This care instructor would give the trainee room manager verbal feedback on her performance and show her the completed checklist. The experimenter also gave feedback to the trainee room manager. From the first training session, both staff conducted the procedure correctly according to the checklist. (see Table 1)

Management

A management procedure termed "positive monitoring" was developed for use by the Unit head. The experimenter discussed this procedure with her and gave her written instructions on how to carry out positive monitoring. When the room management condition was in operation, the head was to observe each room manager for five minutes, once a week, using the portion of the training checklist designed for maintenance (asterisked in Table 1). She was then to give the room manager positive and constructive feedback on her performance. The head was required

ROOM MANAGER CHECKLIST **TABLE 1**

Carestaff: ....

Training: Observe all items.

No. 1 & 2 before the room manager takes over.
No. 3 immediately after she takes over.
No. 4–9 for 5 minutes.

1. After each trial give checklist to carestaff.
2. Once carestaff reaches criterion, file in her folder.

Monitoring: Covertly observe * items for 5 mins.

1. Give verbal feedback.
2. Post checklist for carestaff to initial.
3. File in her folder and re-use.

Score: , 0, or NA (not applicable) Criterion: , or NA for all items.

Did carestaff: Observer: Date:			
1. Tidy the room and make sure materials are convenient?			
2. Tell the previous room manager that she is ready to take over and tell trainees that she will help them now?			
3. Give each trainee a material or opportunity to be busy, i.e. game, song?			
4.* Place other materials within each trainee's reach, if appropriate?			
5.* Make at least 12 contacts to busy trainees? (tally each contact).			
6.* Comment approvingly about the trainees, activities?			
7.* Briefly prompt trainees who do not begin using materials or participating in activity?			
8.* Offer a choice of alternative materials or activity when trainees complete a task?			
9.* Stay in the room unless specifically relieved by another member of staff?			
Write comments on back: (Please date comment) Feedback received:			

to leave the checklist in a specified place so that the room manager could read through it carefully and sign to indicate that she had received feedback. Over and above the feedback provided by the checklist, the head was required to discuss in depth anything the room manager did particularly well, or any problems which arose. If problems had occurred, the head was to offer constructive criticism but only after she had commented on those things the room manager had done well. She was then to observe the room manager during the next day's activity period and repeat the positive monitoring procedure.

2.4 Experimental design

Two different procedures, "room management" and "no distraction" were compared. An ABCB reversal design was used, where the C condition required staff to follow written procedures based on their performance during the baseline phase. Baseline observations were made for three days. After an interval for training staff, the room management procedures were introduced for five days. For the next six days, the "no distraction" procedure was followed. The room management procedures were then reintroduced for five days. Follow-up observations were made at varying intervals in the following four months, during which time the room management procedures were being followed. All observation periods took place for an hour, between 2.30 and 3.30 pm on weekdays.

2.5 Experimental conditions

* Baseline

During baseline, staff were aware of the nature of the study, but no specific procedures had been discussed. They conducted activities of their choice within three curriculum areas - object perception, manual dexterity, and singing action songs - allowing 20 minutes for each area. There did not appear to be an established pattern for working with clients within this hour and the frequency and type of staff/client contact varied considerably throughout the hour. Staff were faced with many distractions during this time, such as being called upon to deal with incontinence or behavioural problems in other parts of the Unit, or to discuss something with the Unit head or her deputy.

Room Management

In the room management condition the two care instructors alternated as room manager, following the procedures described in the "interventions" section above.

No-distraction condition

The staff were not given any specific training for this condition, but they were provided with written instructions on the "no-distraction" procedures. These were a systematised version of some of the staff activities which had been observed before the introduction of room manager procedures. In particular, the different roles of room manager and individual helper were abandoned in this condition, clients did not have a range of materials within reach, but were provided with items one at a time by staff and attention was not given to clients who were engaged in activities. In order to make the change of procedures required by the reversal design more credible to staff, it was suggested in the written instructions that talking to busy clients might distract them, and so it would be avoided in this phase of the study (hence the name of the procedures).

The performances required of staff in this condition included:

a) giving each client one material which he or she enjoyed using;

b) prompting clients to start working;

c) leaving clients who were working with materials to continue undisturbed;

d) dealing with disruptive behaviour.

2.6 Measures

Risley and Cataldo's (1974) measure of client engagement, the Planned Activity Check (PLA-Check), was used as the dependent variable in this study. The measure defines clients as engaged if they are

- manipulating materials;

- looking at pictures, T.V., etc;

- looking at demonstrations or performances by staff, clients or others;
- communicating with staff or clients;
- helping other clients with activities;
- participating in group activities;
- following instructions;
- listening to staff talking;
- eating or drinking.

Further details are available in Porterfield et al. (1980).

Observations were made at one-minute intervals throughout the activity hour. At the beginning of each minute the observer counted the number of clients present and then the number who were engaged. Engagement was expressed as the percentage of clients present for the observation. This percentage disagreement was subtracted from 100 to give a percentage agreement figure. This procedure was repeated for each observation and a mean percentage agreement was then calculated for all sixty observations. Agreement on engagement for the study as a whole was 94 per cent (range 88-99 per cent).

Agreement on the number of clients present was calculated by dividing the number of observations in which primary and secondary observers agreed by the total number of observations and expressing this figure as a percentage. The average for the study as a whole was 99.5 per cent (range 96 per cent-100 per cent).

2.7 Results

Figure 1 shows the average percentage of clients engaged on each day observations were made. In baseline, the mean level of engagement was 31.2 per cent (range 25.7 per cent-37.9 per cent). With the introduction of the room manager procedures, engagement increased to a mean of 80.5 per cent (range 72.9 per cent-90.9 per cent). In the no-distraction (reversal) condition, it decreased to 31.7 per cent (range 21.5 per cent-48.0 per cent). When room manager procedures were reintroduced engagement increased to a mean of 85.7 per cent (range 84.7 per cent-88.1 per cent). Data from the follow-up period, during which the room manager procedures were continued for four months, show that engagement remained high, with a mean level of 82.8 per cent (range 71.5 per cent-91.1 per cent).

The only data on staff performance were those derived from the Unit head's checklists. These indicated that both room managers performed the procedures correctly on each occasion on which they were observed, both during the formal study and the subsequent follow-up.

2.8 Discussion

The results of this experiment suggest that the combination of training methods used - written and verbal instructions, modelling, practice and feedback - are an effective means of changing staff behaviour such that engaged behaviour by clients is encouraged and increased. Unfortunately the measures of staff behaviour used in this study were not as comprehensive as those on client behaviour, being collected only for five minutes per week on each room manager and with no inter-observer agreement checks. A further deficiency in the data is that they were collected only in the room management condition and so although they indicate that staff were implementing the room manager procedures correctly, they cannot indicate whether a true reversal took place. However, although it can be stated unequivocally that the relevant staff behaviours increased as a result of training, the drastic changes in the level of client engagement across conditions suggest that staff behaviour must have changed accordingly.

Although one of the purposes of this study was to assess the effect of the management contingencies (positive monitoring), the use of this procedure by the Unit head was not manipulated as an independent variable. If data on staff behaviour had been collected independently of the monitoring checklists, such a manipulation would have provided valuable information on the functional relationship between the management procedures and staff performance. Indeed, informal observation after the follow-up period suggested that problems in the delivery of positive monitoring led to a decline in the frequency

Figure 1. **Average percentage of trainees engaged during the Activity Hour.**

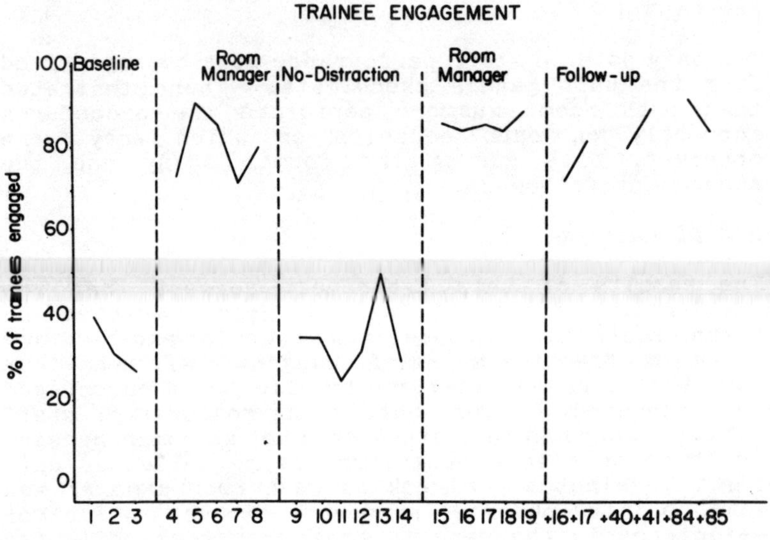

and quality of activity periods at the Special Needs Unit. A further indication of the contribution of the management procedures was the size of the reversal in the second room management condition. The change in clients' level of engagement from baseline to the first room management condition were a function of staff use of the new procedures which in turn seem most likely to be a result of the training staff received immediately before their introduction. No such training preceded the second room management phase and so it can be inferred that the management contingencies (i.e. verbal instructions to use the room manager procedures, coupled with positive monitoring by the Unit head) were the key variables responsible for the acceptable performance of staff during this phase.

3. THE INTRODUCTION OF ACTIVITY PERIODS TO A HOSPITAL WARD

3.1 Background

The work described in this section (Coles and Blunden, 1979, 1981) began as a replication in a hospital setting of the study just described. The initial invitation to carry out the research came from the hospital staff who were concerned with the problem behaviour of one resident. Subsequent observations showed that a number of residents of the ward in question presented a variety of inappropriate behaviours. Discussion between researchers and ward staff resulted in a decision to introduce "activity periods" (as described in the previous study) to increase group engagement in appropriate activities rather than only attempts to eliminate the problem behaviours. However, although introducing activity periods did lead to an increase in client engagement, follow-up observations showed that these improvements were not maintained. Consequently, a second study was undertaken in which a variety of staff management procedures for maintaining the activity periods were employed in addition to the training methods used in the preliminary study.

PRELIMINARY STUDY: TRAINING WARD STAFF TO RUN ACTIVITY PERIODS

3.2 Participants

The study involved 13 profoundly handicapped young

adults who lived in one part of a ward in a large mental handicap hospital (with a total of approximately 400 residents). Their ages ranged from 17 - 24 years. Staff assessed the clients using the SPI and SSI scales (Kushlick et al., 1973). Ten of the residents could not use spoken language as a means of communication; three were non-ambulant; six were incontinent and five were regarded as having severe behaviour problems. Inappropriate behaviours observed by researchers included stereotyped rocking, hitting or biting other residents or staff, eating faeces, tearing clothing and licking walls and windows.

3.3 Intervention

The intervention consisted of training staff in the procedures necessary to run activity periods. The room manager and individual helper procedures were first explained and demonstrated to the staff. This was followed by a period of practice, after which researchers gave staff feedback based on the training checklist, as used in the previous study. No specific management procedures were incorporated at this stage.

3.4 Experimental Design

A modified reversal design was used in this study. A six day baseline was to be followed by a week in which staff were trained in the room manager and individual helper procedures. For the next five days the staff were to revert to their previous routine, after which activity periods were to be reintroduced for a further five days. In practice, on the fourth day of the reversal phase, staff introduced new toys to the ward and encouraged residents to use them while the observations were taking place. Eight days' data were collected under these conditions, and then seven days' data during which staff reverted to following the specified roles of room manager and individual helper in a modified version of the original activity period procedures (see Figure 2).

Experimental Conditions

Baseline

No special activities were required of staff or residents in this condition. Residents usually stood

Figure 2

Experimental Design

Baseline No Activity Period	Activity Period Introduced	Reversal No Activity	New Toys Period	Modified Activity Period Introduced
1 2 3 4 5 6	7 8 9 10 11	12 13 14 15 16 17	18 19 20 21 22	23 24 25 26 27 28 29

or sat around the edge of their living area. Recreational or educational materials were not generally available.

Activity period

In this condition, a modified version of the room manager procedure as described in the previous study was to be implemented. The chief modification was that in this setting, the room manager was to ignore disruptive behaviour as far as possible.

Reversal

Conditions were the same as those of the first baseline phase.

New Toys

In this phase, staff introduced a number of new toys, colouring books, etc, to the ward. They also implemented the room manager procedures to an extent, but inconsistently. Tables were set out for some of the residents to work at. On some occasions staff gave a great deal of positive attention to residents who were engaged, but at other times they did not. Sometimes one staff member would move among the residents but at other times all the staff present would give individual attention to residents for periods of up to 20 minutes. Because of the inconsistency of staff behaviour in this phase, it did not constitute a return to the "activity period" conditions.

Modified activity period

In this phase, staff reverted to the specified roles of room manager and individual helper. The chief modification to the procedure was that staff tried out alternative seating arrangements to those specified in training, as they considered that more suitable ones could be found.

3.5 Measures

Baseline observations took place on weekdays between 9 and 10 a.m.; all subsequent observations took place on weekdays between 9.30 and 10.30 a.m. Each resident was observed in turn at fifteen-second intervals, and his or her behaviour at each instant of observation was classified as engaged, neutral or inappropriate. Definitions of engagement were similar to those used in the previous study. Inappropriate behaviour included activities such as screaming, aggression towards residents or staff, self-injury, smearing or eating faeces, etc. Any behaviour which was not assigned to these two categories was coded as neutral. Further details of the behaviour definitions may be found in Coles and Blunden (1979).

3.6 Inter-observer agreement

Inter-observer agreement was assessed on eleven of the twenty nine days of the study. Agreement was calculated as the number of intervals in which observers made the same coding, divided by the total number of observation intervals, expressed as a percentage. The mean level of agreement throughout the study was 85.4 per cent (range 77.2 per cent-89.4 per cent).

3.7 Results

Figure 3 shows for each phase of the study the percentage of observations in which residents' behaviour was classified as engaged, neutral, or inappropriate.

Engagement was very low in baseline (mean, 6.5 per cent, range 0-10.4 per cent). In the first activity period phase, engagement increased to a mean of 49.5 per cent (range 40.9 per cent-59.85 per cent). In the reversal phase, engagement fell to a mean of 8.3 per cent (range 2.7 per cent-13.2 per cent). The introduction of new materials led to an increase in engagement to a mean of 32.9 per cent (range 23.4 per cent-45.8 per cent). The reintroduction of the activity periods resulted in a further increase in the mean level of engagement to 49.9 per cent (range 34.0 per cent-58.5 per cent).

In appropriate behaviour showed corresponding changes, although the fluctuations were not so marked. In baseline the mean percentage of observations coded as inappropriate was 46.1 (range 37.0 per cent-54.1 per cent). In the first activity period phase, this fell to a mean of 29.3 per cent (range 21.8 per cent-35.8 per cent). In the reversal phase the mean level was 43.1 per cent (range 40.7 per cent-46.7 per cent). In the "new toys" phase, the mean was 29.8 per cent

(26.2 per cent-42.7 per cent) and in the second activity period phase the mean level of inappropriate behaviour was 31.6 per cent (range 24.6 per cent-37.4 per cent).

These results suggest that holding activity periods tends to reduce inappropriate behaviour slightly, and has a much more marked effect in increasing engagement and reducing the amount of time clients spend unoccupied. It is difficult to ascertain how much of this is due to the availability of materials in the activity period phases and how much to the behaviours of staff intended to encourage client engagement. The unexpected "new toys" phase of this study might have provided a control for this except that staff were also using some of the procedures from the activity periods in this phase. Overall, it could be argued that the availability of material was the crucial variable, since although no direct measures of staff behaviour were taken, staff were observed to be using the activity period procedures inconsistently in the original and modified phases of the study and carrying over some of the behaviours associated with activity periods into the supposed reversal phase when they introduced new toys.

In the first activity period phase, room managers found it difficult to move quickly from one resident to the next and would spend up to five minutes with an individual client. Thus the contact which residents received was not as frequent as planned. Also a larger proportion of staff contact was with residents who were not engaged. This contact ranged from the brief prompts specified in the procedures to shouted orders. Subsequent discussion revealed that staff had some misunderstanding about the performances required of them. This led to the minor modifications incorporated in the second activity period phase. However, in this phase several departures from the agreed procedures occurred. On some occasions, as planned, the room manager made frequent positive contacts with the engaged residents and the individual helper spent time working with individuals. At other times both staff members were seated with individual residents for long periods and it was not possible to discriminate between the two roles. On some occasions as planned, the room manager made frequent positive contacts with the engaged residents and the individual helper spent time working with individuals. At other times both staff members

Figure 3. Resident behaviour classified as engaged, neutral and inappropriate across phases of the study.

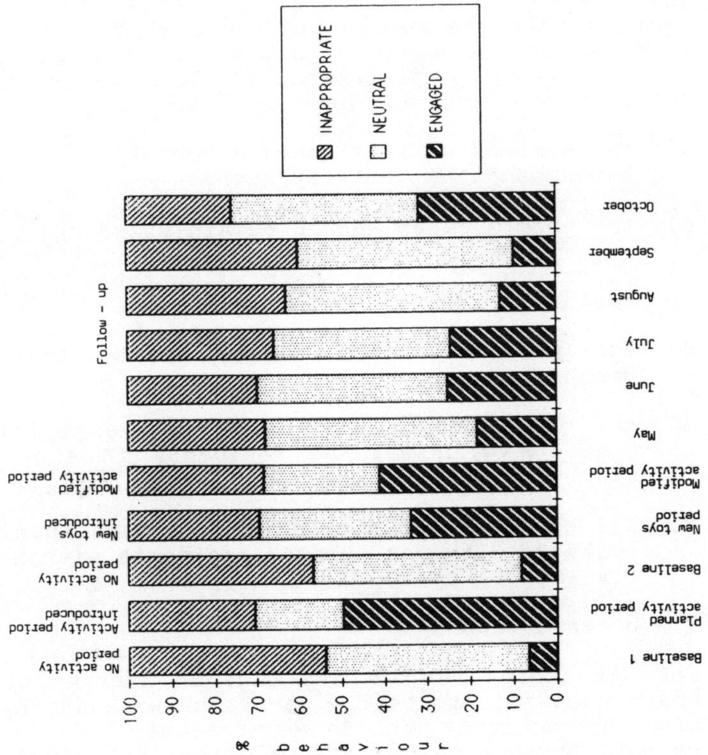

were seated with individual residents for long periods and it was not possible to discriminate between the two roles. On some occasions also, a large proportion of staff contact was with residents who were not engaged and was negative in tone rather than the brief prompts to use materials specified in the procedures.

FOLLOW-UP TO PRELIMINARY STUDY

3.8 Background

At this stage of the project, discussions were held between ward staff, senior nursing staff and the researchers concerning the results presented above. All parties agreed the activity periods had benefited the clients and that the staff should continue to run them. It was decided that the researchers should carry out a follow-up study to see whether the activity period procedures were maintained by staff and whether client engagement was maintained at a high level. Criteria by which maintenance of the activity periods should be assessed were agreed. These criteria were:-

a) two members of staff should normally be present throughout the activity hour;

b) the room manager should remain standing;

c) there should be a chair at a table for each resident;

d) each resident should have equipment within easy reach;

e) the room manager should make at least fifteen contacts with engaged residents in each five minute period;

f) the room manager should make no more than five contacts with non-engaged residents within each five-minute period.

3.9 Observations

For six months researchers made an average of two unannounced visits to the ward each week during the hour when activity periods were scheduled. On roughly half of these visits, data on client behaviour were collected for an hour as in the preliminary study.

On the other visits, a simple checklist was completed during a fifteen minute period. This provided information on the extent to which the criteria for activity periods were met and on the level of resident engagement. Inter-observer agreement for the behaviour classifications was assessed on two occasions, with 76.2 per cent and 93.7 per cent agreement. Agreement on the 15-minute checklist was assessed on four occasions. The mean level of agreement was 80.9 per cent (range 76.2 per cent-85.7 per cent)

3.10 Results

Figure 3 also shows the classification of residents' behaviour during the follow-up period. Engagement tended to be lower than in the activity periods and 'new toys' phases of the preliminary study (mean 19.1 per cent, range 3.6 per cent-46.9 per cent). Inappropriate behaviour was initially at a similar level to that in the second activity periods phase in the preliminary study, but it increased steadily during the third, fourth and fifth months of the study. The overall mean was 34.2 per cent (range 18.2 per cent-51.3 per cent).

Adequate implementation of the activity period procedures required that six items should be performed to criterion level. Staff did not achieve this on any of the twenty observation days of the follow-up period. The number of items carried out to criterion averaged 33 per cent (equivalent to two out of the six) and on no occasion was the criterion met for more than half the items.

The number of staff present varied greatly. On some occasions no staff were present in the activity area although this was only for brief periods and a member of staff was usually nearby. On one occasion 10 staff were observed in the activity period area at the same time. On most occasions one member of staff did remain standing for five minutes. There were usually insufficient chairs for all residents to be seated at a table. Criteria for materials within reach of residents and positive contacts to engaged residents were never met. However, on six days staff met the criterion for making less than five contacts with non-engaged residents.

3.11 Discussion

The results of the preliminary study indicated that training existing ward staff to run activity periods led to sizeable changes in the level of engagement of the profoundly handicapped residents in this setting. Before activity periods were introduced, very few client behaviours were classified as engaged. When staff were running activity periods, engagement increased considerably. The unplanned introduction of new toys to the ward provided a partial control for the availability of materials (which were not readily available during the two baseline phases): the fact that engagement was higher in the two activity period conditions suggests that staff procedures implemented in these two phases played an important part in raising the level of engagement over and above the availability of materials. Although in the preliminary study no formal data were collected on staff use of the room manager and individual helper procedures, engagement levels were highest when staff appeared to be adhering most closely to the procedures as specified during training.

The lack of adherence to the activity period procedures in the six month follow-up period was due to a number of factors. These included staff shortages; staff meetings being held during the hour when activity periods should have been held; and during spells of warm weather, residents being moved to an outside play area where activity periods did not take place.

The marked improvement in the clients' behaviour during the main study was sufficient for staff to wish to continue to carry out the activity periods. However, these improvements in the clients' behaviour did not appear to be sufficiently reinforcing to staff to maintain long term performance of the behaviours which brought them about. This finding is consistent with those of other researchers (e.g. Woods and Cullen, 1983). Consequently, further work was undertaken in order to develop management procedures for maintaining the improvement in client behaviour associated with the running of activity periods.

MANAGEMENT STUDY: A HIERARCHICAL FEEDBACK SYSTEM FOR LONG TERM MAINTENACE

3.12 Participants

The total package of interventions introduced in this study consisted of the following:-

Training Care Staff

Because all but one of the staff originally trained in the activity period procedures had now left the ward, the six staff now responsible for this group of residents were taught how to organise them. The same method of training was used here as in the preliminary study, except that, in addition to demonstrations by researchers and practice with feedback, staff were also prompted to contact residents appropriately during their periods of practice, and were given written descriptions of the procedures.

Training senior nursing staff in positive monitoring

The senior nursing staff associated with the ward (Nursing Officer and Senior Nursing Officer) were trained in the use of "positive monitoring". This training consisted of discussion with the researchers who also demonstrated the technique and provided the senior staff with written guidelines for carrying it out. In addition, the Nursing Officers observed positive monitoring being carried out at the Special Needs Unit described in section 2 of this chapter.

Training charge staff to collect data

The ward Charge Nurses and their deputies (two State Enrolled Nurses) were trained to collect behaviour classification data on the residents involved in the activity periods. A written description of the observation techniques was provided by the researchers who discussed it with the staff concerned.

3.13 A hierarchical system of reporting and feedback

A hierarchical system of reporting and feedback involving the ward charge staff, Nursing Officer, Senior Nursing Officer and Sector/Health Care Team was instituted. Written descriptions of the performances required by this system were drawn up by the researchers: these were circulated to all parties involved, and discussed with them by the researchers.

The various components of this monitoring system were introduced sequentially, but when it was fully operational the following procedures occurred. Each day charge staff calculated and graphed engagement levels during the activity hour and each week three copies of the graph were forwarded to the Nursing Officer along with a summary of the Behaviour Classification Data (engaged/neutral/inappropriate) for the week. Once a fortnight, the Nursing Officer made an unannounced visit to the ward at the time when the activity period was scheduled. He completed the monitoring checklist and then gave feedback to the staff on the basis of his observations. Each month, he sent to the Senior Nursing Officer a monthly data sheet, combining the Charge Nurses' weekly summaries and his own fortnightly observations, along with notes of any actions taken on the ward to ensure the correct implementation of the procedures. In addition, he forwarded two copies of the weekly engagement graphs to the Senior Nursing Officer as he received them from the Charge Nurse.

The Senior Nursing Officer was responsible for making an unannounced visit to the ward during the activity period, once each month, to complete the monitoring checklist and give the staff feedback. He then prepared a report which combined his own review of the activity period, based on his checklist observations, with the Nursing Officer's monthly report. This was forwarded to the Sector Health Care Team along with a copy of each of the four weekly engagement graphs. At their monthly meetings, the Sector Health Care Team gave their comments to the Senior Nursing Officer, and these were relayed to the ward staff themselves by the Nursing Officer. These arrangements are summarised in Table 2.

3.14 Experimental Design and Conditions

The study took the form of a seven-phase time-series design in which the various training and management procedures were deployed sequentially. The phases, their duration and conditions, were as follows:-

TABLE 2 REPORTING ARRANGEMENTS FOR MONITORING SYSTEM

PERSON MAKING REPORT	FREQUENCY	DAY	DUTY	PERSON RECEIVING
CHARGE NURSE	Weekly	Wednesday	Sends a) 3 copies of the Graph) b) Weekly Summary Sheet) TO	NURSING OFFICER
NURSING OFFICER	Weekly	Wednesday	Receives Graphs & Weekly Summary Sheet	
			Sends 2 Copies of Graph TO	Sen. NURSING OFFICER
	Fort-nightly	Beginning of Fortnight	Decides and Notes Random Date on Which Will Complete The Activity Period Checklist	
		Date	Completes The Activity Period checklist	
	Monthly	End of Month	Completes The Monthly Data Sheet	
			Sends The Monthly Data Sheet TO	Sen NURSING OFFICER
SENIOR NURSING OFFICER	Weekly	Thursday	Receives The Graphs	
		Beginning of Month	Decides & Notes The Random Date on Which Will Complete the Activity Period Checklist	
	Monthly	Date Decided	Completes The Monthly Checklist	
		End of Month	Receives Monthly Data Sheet	
			Gives Comments About Monthly Data Sheet TO	NURSING OFFICER
			Constructs A Monthly Report	
			Sends The Monthly Report & Graphs to	HEALTH CARE TEAM
HEALTH CARE	Monthly	Day of Meeting	Gives Comments about Activity Period to	Sen. NURSING OFFICER S. N. O.

Evaluating the Impact

1) First baseline (6 months)

This was the follow-up period to the preliminary study, when no maintenance procedures were in operation but when activity periods were supposed to be held.

2) Modified baseline (5 days)

In this phase, no maintenance procedures were in operation but staff were aware they would be introduced at a later time.

3) Stage 1 training (20 days)

Staff were trained in the activity period procedures by a researcher, to a criterion (for Room Manager) of ten contacts to engaged residents per five minutes. The charge staff assigned staff to the two roles. The monitoring procedures were used by the Nursing Officer and Senior Nursing Officer from this phase onwards through the study.

4) Stage 2 training (32 days)

The charge staff were trained by the researchers to use positive monitoring; staff were given feedback using a more stringent criterion (15 contacts to engaged residents per five minutes).

5) Daily monitoring (5 weeks)

Charge staff took over responsibility for positive monitoring from the researchers and carried this out first daily, then weekly; the researcher trained the charge staff to collect behaviour classification data.

6) Partial monitoring (6 weeks)

This was a transitional phase during which researchers withdrew their close involvement and the charge staff took complete responsibility for running and monitoring activity periods. Staff should have assumed this responsibility at the start of this phase: however, training staff in the activity period procedures took longer than expected as not all staff were trained to criterion by the end of phase 4. Charge Nurses took over responsibility for training them from the researchers. This led to delays in training charge staff in collecting behaviour classification data, which carried over from phase 5 into phase 6.

7) Weekly monitoring

In this phase charge staff were completely responsible for running and monitoring the activity periods.

Data were collected by a second observer on three days of phase 2, weekly in phases 3-5, on two days in phase 6 and on three days in phase 7. Inter-observer agreement for behaviour classification was calculated as in the preliminary study. The mean percentage agreement was 89.7, ranging from 81.5 per cent - 98.0 per cent. Agreement for the frequency of positive contacts was calculated for each minute, using the formula below:-

Total contacts recorded by 1st observer minus disagreements multiplied by 100 divided by total contacts recorded by 1st observer.

An average agreement figure was then calculated for each day. The average daily agreement was 77.1 per cent, ranging from 55.5 per cent - 90.2 per cent. There were some difficulties at first in agreeing on positive contacts: low agreement figures occurred on three of the 21 observation days.

3.15 Results

1) Resident behaviour

For the six months of the follow-up period of the preliminary study, which constituted the baseline of this study, the mean level of engagement was 19.1 per cent. In the four weeks of the modified baseline, when no management procedures were in operation but the nature of the study had been revealed to the staff, engagement rose to a mean of 41.2 per cent (and adherence to the activity periods procedures was generally greater). The training of staff, coupled with the management procedures implemented by the Nursing Officer and Senior Nursing Officer, was associated with an increase in the level of engagement to 61.6 per cent. The subsequent interventions did not lead to any further increase in the level of engagement but did appear to maintain it: the average level for phases 3-7 was 60.1 per cent, with a range

TABLE 3 RESIDENT BEHAVIOUR CLASSIFIED AS ENGAGED, NEUTRAL AND INAPPROPRIATE

PHASE	Engaged % Mean	Engaged % Range	Neutral % Mean	Neutral % Range	Inappropriate % Mean	Inappropriate % Range
I (First Base-line)	19.1	3.6-46.9	46.7	25.3-58.4	34.2	18.2-51.3
II (Modi-fied Base-line)	41.2	37.8-48.7	35.3	27.5-41.0	23.5	19.6-29.8
III (Stage I Train-ing)	61.6	43.4-75.7	21.5	14.0 28.6	16.9	10.3 30.3
IV (Stage II Train-ing)	59.3	47.7-75.2	24.7	8.4-38.0	16.0	5.5-26.4
V (Daily Moni-toring)	60.7	50.0-71.1	25.9	16.5-36.7	13.3	2.3-28.5
VI (Par-tial Moni-toring)	58.7	41.5-72.5	27.1	12.0-41.5	14.2	5.1-30.7
VIII (Week-ly Moni-toring 16 weeks)	60.3	47.3-73.3	19.5	10.3-30.3	20.2	10.4-33.6

of 41.5 per cent - 75.7 per cent. Full details are given in Table 3.

2) Staff behaviour

Table 4 shows the mean number of positive contacts per five minutes made to engaged clients by the room manager, from phase 3 onwards. The criterion in phase 3 was 10 contacts, and 15 thereafter. The table includes data from sessions when staff were being trained, which accounts for the figures being below criterion.

Unfortunately, these data were not collected during the modified baseline phase, and so it is not possible to ascertain the effect on this variable of staff being informed that procedures were to be introduced to produce better maintenance of the activity periods. The results which are available, though, indicate a gradual increase in the frequency of positive contacts, and in phase 7, when all staff had been trained to criterion, the average for the phase was above the criterion level. (See Table 4)

3.16 Discussion

A number of points deserve discussion. Firstly, there are several limitations to the design of this study. The chief dependent variable is that of client engagement: the rationale for this, as in the previous study, is that changes in staff behaviour must produce changes in client behaviour if they are to be justified. While this is a valid argument, there is little quantitative evidence that staff's use of the activity period procedures increased. Data taken during the six months' follow-up to the preliminary study showed generally low levels both of compliance with the procedures and client engagement. While the room manager and individual helper procedures include a large number of identifiable behaviours (six were specified in the checklist used in the six-month follow-up), in the management study data were only collected for one of these - the frequency of the room manager's contacts with engaged residents. Data collected for this variable during the post-baseline phase of the management study show that on average the frequency of such contacts was below the criterion set in all the phases except the final one: but these averages include data from sessions before staff had been trained to criterion.

TABLE 4

Mean number of room manager's contacts with engaged residents per five minutes.

Phase	Contacts
1. Baseline	4.0
2. Modified Baseline	not observed
3. Stage I training	7.7
4. Stage II training	10.4
5. Daily monitoring	14.4
6. Partial monitoring	13.2*
7. Weekly monitoring	16.0

*includes data from four days when neither staff member was trained.

In the light of these limitations, it is only an assumption that the changes in client behaviour are a result of increased use by staff of the specified procedures. However, within these limitations, the results of this study suggest that, given a comprehensive system of monitoring, it is possible to maintain new procedures which without such monitoring were not maintained by staff who had been trained in their use.

Because of the complexity of the monitoring system used, it did not seem feasible to carry out any experimental manipulations, such as reversals, to establish which aspects of the system contributed most to the improved level of engagement. Nor is it possible to separate the effect of training from the introduction of the monitoring by Nursing Officer and Senior Nursing Officer, since the two components of the intervention were introduced simultaneously. In the preliminary study, training resulted in a mean client engagement level of 49.5 per cent, an increase of 43 per cent, so it seems reasonable to attribute the increase in engagement from phase 2 to phase 3 of the management study to the effects of the training provided for staff. However, the training provided in the "management study" included some extra components not used in the preliminary work. In the earlier study, the procedures were first explained and demonstrated to the staff. This was then followed by a period of practice, after which the staff received feedback based upon a training checklist. In the management study, staff were trained using written procedures, modelling, prompts to contact residents appropriately, and by using positive monitoring checklists. It is quite possible that the additional components of training, especially the written descriptions of the procedures, played a large part in the improved maintenance of the activity periods. Or, to put it another way, it is quite possible that if staff had had written procedures to refer to in the preliminary study, maintenance during the six-month follow-up period would have been much greater. Although previous research on the effects of feedback leads one to predict that it would contribute to the effects observed in the "management study", its impact cannot be disentangled from that of the training, which in the later study was probably more efficient.

It is interesting to note that the transfer of responsibility for regular monitoring and feedback from the researcher to the charge nurses did not lead to any major changes in the dependent variables. It might have been surmised that positive feedback from the charge nurse would have been more reinforcing than feedback from the researcher, who occupied only a marginal place in the reward hierarchy of the hospital organisation. However, informal observations showed certain improvements in the running of the activity periods once the charge staff assumed responsibility for monitoring. Because of the increased amount of time they spent with the group of residents involved in the activity periods, the charge staff were able to point out to the care staff the progress made by individuals, and practices which were particularly effective for individual residents. This additional positive interaction between charge staff and care staff appeared to improve staff morale and the consistency with which staff interacted positively with individual residents.

Because of the various limitations of the two studies, their results can only be regarded as suggestive rather than conclusive. However, the implications are as follows:-

1) Staff can be trained through a combination of verbal instructions, modelling, and practice with feedback, to use activity period procedures which lead to an increase in purposeful activity on the part of their severely handicapped clients. The addition of written procedures to this training package may contribute to improved long-term maintenance.

2) In the absence of specified management procedures, the changes in staff's use of activity period procedures, and the associated improvement in client engagement, are likely to decline over time.

3) The introduction of a system of regular reports by charge staff on client behaviour, which are circulated to senior nursing staff for carrying out positive monitoring of the activity periods, appears to maintain the running of activity periods after training.

4) The responsibility for regular monitoring and training, initially taken by the research team, can be transferred to the ward's charge staff

without detriment either to staff's performance or the clients' level of engagement.

4. INTRODUCING A SYSTEM OF PROMPTS TO A HOSPITAL WARD

4.1 Background

The work described so far in this chaper has involved a combination of training and management procedures which appeared to be of varying effectiveness in different settings. In these studies, considerable emphasis was given to training as well as to management procedures. The research described in this section, however, was undertaken to establish whether a set of staff procedures could be introduced with a minimum amount of formal training but maintained through a management procedure which had been shown to be effective in other settings.

A number of studies have shown that when coupled with reminders of what staff performance should be, feedback alone is an adequate method of changing staff behaviour in the absence of any other form of behavioural control (such as training or monetary rewards). Examples are provided by Hutchinson, Jarman and Bailey (1980) where the behaviour of concern was attendance by professionals at weekly team meetings; Prue, Krapfl, Noah, Cannon and Maley (1980), where the behaviour of concern was keeping records of the implementation of training programmes in a psychiatric hospital; and Repp and Dietz (1979), where the target behaviour was the submission of progress reports on clients. Such management techniques have been shown to be effective not only on administrative behaviours but also on a number of different types of staff-client interactions, for example, conducting or completing training sessions (Kreitner, Reif and Morris, 1977; Welsch et al, 1973) or toileting residents (Greene, Willis, Levy and Bailey, 1978).

Whereas early studies of staff management techniques used feedback which was provided by researchers or supervisory staff of the setting concerned, later research in the field concentrated on feedback provided by staff recording their own behaviour. Albuquerque-Williams and Martin (1979) carried out a study in which care staff of a mental handicap hospital were required to record the quantity and appropriateness of their interactions with severely and profoundly handicapped clients. Although the short time available for training did not allow enough manipulations to demonstrate complete experimental control, they reported that this self-monitoring increased the quality of staff-client interactions and that it probably helped to maintain the high percentage of these interactions which were appropriate. Burg, Reid and Lattimore (1979) found that requiring carer staff to record the frequency of their contacts with clients increased the frequency of such contacts. Follow-up observations seven and eleven weeks after regular data collection had ceased showed that, as self-recording continued, the behaviour change was maintained. Unfortunately, the design used by Burg et al did not separate the effects of self-monitoring from the initial effects of instructions to interact with clients. However, results from the other studies cited would suggest that the maintenance of a high level of staff-client interaction was largely attributable to the feedback provided by self-recording.

Burgio, Whitman and Reid (1983) also studied the effects of self-monitoring procedures on staff's interactions with clients. Staff were briefly reminded of the necessity to make attention contingent upon appropriate behaviour, and then trained in the following activities: setting their own appropriate criterion levels for contingent attention, rather than using criteria determined by supervisors or researchers; recording and graphing their own behaviour; and administering self-praise for meeting or exceeding their own daily goal. Using a multiple baseline across settings design, Burgio et al. found that once the self-control procedures were instituted, there was an increase in staff interaction contingent upon appropriate client behaviours.

If staff behaviour can indeed be reliably changed by low-key management intervention such as self-recording in the absence of a period of intensive training, this represents a considerable advance over more traditional approaches to changing staff behaviour. Changing behaviour through management techniques requires less investment of time by supervisory staff or by training specialists, and as a result the techniques involved can be more easily replicated than those which require a great deal of input from external professionals. Also, as Burgio et al. point out, self-monitoring may provide staff with more accurate feedback than that given by supervisors, since staff can record their own behaviour continuously and at first hand. Finally, an effective strategy for changing staff behaviour which consists of a simple method of providing feedback has greater possibilities for dissemination than an approach which relies upon individual tuition for staff.

The work reported in this section (Jones, Evans and Blunden, 1982, 1984) was an evaluation of the effect of just such a low-key intervention as a means of introducing new staff procedures to a ward of a mental handicap hospital. The procedures concerned constituted a system for making requests and giving graded prompts and instructions to clients in order to increase their level of independence in various skills. This system, known as "Ask-Tell-Help", was based on the "Ask-Say-Do" method described by O'Brien, Porterfield, Herbert-Jackson and Risley (1979) which was developed as a means of using naturally occurring events to teach skills to toddlers. "Ask-Tell-Help" applies the same approach to mentally handicapped adults. It requires staff to use different levels of prompting to encourage clients' use of skills. Clients who are not engaged in an appropriate activity are initially asked what they should be doing, that is, given a non-specific verbal prompt (for example, "What do you have to do now that you've finished breakfast?"). If this level of prompting does not lead to clients carrying out the activity, they are then told what to do, that is, given verbal instructions: for example, "take your dishes to the sink". If verbal instructions are ineffective, clients are then physically guided through the action.

The method is a general approach which can in theory be applied to any skill or set of skills which clients might need to use during the day. Preliminary observations in the setting concerned suggested that the early morning period, between residents waking and leaving the ward for their morning's activities, provided a number of opportunities for the development of skills, and so the material prepared for staff was geared to using Ask-Tell-Help at this time of day.

4.2 Setting and participants

The work was carried out in one ward of a mental handicap hospital. The ward concerned was divided into two halves each with twelve residents. This study took place in one half of the ward which consisted of a day room, dining room, kitchenette, dormitory, toilets, washbasin, nurses' office and staff locker room.

The staff involved in this study consisted of two Charge Nurses, two State Enrolled Nurses (one of whom was transferred to another ward during the course of the study) and a number of unqualified nursing assistants. The clients involved were the twelve severely mentally handicapped men who lived in one half of the ward concerned. Their ages at the start of the study ranged from 27 to 66 years, with an average of 40 years. The average length of their residence in the hospital was 23 years, ranging from 12 years to 49 years. One of the Charge Nurses assessed the residents on the SPI and SSL scales. All twelve were fully ambulant; three were mildly incontinent; two were rated as presenting severe behaviour disorders and three as presenting mild behaviour disorders. All of the residents were scored as "partly able" on the self-help section of the scale. Typically this meant that they could feed themselves independently but needed help with dressing and/or washing.

4.3 Intervention

Three interventions were used in the course of this study: a staff interview, training leaflets describing the "Ask-Tell-Help" procedures, and checklists on which staff recorded the amount of assistance residents were given in various activities.

Staff Interview

All members of the ward staff responsible for the twelve residents were interviewed by the researchers. The questions concerned the staff's opinion of their role on the ward and the activities necessary to this role; the priorities they defined for their clients, both in general terms and in terms of specific skills which the residents needed to acquire; and what help the staff would need to achieve these goals for their clients. The interview had two functions. Firstly, it allowed for the possibility of using staff's suggestions about ways of achieving client goals in subsequent interventions. Secondly, it allowed for the possibility that, having considered the abilities and disabilities of the residents, staff would begin to work on developing their clients' skills before they had been given any specific procedures for this.

Ask-Tell-Help training leaflets

A three-page leaflet describing the "Ask-Tell-Help" method was distributed to all staff on the ward. Another leaflet was prepared for the charge staff alone, summarising the procedure and describing various ways it could be used on the ward. The Charge Nurses were asked to distribute the "Method" leaflets at one of the regular staff meetings and ask staff to read them. The charge staff were then to read the leaflet aloud and lead a discussion of ways in which the procedures could be used on the ward based on the suggestions in the "Charge Nurse" leaflet. Staff were asked to read the "Method" leaflet again and to use the "Ask-Tell-Help" method on the ward each morning thereafter.

Checklist and recording system

A series of checklists were introduced on which staff recorded, each day, whether each resident had carried out particular skills independently, when asked, when told, when helped, or whether the resident did not carry out the task or it was done for him. Definitions were provided on the checklists. Checklists were introduced sequentially at two week intervals over a period of eight weeks. Each time a checklist was introduced, the Charge Nurse was asked to show a copy to staff and discuss it with them at the ward's weekly meeting; the checklist would then be introduced on the following morning. The Charge Nurse was to give out the checklists to staff each morning before they began working with the residents, and to collect the checklists from them when the residents left the ward for their morning activities. He was then to transfer the information from the checklists to a summary sheet for each individual resident. This information was to be recorded for each resident each day, for each skill on which checklists were currently being used.

This self-recording system therefore differed from those used in other studies in that it focused on clients and did not require staff to monitor their own behaviour directly. However, existing ward contingencies appear to maintain the keeping of client-focused records (drug charts, etc.) and so it seemed feasible that another client-focused record system might be maintained as a permanent part of the ward routine. Furthermore, although the checklists did not provide staff with direct feedback on their own behaviour, in listing the possible types of assistance which staff might give residents, they performed the cueing function regarded as an important part of self-monitoring procedures (Nelson and Hayes, 1981).

4.4 Experimental design and conditions

The study used a four-phase time-series design with a multiple baseline across behaviours in the final phase. It was intended that each phase should last for two weeks (i.e. six data points) but this was modified in practice. Continued variation in the residents' level of activity in the "post interview" phase led to it being extended to nine weeks in order to ascertain the limits of this variability. The "leaflets" phase was scheduled for four weeks but was extended to seven to allow sufficient observations of new staff who arrived on this half of the ward during the phase.

The experimental conditions were as follows:

Baseline

Staff and clients were observed by the researchers before any intervention.

Post-interview

Staff and clients were observed after the staff had been interviewed by the researchers.

Leaflets

Staff and clients were observed after the charge staff had been given the "Method" and "Charge Nurse" leaflets and asked to lead discussions with staff on how to use the method on the ward and give each staff a copy of the "Method" leaflet for guidance.

Checklists

Checklists were introduced at two week intervals. For the first two weeks, staff were to complete the "dressing" checklist and for the second two weeks, the "shaving checklist" as well. From the fifth week of this phase, staff had to complete checklists on laying the table and washing, and from the seventh week, checklists on cleaning teeth and bedmaking.

Follow-up

Staff were asked to continue to use "Ask-Tell-Help" and all six checklists for the nine week period during which follow-up observations took place.

4.5 Measures

All observations took place between 7.15 and 9.15 a.m. on three randomly selected weekdays each week. In the follow-up phase, one set of data was collected on a randomly chosen weekday once in each three week period. Data were collected using a 30-second momentary time-sampling procedure in which residents were observed sequentially. On the instant of observation the observer had to decide what activity the resident was engaged in. Thirteen activities were given on the recording form: dressing, eating, washing, cleaning teeth, brushing/combing hair, shaving, laying table, bedmaking, clearing up, other, neutral, inappropriate or out of room. The following categories of assistance were used: (a) independent; (b) supervised (a member of staff was observing the resident carrying out an activity but not giving physical or verbal help); (c) giving materials (a member of staff was giving the resident materials necessary to carry out an activity but no other physical or verbal help); (d) physical guidance; (e) verbal instructions; (f) off-task talk (the resident was engaged in an activity and a member of staff talked to him about some other topic); and (g) doing something for the resident.

Insofar as these were measures of staff/client interaction, they acted both as a measure of client progress and staff use of the procedures, thus overcoming one of the limitations of the previous studies detailed in this chapter. The frequency of occurrence of these observations was expressed as a percentage of the total number of observation intervals, excluding observations coded as "other engaged" or "out of room". In addition to these measures, the percentage of the checklists which staff completed in the checklist and follow-up phases was calculated, as a further measure of staff compliance with the procedures. Because the research measure sampled behaviour momentarily but the checklists required staff to make judgements about whole tasks, it was not possible to assess how acurately staff completed the checklists.

4.6 Inter-observer agreement

Once a week two researchers carried out observations simultaneously but independently in order to assess inter-observer agreement. Percentage agreements were calculated separately for each category of client activity, degree of assistance, and for a combination of these, where observers had to agree on both activity and degree of assistance. In addition, Cohen's Kappa coefficient of agreement (Cohen, 1960; Hollenbeck, 1978) was calculated for degree of assistance and type of activity. This statistic corrects for chance agreement and is especially appropriate when the distribution of observations between categories is markedly uneven, as in this study.

Table 5 shows the mean agreement scores for each set of data and the range over the 24 reliability observations. It will be seen that throughout the study agreement was acceptably high.

4.7 Results

Assistance given to residents

Figure 4 shows, for each phase of the study, the mean percentage of observations in which type of assistance was recorded (since the percentage of some types of assistance were often extremely low, some categories have been amalgamated for ease of presentation).

The introduction of the "Ask-Tell-Help" leaflets and the checklists would have been expected to bring about an increase in the level of physical and verbal prompts and giving residents materials, in independent activity and "semi-independent" activity ("supervised" and "off-task talk" categories) and a decrease in the frequency with which staff carried out tasks for residents. The table shows that prompts remained at a very low frequency throughout the study; that there was only a very slight reduction in the frequency of "done for" codings (which were low in any case); and that independent activity increased steadily throughout the study.

TABLE 5

PERCENTAGE AGREEMENT AND KAPPA COEFFICIENT OF AGREEMENT: AVERAGE AND RANGE FOR EACH SET OF OBSERVATIONS

	PERCENTAGE	KAPPA
Client activities	92.5 (87.5-96.9)	88.7 (78.0-95.7)
Degree of assistance	94.7 (89.6-97.9)	86.1 (74.2-94.5)
Overall agreement (activity and assistance)	(86.1-95.3)	91.7

Figure 4. Percentage of observations coded as "independent" and "done for residents" across phases of the study.

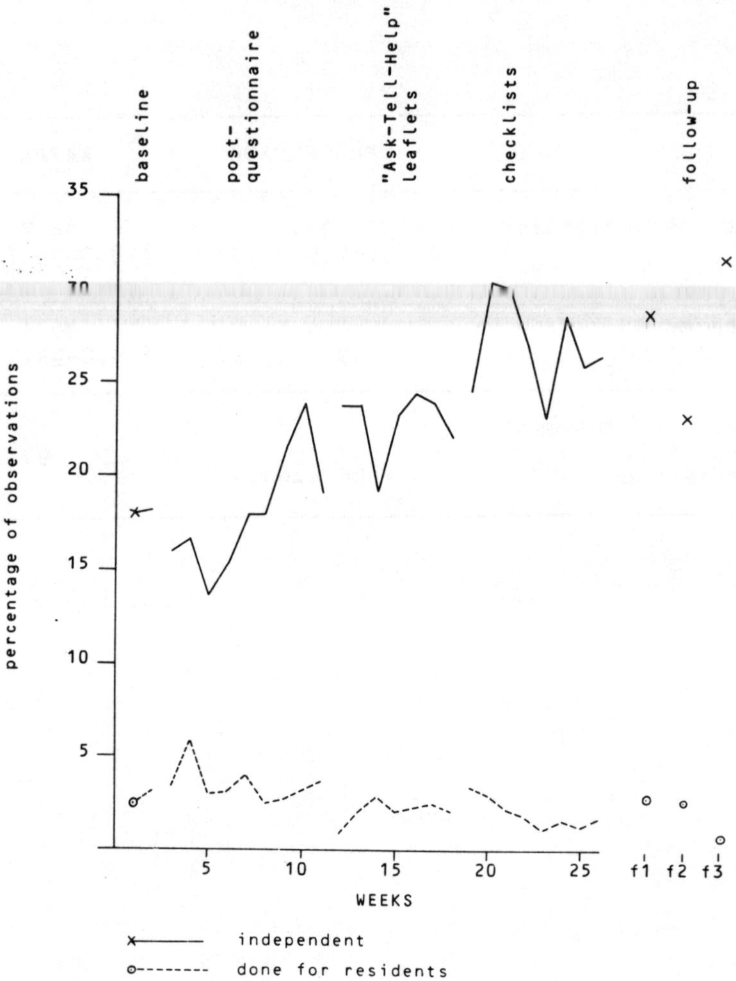

Figure 4 shows the weekly results for the two variables showing the greatest changes - independent activity and activities done for residents by staff. The percentage of intervals in which residents were seen to be independently engaged in any of the nine activities named on the observation schedule rose throughout the study from 17.9 per cent in the first week to a peak of 30.3 per cent in the second week of the checklist phase. Although this represents a considerable improvement, given the initial low level of independent activity, the changes did not occur in response to the components of the intervention which were expected to affect the level of independent activity. The most obvious change was a steady increase in independent activity during the post-interview phase, although it was not expected that the interview would have a major effect on the staff or client behaviour. The introduction of the "Ask-Tell-Help" leaflets did not lead to any further increase in the level of independent activity: the seven data points for this phase were almost entirely within the range of the last five points of the post-interview phase. During the checklist phase there was a slightly higher level of independent activity, but the lower scores in this phase were within the range of the two previous phases.

"Done for" codings were most frequent in the second week of the post-interview phase and least frequent in the week that the leaflets were introduced. However, they increased in frequency in subsequent weeks. There was a gradual reduction in this category after checklists were introduced, but this effect did not persist in the follow-up phase.

In addition to these overall results, the frequency of different types of assistance given for each skill was calculated, in order to assess the differential impact of the checklists during the multiple baseline phase. No overall pattern was found in the results. The clearest data, and the only set consistent with the results expected, were those for shaving.

In the first two phases, virtually all shaving observed was done by staff. The introduction of the leaflets and the brief "training" was followed by an increase in the proportion of observations of shaving where residents received prompts, but this effect did not last throughout the phase. After the shaving checklists were introduced, however, staff were once more observed using prompts; the percentage of observations of residents shaving independently or with supervision increased; and the percentage of observations of shaving carried out by staff decreased. These effects were maintained throughout the six weeks of the phase.

Staff had been completing dressing checklists for two weeks before the introduction of shaving checklists. However, with the exception of a single observation of shaving with supervision, changes observed in assistance with shaving only occurred after the shaving checklist itself had been introduced. This suggests that it was indeed the checklist specific to shaving which was responsible for the change and that requiring staff to record their use of the "Ask-Tell-Help" method with one skill does not affect the type of assistance they give residents in other skills. Data for other skills do not give a clear picture of their responsiveness to the interventions, but this may be due as much to methodological limitations of the data collection procedures (discussed in Jones et al, 1982) as to any ineffectiveness of the intervention.

Staff completion of checklists

During the eight weeks of the checklist phase, staff completed 71.4 per cent of the checklists they were given. There was no suggestion that the presence of observers affected staff filling in checklists: the percentage completed was 70.5 on days when observers were present and 72.1 on days when they were not. In experimental terms this meant that one of the independent variables was not in operation consistently during the period when its effect was being evaluated. Therefore the inconclusive results in terms of assistance given to residents might be partly due to staff's inconsistent use of checklists. In order to test this hypothesis, a comparison was made between observational data from days when checklists were completed and days when staff did not fill them in. There was no appreciable difference between the two sets of data.

4.8 Discussion

The overall conclusion to this study is that a minimal training intervention backed up by self-administered feedback was not an effective way of changing the interactions between staff and mentally handicapped clients. This is surprising when reports elsewhere in the literature of the success of such an approach in changing staff behaviour are considered. However, where feedback (as opposed to training or some other set of contingencies) has been the main form of behavioural control, the behaviours concerned have usually been administrative (Hutchinson et al., 1980; Prue et al., 1980; Repp and Dietz, 1979) or defined in fairly gross terms such as "positive interactions" (Burg et al., 1979; Burgio et al., 1983) or "toileting" (Greene et al., 1978). It may be that the successful introduction or a relatively complex staff practice such as using a hierarchical system of prompts does require intensive training. Studies which have used self-monitoring of more complex staff behaviours have done so in conjunction with intensive training strategies (Burgio et al., 1983; Kissel, Whitman and Reid, 1983). In the ward on which this study took place, though, it seemed likely that three other specific factors contributed to the ineffectiveness of the intervention: the type of activity occurring before the intervention, the format of the checklists, and the involvement of the charge staff. These are considered below.

Existing type of ward activity

The "Ask-Tell-Help" intervention was intended to increase the frequency of clients' independent behaviour and staff's use of prompts and to reduce the frequency with which staff carried out tasks for clients. However, a sufficiently thorough analysis of conditions on the ward prior to the study would have suggested that this was not the area in which change was most needed. The frequency with which staff carried out tasks for residents during baseline was very low, and so no major reduction in this type of behaviour could occur. However, all types of interaction with clients were infrequent during baseline (amounting to approximately 4.5 per cent of observation intervals) and the overall level of engaged behaviour including all types of assistance, was also low (approximately 22.7 per cent of intervals). Most of the engaged behaviour during baseline consisted of dressing and eating (approximately 19 per cent of intervals), activities which were largely carried out independently.

A beneficial impact of the intervention would

therefore be most likely to be shown in the application of "Ask-Tell-Help" to skills which did not frequently occur at the start of the study: any other large scale increase in the use of prompts would mean that residents were being prompted to carry out activities which they were capable of performing independently. However, although the leaflets and checklists did suggest areas other than dressing and eating in which "Ask-Tell-Help" could be applied, staff did not consistently attempt to develop residents' abilities in these areas. Although the intervention did have its expected effect on shaving, it did not lead to similar changes in other areas. It is uncertain why this should have been so. Both before and after the introduction of leaflets and checklists, staff and clients engaged only sporadically in such activities as washing and cleaning teeth. There were several days in the course of the study when the observers did not see these activities occur at all; and on days when they did occur, they tended to be completed very quickly so that it was not unusual for the time-sampling observations to miss clients and staff when they were engaged in these activities.

It is possible that a change in the way "Ask-Tell-Help" was presented to staff, so that it emphasised the use of the method in developing specific skills, rather than as a general means of encouraging clients' independence, would have led to a corresponding increase in residents' participation in a wider range of activities. Some of the staff suggested that the procedures might have been introduced for one resident or one skill at a time, so that they could have achieved competence in using "Ask-Tell-Help" in a limited area before applying it more generally. It is possible that such an approach might have resulted in greater use of the procedures by staff, and that in this study new skills became the targets for intervention (on the introduction of the relevant checklist) at too rapid a pace for staff.

Format of checklists

The self-recording checklists used in this study required staff to record assistance which all clients received, irrespective of which member of staff gave that assistance. In effect, staff members were therefore recording the group behaviour of staff rather than their own individual behaviour as in other studies of self-monitoring. Feedback on group performance when data are collected and displayed by supervisors or researchers (e.g. Panyan et al., 1970; Welsch et al., 1973) has been shown to be effective. However, it appears that having staff collect such data is less effective, possibly because of the lack of immediacy compared to systems in which staff members monitor only their own behaviour. A system in which staff members only recorded their own use of prompts might well have had more impact than the one employed here.

It became apparent during the study that the checklists were not functioning in the manner intended. Firstly, carrying and completing checklists involved considerable response cost to staff. Charge Nurses had been given written instructions to distribute checklists to staff at the beginning of the early morning period. When they were interviewed after the study, they reported that when they gave checklists out at this time, staff complained that they could not carry out their duties while carrying checklists and quickly returned them to the nurses' office. As a result checklists had to be completed at the end of the early morning period, and so did not cue staff to use "Ask-Tell-Help" throughout the morning.

Some staff indicated that they were unsure about how to complete the checklists. In order to keep the checklists relatively small and easy to complete, the target skills were not broken down into their constituent parts. Staff had to make decisions about whether whole tasks were carried out with the specified degrees of assistance. Some of them found this difficult, especially when residents only required brief amounts of assistance in one part of an activity. Thus they were not sure how the information they recorded on the checklists related to their appropriate use of the new procedures; whether for example, a brief physical prompt in one part of an activity allowed the client less independence than a number of verbal prompts at different stages of the task. Furthermore, the checklists were not sensitive to small degrees of progress that the residents might make, and so a possible source of reinforcement to staff for using the procedures - that of observing and recording their clients' progress - was absent.

Involvement of Charge Staff

The "low-key" approach as adopted in this study requires that, wherever possible, all functions of training and management should be carried out by staff of the setting rather than external agents. Consequently the researchers delegated several important responsibilities to the charge staff of the ward but did not attend the staff meetings at which the new methods were introduced. It is not, therefore, known how closely these instructions were followed. Charge Nurses were not seen to give feedback to care staff on their use of the "Ask-Tell-Help" procedures as they used them, although the "Charge Nurse" leaflets explicitly instructed them to give this kind of feedback. Finally, for a variety of reasons, charge staff rarely took part in the early morning activities on this half of the ward. However, research suggests that such participation may have beneficial effects both at a general and specific level. Raynes et al (1979) noted a better quality of staff-resident interaction in wards where supervisors were involved in daily activities with residents; and a study by Wallace, Davis, Liberman and Baker (1973) showed that ordinary care staff increased their use of new procedures when the ward supervisor began to carry out the new routine. Although the charge staff had not been specifically requested by the researchers to use "Ask-Tell-Help" on the ward during the early morning period, it is possible that if they had been seen to do so, the ordinary staff might have increased their use of this system of prompts.

4.9 General Conclusion

Taken together, the results of the study described here suggest a particular strategy for future developments of this approach to staff training and management. The factors which may have limited the effectiveness of the "Ask-Tell-Help" package include a failure to present the procedures in a way which would have had most impact on the particular conditions prevailing on the ward; a system of self-monitoring which was not as effective in providing feedback to staff as it might have been; and the possible failure of the supervisors of the setting to carry out certain activities likely to encourage the use of new staff procedures. These deficits suggest a strategy which makes specific attempts to overcome them.

First, such an approach would involve greater collaboration between innovators and the supervisors and staff of the setting in order to develop interventions which can achieve particular goals within certain constraints of the setting.

Second, the role of supervisors would need to be more clearly delineated, so as to cover their participation in staff training, their own use of the new procedures in the setting, and providing feedback to the ordinary staff of the setting on their implementation of the new procedures.

Third, just as ordinary staff require monitoring and feedback during the introduction of methods of working, so the supervisors' behaviour may need to be monitored, and feedback provided, if they are to perform adequately their role of training and supervising staff in the use of new procedures. The final study described in this chapter goes some way to establishing the feasibility of such an approach.

5 CHANGING STAFF BEHAVIOUR THROUGH COLLABORATIVE GOAL-SETTING AND FEEDBACK

5.1 Introduction

The methods employed in the studies reviewed so far have been examples of "internal controls" - that is, methods by which services are monitored and improvement is attempted from within. However, it is also important that there should be some influence on the behaviour of service providers which operates in the best interests of the clients of that service (Skinner, 1972; Boles and Bible, 1978). Such "counter-controls" are especially important in services for very dependent clients such as mentally handicapped people, who can usually exert little influence themselves over those who provide services to them. One form of external control which has been widely recommended (DHSS and Welsh Office, 1971; National Development Group, 1976, 1978, 1980; Tyne and Wertheimer, 1980) is that clients and their families or advocates become more actively involved in planning and developing services. It has also been suggested that involving all levels of direct-care staff in planning such decision-making is likely to make mental handicap services more responsive to the needs of their clients (Raynes et al.; 1979; Towell, 1982).

The study described here (Porterfield, Evans and Blunden, 1982) was intended to evaluate this approach to improving services. It was an adaptation of earlier work by Boles and Bible (1978). The aims of the study were:

a) to involve clients' families, staff and supervisors with researchers in identifying aspects of the service which presented problems;

b) to develop specific staff procedures designed to improve these aspects of the services;

c) to develop a monitoring system for these procedures;

d) to evaluate the effect of these interventions on staff and client behaviour.

5.2 Setting and participants

The setting for this study was a Health Authority mental handicap unit which provided long and short-term residential and day care. The Unit consisted of four bungalows and an industrial therapy unit and was situated in the grounds of a geriatric hospital. The study took place in one of these bungalows. As well as day care, the bungalow provided residential accommodation for a maximum of eight clients. It contained six bedrooms, a kitchen, dining room, lounge, utility room, toilets, shower and bathroom. There were also toilets and a small cloakroom for staff.

During the study, the bungalow provided services for a total of 27 clients. Some of the short-term care clients only used the bungalows for brief periods, and few data were collected for thirteen of these clients. Results presented in section 5.7 below are based on data from the fourteen clients (eleven women and three men) who were present for at least two observations before, and two observations after, the introduction of new procedures. Their mean age was 26 years, ranging from 15 to 64 years.

The clients' abilities were assessed using a modified version of the Behaviour Assessment Record (Hope, 1977). Ten of the fourteen were able to walk without assistance and thirteen could eat without help. Six toileted themselves with only occasional or no accidents and six (not entirely the same individuals) were "dry all night". None of the clients could dress themselves completely, although three could put on one or two items by themselves. The receptive language skills of the group were fairly well developed, but only five clients could use "simple sentences to describe activities" and none could "carry on a simple conversation".

The staff of the mental handicap unit consisted of a Nursing Officer, one Charge Nurse, one Staff Nurse and three State Enrolled Nurses (SENs). All other staff working on the bungalows were unqualified care assistants.

Eight care assistants were assigned to the bungalow in question. Two worked full-time (37 hours per week), three for thirty hours per week, and three for twenty hours. Staff from the children's bungalow in the unit usually assisted the staff of this bungalow while the children were attending school so that a total of twelve staff worked there regularly. Of these, three had worked at the unit for less than a year and the remainder up to three years (i.e. from the opening of the unit). All had received some form of in-service training; in addition, two care assistants had been trained as nursery nurses.

Thirteen families participated in the study, those of the clients resident in or regularly attending the bungalow (one of the fourteen clients had no close relatives). In each case clients were represented by their parent or parents.

5.3 Intervention

The intervention took place in two stages.

Preliminary Interviews

The researchers interviewed all direct care staff, domestic staff and supervisory staff involved with the bungalow, and the families of clients who were resident in or regularly attended the bungalow. The interviews were intended to ascertain each person's opinion about various aspects of the services provided by the unit, including its aims and how far these were being met. The interview also presented a list of eight aspects of the unit's services and each person was asked to select the three aspects which he or she felt was most in need of development in the bungalow. In addition, interviewees were also asked to suggest ways in which they would like to see these service areas developed.

New procedures for priority areas

The three areas selected most often by families and staff were **a)** organisation of staff, **b)** family-staff communication and **c)** client recreational activities. On the basis of comments made in the interviews, the researchers developed procedures designed to produce change in these areas and checklists which supervisors could use to provide feedback to their staff on the extent to which change was being achieved. The specific procedures were as follows.

a) **Organisation of staff** The procedures for this priority area required one member of staff to supervise the main group of clients while other members of staff worked with individual clients. The SEN responsible for the bungalow was required to assign staff to either group or individual work for one-hour periods, and to prepare and display this rota a week in advance.

Staff did not receive any formal training in these procedures, but were given a leaflet which described the specific duties involved. The supervisors (Nursing Officer, Charge Nurse and SENs) were asked to complete a brief staff feedback checklist. This covered the following aspects of the procedures - whether two staff were present, whether one was doing individual work and one working with the remainder of the group - and if not, for what reason. On completing the feedback checklist, the supervisors were to discuss the checklist their observations with the staff concerned. The completed checklist was then posted next to the rota.

b) **Family-staff communication** The intervention devised for this aspect of the unit's services consisted of a "client report book" which served as a two-way channel of communication between staff and families about the clients. The report book consisted of a loose-leaf folder with specially printed pages to be completed by staff or families, as appropriate. The pages to be completed by staff were divided into sections

Figure 5. Sample page of client report book

CLIENT REPORT

From Bungalow 2 Staff to Client's Family

NAME : ....

DATE : ....

	MORNING (7.15am–1pm) Staff completing report:		AFTERNOON/EVENING (1pm–9pm) Staff completing report:	
ACTIVITIES	TRAINING/ TEACHING		TRAINING/ TEACHING	
	SPECIAL INDIVIDUAL		SPECIAL INDIVIDUAL	
	DOMESTIC		DOMESTIC	
	OUTING		OUTING	

EATING		B'fast	Lunch	Comments :		Dinner	Comments :
	Ate well				Ate well		
	O.K.				O.K.		
	Ate little				Ate little		

PERSONAL CARE		Indep	Helped	Done for			Indep	Helped	Done for	
	Bathing					Bathing				
	Hair washing				Toiletting Accident	Hair washing				Toiletting Accident
	Toiletting					Toiletting				
	Other					Other				

BEHAVIOUR			If problem – describe			If problem – describe
	very good			very good		
	good			good		
	problem			problem		

OTHER COMMENTS (fits, items needed, etc)		

NIGHT (9pm – 7.15am) Staff completing report: ....

Slept well		Awake from .... to ....
Woke – no problem		If problem – describe :
Woke – problem		
Incontinent		

NOTE TO CLIENT'S FAMILY/FRIENDS: Please initial this page so that we will know that you have seen this report. Thank you.

Initials : ....

covering morning, afternoon and night. Staff working during each period were to complete the appropriate section describing client activities, eating, personal care and behaviour (see Figure 5). The pages to be completed by families allowed them to record details of special activities their relative had participated in, any problem behaviours, illness or injury, or any other comments (e.g. new skills learnt). These report books replaced the existing method of record keeping on the bungalow and travelled with the clients between the unit and their homes.

As with the "staff organisation" intervention, there was no formal training for staff or families in the use of the report book. The researchers discussed the report books and how to complete them, at one of the family-staff meetings and brief instructions were included in the book. However, questions concerning the completion of the staff section were added to the supervisors' checklist. These covered the following aspects of the procedures:

(a) whether there was a report book present for each client in the bungalow at the time of the supervisor's visit;

(b) whether all the report books had been completed by the previous shift;

(c) whether the activities recorded for the clients were appropriate.

After completing the expanded checklist, supervisors were to give staff feedback on the extent to which they were complying with the report book and staff organisation procedures.

c) **Client recreational activities** The intervention for this area of service provision consisted of assigning to each client a "key worker" - a member of staff with particular responsibilities to that client. When that member of staff was scheduled to carry out individual work, she was to spend some of this time working with her "key clients" on recreational activities. In addition, the staff member assigned to work with the main group of clients was now required to see that all members of the group had materials in reach, and to talk to clients who were engaged. At the third family/staff meeting, a leaflet was distributed describing the duties of staff assigned to work with the group and with individuals in this area.

Questions concerning client participation in recreational activities were added to the supervisors' feedback checklist. Supervisors had to record whether each client had recreational materials within reach, the proportion of clients present who were engaged and the number of contacts made by the "group" staff member to each client in a ten-minute period. Supervisors were now required to complete the checklist and give feedback twice daily. A graph showing client activity levels and the extent to which staff were completing their assigned roles was displayed in the bungalow. In addition, the results of the checklists were reported at the weekly meeting of the external professionals who worked at the unit (e.g. community nurses, social workers, psychiatrists).

5.4 Experimental Design and Conditions

The study used a five-phase time-series experimental design.

It was conducted in the following sequence:-

Phase 1: Baseline (4 weeks)

The regular procedures of the bungalow were in operation and general observations were made on client and staff behaviour.

Interviews

Interviews were conducted with staff and clients' families to determine priority areas for service development.

Phase 2 (4 week)

General measures of staff and client behaviour were continued and research checklists on specific aspects of staff behaviour in the three "priority areas" were completed.

Evaluating the Impact

Phase 3 (6 weeks)

The procedures for the first priority area where staff were assigned responsibility for group or individuals, were introduced.

Phase 4 (5 weeks)

The procedures for the second priority area (client report books) were added.

Phase 5 (5 weeks)

The procedures for the third priority area (individual key workers with responsibility for client recreational activities), were added to the two sets of procedures already in operation.

Post-study interviews

Clients' families and staff were interviewed again to determine any changes in their stated opinions about the service and the impact of the interventions.

Follow-up

Data were collected for one week 14 weeks after the end of the study.

This design allowed the researchers to collect general data on key aspects of client and staff behaviour for the duration of the study. In addition, after the initial interviews, the researchers devised the experimental interventions and prepared checklists covering key aspects of the specific procedures to be introduced. The post interview phase allowed for collection of baseline data on these specific behaviours, and also for the assessment of the impact of the interviews on the more general aspects of staff and client behaviour. Finally, the sequential introduction of the interventions in phases 3 to 5 constituted a multiple baseline analysis of staff and client behaviours under the different conditions.

5.5 Measures

Three measures were used to evaluate the effectiveness of these interventions - the Staff Behaviour Measure and Client Behaviour Measure (Porterfield, Evans and Blunden, 1981) and a checklist covering the specific procedures involved in the interventions.

1) Staff Behaviour Measure (SBM)

Using this measure, researchers observed staff sequentially at 30-second intervals. Staff behaviour was coded according to the following categories:

a) negative contact with clients

b) positive contact with clients

c) dealing with clients' recreational or educational materials

d) dealing with domestic materials

e) administrative tasks

f) in office

g) staff-staff contact

h) other (e.g. supervising clients, drinking tea)

i) away or in private room

2) Client Behaviour Measure (CBM)

Using this measure researchers observed clients sequentially at thirty-second intervals and coded their behaviour according to the following categories:

a) Engaged in
- recreational or educational activity
- looking or listening activity (e.g. watching TV)
- personal activity (e.g. eating, combing hair)
- domestic activity (e.g. washing up)
- contact with another person

b) Inappropriate
- self stimulation
- self agression
- other agression

other (e.g. swearing, food stealing)

c) Neutral

Detailed definitions of these categories and of the observation procedures can be found in Porterfield, Evans and Blunden (1981). In this study, observations of staff and client behaviour were made for two hours on five days of each week (Sunday to Saturday), so that the hours 9 a.m. to 7 p.m. were covered each week. Forty-five minutes of CBM data and fifteen minutes of SBM data were collected each hour. For reasons of privacy, observations were confined to the communal living areas of the bungalow and were not carried out in the bedrooms, bathrooms or toilets.

3) Research checklists

Once the priority areas for service development had been established, the researchers devised checklist for their own use in assessing staff compliance with the new procedures, distinct from the supervisors' feedback checklists. These checklists covered the following aspects of the procedures:

a) one staff member working with group and one with individuals;

b) percentage of clients present in bungalow for whom report books were present;

c) percentage of shifts for which report books had been completed;

d) at least ten recreational/educational materials present;

e) percentage of clients with at least one material within reach;

f) percentage of clients contacted in ten minute period

g) number of contacts to clients made by one staff member in ten minutes.

The information required to complete these checklists was obtained from bungalow records and by direct observation. Checklists were completed on each day that CBM and SBM data were collected (except in the pre-interview baseline when the priority areas had not been decided).

5.6 Inter-observer agreement

The majority of observations were shared between two researchers. Approximately once a week (19 of the 24 weeks of the study) the two researchers observed simultaneously in order to assess inter-observer agreement.

Percentage agreement was established in the same way for both staff and client measures and was calculated on the basis of each observation interval. In each interval, a number of observation codes may have been recorded. For an agreement to be scored, there had to be agreement on every code recorded in that interval. Percentage agreement was calculated as the Number of intervals on which the observers agreed multiplied by 100 divided by total number of intervals. Agreement was calculated only for intervals in which both researchers had observed the client or staff member, i.e. not for intervals in which one or both observers had recorded "out of room" or missed an observation.

The mean inter-observer agreement scores were 93.9 per cent (range 85.7 per cent - 100 per cent) and for staff behaviour 93.0 per cent (range 83.7 per cent - 97.6 per cent) for client behaviour.

To obtain agreement measures for checklist data, both researchers completed a checklist simultaneously but independently. Agreement was calculated on the basis of each checklist question and the percentage was calculated by multiplying the number of questions on which the observers agreed by 100 and dividing by the number of questions.

The mean agreement score for the checklists was 94.6 per cent (range 81.8 per cent - 100 per cent).

5.7 Results

1) Research Checklist Data

Table 6 shows, for each phase of the study, the mean value of the data collected on the research checklist. No data are given for phase 1 because checklists had not been drawn up at that time.

Procedures aimed at improving staff organisation were introduced at the start of phase 3. The table shows

TABLE 6

PERCENTAGE OF INTERVALS IN WHICH CLIENTS RECEIVE DIFFERENT LEVELS OF ASSISTANCE - AVERAGE FOR PHASES

	Phase of Study				
	Baseline	Post-interview	Leaflets	Checklists	Follow-up
Level of	2.8	3.5	2.1	2.0	2.1
Physical prompt, task talk, given materials	1.2	1.0	1.6	2.0	0.9
Supervised, off-task talk	0.5	0.3	0.3	0.9	0.5
Independent	18.2	17.8	22.9	27.0	27.6
Total Activity	22.7	22.6	26.9	31.9	31.1

Figure 6. Staff behaviour as coded across phase of the study.

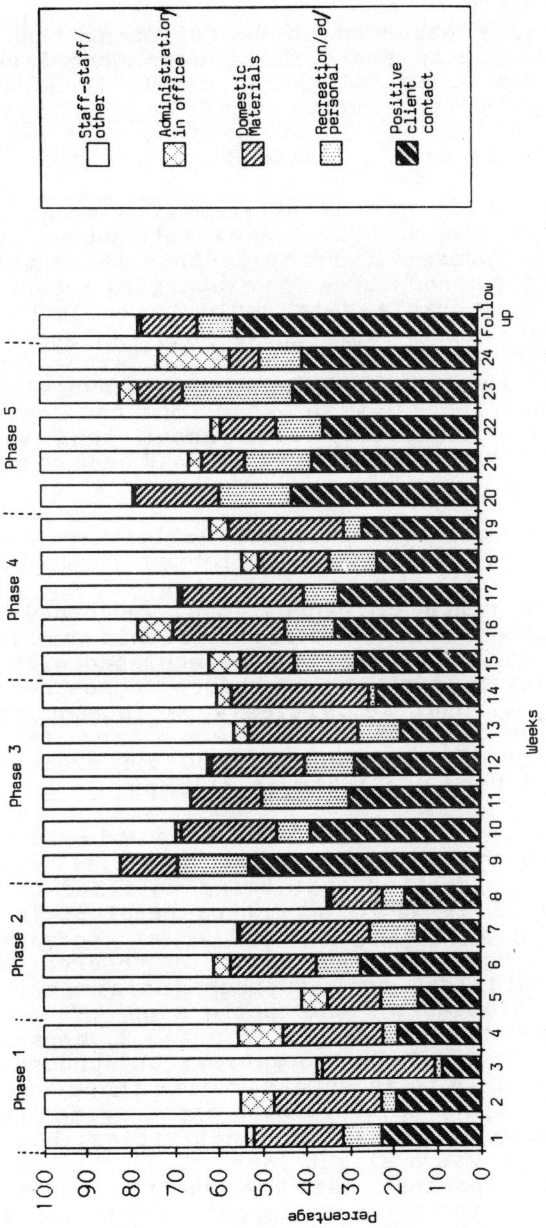

that following the introduction of the procedures assigning staff to group or individual work, staff were generally observed to be following the roles specified. During phase 4, however, the level of adherence was lower and varied widely (from 42 per cent - 100 per cent). Because staff were not assigned to any roles prior to phase 3, it was not possible to collect this data in phase 2.

Procedures to improve staff-family communication (i.e. client report books) were introduced at the beginning of phase 4. Prior to this there were no clearly defined procedures for exchanging information and so no comparable data could be collected for phases 2 or 3. The table shows that, subsequent to the introduction of report books, an average of 91 per cent of the clients attending the bungalow had their report books with them on the days of observation. The table also shows that a high percentage of the relevant sections had been completed by staff.

Checklist data on recreational activities and the associated procedures were collected from phase 2 onwards. The table shows that there were few occasions when a wide range of recreational or educational materials were available to clients. This was largely due to the bungalow being poorly equipped with such items. However, once the procedures concerned with client recreational activities were introduced, at the beginning of phase 5, there was a large increase in the number of occasions when 10 different types of materials were available to clients.

The percentage of clients with materials in reach increased in phase 3 and remained at a similar level in phase 4, suggesting that being assigned to work with either individuals or groups resulted in more clients gaining access to some form of recreational material. However, the specific "recreational" procedures did lead to a further increase in this measure. Similarly, the proportion of clients contacted by staff increased in phase 3, apparently in response to the "staff organisation" procedures. It is not possible to ascertain how far these contacts were specifically concerned with encouraging clients to participate in recreational activities, however. Although there was a slight increase from phase 4 to phase 5, it appears that the staff organisation procedures had the greatest impact on this variable.

The number of contacts to each client also showed a similar pattern of a large increase from phase 2 to phase 3, concurrent with the introduction of staff organisation procedures, followed by a slight reduction in phase 4 and a further increase in phase 5 when "recreational" procedures were introduced.

2) Staff Behaviour Measure Data

Figure 6 shows the percentage of observed staff behaviour assigned to each category of the SBM for each week of the study. For ease of presentation, the "staff-staff" and "other" categories have been combined, as have "administration' and "in office". Negative contacts to clients occurred so infrequently (0.04 per cent of total observations) that they are not included.

The data presented in Figure 6 support those derived from the checklists, indicating that staff contact with clients increased over the course of the study, from a mean of 17.7 per cent in baseline to 39.9 per cent in phase 5 (55 per cent in follow-up). Staff's use of recreational/educational or clients' personal materials also increased from 4.3 per cent in baseline to 16.1 per cent in phase 5. The mean percentage of "staff/staff and other" codings dropped from 49.3 per cent in phase 1 to 27.2 per cent in phase 5 (23 per cent in follow-up) and that of domestic activity from 23.5 per cent to 11.9 per cent. The percentage of "administrative/in office" codings did not change appreciably.

3) Client Behaviour Measure Data

Figure 7 shows the percentage of observed client behaviour coded as engaged, neutral or inappropriate for each week of the study. This category never accounted for more than 1.5 per cent of observations in the entire study. The mean level of client engagement increased from 26.9 per cent in phase 1 to 59.5 per cent in phase 5. Neutral codings decreased correspondingly from 65.9 per cent to 36.7 per cent. The mean level of inappropriate behaviour decreased from 6.8 per cent in baseline to 3.3 per cent.

5.8 Conclusion and discussion

The main results of this study were that:

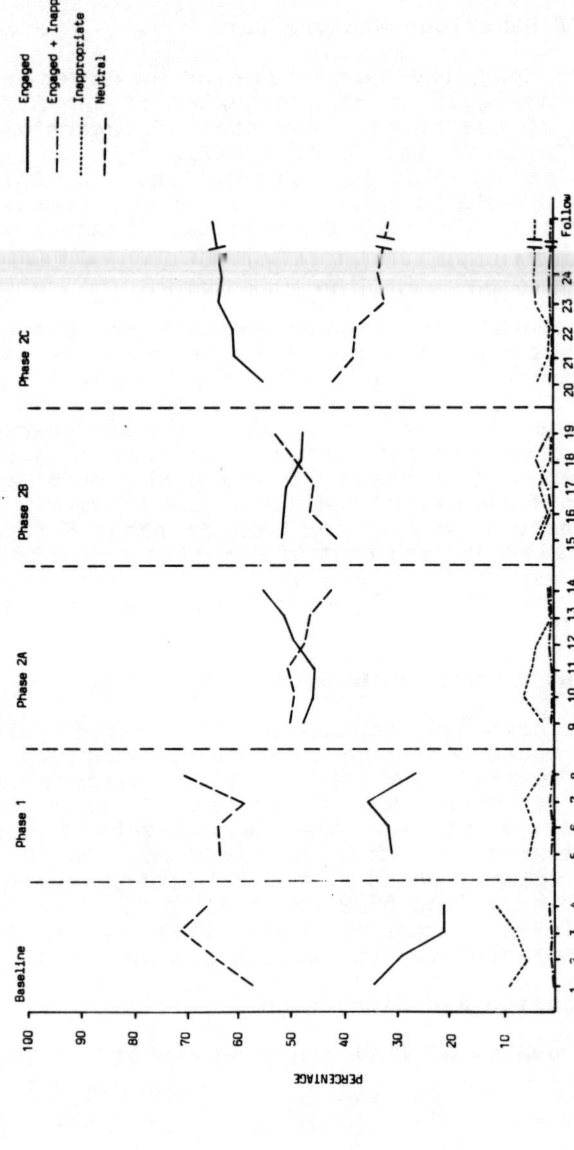

Figure 7. Client behaviour as coded across phases of the study.

a) as procedural interventions relevant to particular service areas were introduced in turn, staff behaviour consistent with the new procedures increased;

b) a number of beneficial changes occurred during the phases of the study following the first intervention which remained relatively stable as subsequent interventions took place. These changes included:

- an increase in staff contact with clients, and a decrease in the proportion of staff time spent interacting with other staff and working on domestic tasks without clients present;

- a large increase in the number of clients with recreational materials to hand;

- an increase in engaged behaviour by clients with a corresponding decrease in neutral behaviour.

The conclusions should be considered in the light of the limitations of the experimental design. Three of the measures of those staff behaviours directly associated with particular interventions could not be recorded at all before the introduction of those procedures, so baseline measures could not be taken. For example, it would be meaningless to record that 0 per cent report book sections were filled in in the phases before staff were given these books. Nevertheless, the high compliance with these procedures, as recorded on the research checklists in the weeks following their introduction, indicates the impact of the combination of procedures used to introduce these new staff routines.

The checklist measures with which it was possible to collect baseline data were those associated with the "recreational activities" intervention of phase 5. The data indicate that substantial changes in these variables occurred upon the introduction of the "staff organisation" procedures, two phases earlier. However, introduction of the specific "recreational activities" procedures did lead to a further increase in the associated staff behaviour. The SBM data on staff contact with clients also indicated this effect: Figure 6 shows that there was a dramatic increase in staff contact variable in the first week of phase 5.

However, this effect was not maintained throughout the phase. This suggests that although the novelty of using the new procedures, and their introduction at the family-staff meetings, contributed to this effect, their impact was not sufficient to maintain performance throughout the phase. With the introduction of the "recreational activities" procedures, greater emphasis was placed on client contact by the staff member responsible for the group and staff were given specific feedback on their level of contact with clients.

Unfortunately it is not possible to separate the effects of the instructional leaflets which staff received from the feedback which they were given. However, the researchers informally observed that in phase 4 the supervisors were not consistent in their use of the feedback procedures, and the checklist data show that the majority of behaviours in this phase were at lower levels than in the previous phase. In phase 5 more emphasis was given to the feedback procedures. Monitoring occurred more frequently, staff received feedback more promptly, client engagement levels were displayed publicly, and external professionals were provided with information derived from monitoring. The checklist data for phase 5 showed improved compliance with the procedures for two of the three behaviours targeted in the previous phases. Although these factors were not systematically varied, the data suggest that the improved feedback was at least partly responsible for improved staff performance.

Considered as a whole, these results indicate the effectiveness of a strategy for introducing new procedures to mental handicap settings based on:

(a) involving clients' families and staff in selecting areas for improvement in services;

(b) developing procedures for these priority areas based on suggestions offered by clients' families and staff;

(c) a minimal "training" intervention consisting of discussion of new procedures at a meeting between clients' families and staff, and written descriptions of procedures for staff;

(d) daily feedback to staff on their use of new

procedures, given by the supervisor of the setting or his/her deputy.

6. OVERALL DISCUSSION AND CONCLUSIONS

6.1 Principal findings

Five studies of various approaches to staff training and management are reported in this chapter. The conclusions of these studies are as follows.

Study No.1: Establishing activity periods in a day care setting

A combination of training relying on written and verbal instructions modelling practice and feedback, followed by on-the-job feedback from a supervisor, led to changes in client behaviour consistent with staff applying the procedures in which they had been trained.

Studies No. 2 and 3: Introducing activity periods to a hospital ward (preliminary and management studies)

A replication of this approach which omitted written instructions and without specified monitoring by supervisors, led to initial changes with poor long-term maintenance. A further replication suggested that with these features included, both initial changes and long-term maintenance can be achieved, and that responsibility for providing staff with feedback can be transferred from researchers to supervisors of the setting with no ill effects.

Study No. 4: Introducing a system of prompts to a hostel ward

An attempt to introduce new procedures by a minimal training intervention, i.e., discussion of new procedures by charge staff and circulation of written descriptions of these procedures, coupled with staff self-recording these procedures did not lead to major changes in staff behaviour.

Study No. 5: Collaborative goal setting and feedback

Introducing procedures based on suggestions made by clients' families and staff by a similar combination of brief discussion and written procedural guides, coupled with feedback provided by supervisors, did lead to substantial changes in staff behaviour.

6.2 Implications of these findings

The results of these studies indicate that the behaviour of staff in services for mentally handicapped people can be changed through a variety of training and management strategies, and that improvements in clients' quality of life are associated with these changes in staff behaviour. In addition, it appears that certain combinations of the various components of the interventions adopted in this body of work may be most effective where particular conditions are encountered in a service setting.

Unfortunately it has not been possible to evaluate the relative impact of these different combinations: the constraints of carrying out applied research in service settings have somewhat limited the scope of this work. Applied research must appear to offer some possible benefit to the "consumer", in this case the organisation providing the service. While in all these studies the programme of search was undertaken in order to provide a solution to problems in the service identified by staff at various levels of the organisation, the benefit of experimental rigour is not always obvious to care staff; nor is the rationale for frequent variations in work routines arising from different experimental conditions, as witness the problems experienced in instituting reversal phases in the first and second studies reported.

The "solution" provided in the form of an experimental intervention has not always been an intuitively obvious one for the staff concerned: for example, rather than eliminating a particular problem, it may have focused on providing an alternative activity. Furthermore, a "solution" may seem ideal for a given "problem" from a reading of the research literature, but may be inappropriate given the organisational idiosyncracies of the setting in which the problem occurs. For example, involvement by supervisors in the form of carrying out new routines and giving staff feedback on their performance may well be an effective means of changing staff behaviour, but it would not be a feasible intervention in a setting where supervisors are not on duty at the time of the targeted routines or are frequently called away to deputise for others in the management hierarchy.

Because of such organisational constraints and the need to invest the different experimental conditions with some credibility for direct care staff, it has not seemed feasible to mount a programme of research aimed at manipulating all the variables identified as influencing direct care staff's performance in order to discover best combinations of training and management techniques, types of staff and client behaviour, and organisation of the setting.

However, the five studies point to some general conclusions which may be susceptible to more detailed examination in future work.

1) The combination of written descriptions of new staff procedures, demonstrations of these procedures, practice with feedback, and on-the-job feedback from supervisory staff, appears to be an effective way of changing staff behaviour.

   These conclusions, drawn from the first, second and third studies reported in this chapter, are congruent with the results of early work on staff training and management which relied largely on intensive training of direct care staff by professionals. However, subsequent research indicated that changes in staff behaviour could also be achieved through "weak" or "low-key" interventions, such as brief discussions of new procedures, backed up by more powerful techniques such as feedback delivered by researchers, supervisors or self-monitoring. This idea informed the fourth and fifth studies reported in this chapter, which suggest the second broad conclusion.

2) Changes in staff behaviour and its presumed impact on client behaviour equivalent in impact and performance to those brought about by more intensive methods, can be achieved solely through providing staff with written descriptions of new procedures and on-the-job feedback from supervisors. This may depend on these new work practices being decided jointly by researchers, staff and other interested parties, e.g., clients or their relatives.

3) Although feedback was not varied systematically in these studies, informal observations suggested that the factors most closely associated with fluctuations in targeted staff performances and client behaviour was the quality of feedback provided by the supervisor. The desired changes in client behaviour also appeared to be greatly influenced by the simple accessibility of materials. These broad conclusions have implications for three important topics in staff training and management.

Self-management

The investigation of self-management in the fourth study reported in this chapter did not find any consistent increase in the frequency of the behaviours noted by staff. This is in contrast to other studies in which behaviour management through self-recording has been demonstrated to be effective (Burg et al., 1979; Burgio et al., 1983; Kissel et al., 1983). However, the complexity of the behaviours required of staff may have required intensive training, rather than the low-key approach used in this study, to establish them in the staff's repertoire before self-monitoring could effectively control behaviour. In addition, the cumbersome recording for this and the focus on group rather than individual data, are also likely to have limited the impact of self-recording. In view of these limitations and of the success of self-monitoring reported by other writers, its lack of impact in this study should not weigh against its use in future. Not only has it been shown experimentally to be effective: it is also theoretically respectable from the standpoint of both behavioural psychologists in terms of cueing and reinforcement functions and for organisational sociologists in terms of delegating responsibility as far as possible down the management hierarchy.

Collaborative service development

Various writers concerned with the effectiveness of organisations in general (e.g. Skinner, 1953; Hall, 1967; Paulson, 1974; Davey, 1981) and mental handicap services in particular (Raynes et al., 1979; Towell, 1982) have recommended increased decentralisation so that front-line staff take a part of the responsibility for the planning and delivery of the organisation's services. The collaborative strategy used in the fifth of the studies presented here, which involved not only front-line staff but clients' families as well, provides an effective means of deciding upon what staff behaviours need to be trained. It is also possible that the collaborative approach may expedite the uptake of new procedures. A comparison of the fourth and fifth studies suggests such an effect, although because of procedural and other differences between settings, comparisons between studies cannot be made with complete confidence. The "training" intervention of both studies relied chiefly on presenting staff with written descriptions of new procedures. In the fourth study, the "problem" was defined by the research team and senior nursing staff. Although ward staff were asked for their ideas about how residents' skills might be developed, they were not consulted about whether or not they considered such development a priority for their clients. It may be that in the fifth study the greater relevance of the procedures to the staff who had helped to identify the priority areas to which the new procedures applied and on which they had made suggestions, accounted at least in part for the greater impact of the intervention on staff in that setting.

Role of supervisor

Even when new practices are introduced by such a collaborative approach, it appears that the supervisor of the setting may have a crucial role to play in their implementation. Various writers on mental handicap and other services have commented on the central role of the supervisor or manager. Raynes et al.'s (1979) view of the role of the supervisor as an important delegator of authority, enabling direct care staff to take responsibility for important decisions concerning clients, was discussed in the introduction to this chapter. Hart and Risley (1976) see the supervisor of a setting as the key person in defining and implementing the goals of the setting. The supervisor is the agent through whom external standards, set by parents, administrators or other persons from the world at large, are mediated to the staff of the setting. Along with Boles and Bible (1978), Hart and Risley regard supervisors as responsible for "quality control" within the setting, identifying areas which need improving and defining criteria for measuring the services success.

These theoretical discussions on the influence of the supervisor on the practices of a work setting have been supported by informal observations in the course of the five studies reported in this chapter. The frequency and quality of feedback which supervisors gave to staff on their use of new methods of working appeared to be a very significant influence, but others may be equally important. To the extent to which the supervisor has authority within the service, he or she can also control other factors which may influence the adoption of new procedures. For example, if supervisors of a setting have some control over the resources it receives, they can play a part in ensuring that materials needed for leisure or self-care activities are to hand. They can also, of course, exert an influence on the availability of staff to carry out these new routines and on the scheduling and siting of other activities on the ward which might conflict with the new procedures. Finally, they can be in a position to be a powerful model for other care staff, which may also determine whether or not changes in working practices take root.

One or two studies of the role of the supervisor in service settings have examined these issues with more adequate experimental control. In a study by Wallace et al. (1973), procedures for running leisure activities for psychiatric hospital residents were introduced in response to repeated requests from front-line staff. However, a variety of interventions failed to increase the staff's use of these procedures and only when the ward charge nurse was observed working with clients on the scheduled leisure activities did attendance by regular staff increase. Thus the active participation of supervisory staff in new routines may contribute greatly to their adoption by direct care workers. The importance of the supervisor as a source of feedback to care staff has been demonstrated in many studies, but only recently had the logical development of this been documented in the research literature. Page, Iwata and Reid (1982) examined the effects of a training programme for supervisors on the behaviour of care staff and clients. Three supervisors were trained to give staff appropriate feedback on their use of teaching techniques with profoundly handicapped children. This training led to increases in the appropriate teaching behaviour of forty-five direct care staff. Given the saving in professional time in training three supervisors as opposed to fifteen times as many direct care staff, there seems to be a strong case for research on the development of staff behaviour through direct interventions with the staff's supervisors.

The work described in this chapter, coupled with that which has appeared from other sources since it was carried out, suggests that future research in staff training in mental handicap services should concentrate on developing two aspects of such organisations. The first is the involvement of all levels of staff and wherever possible clients and/or their families in defining priorities for service development and, by implication, the procedures in which staff are trained. This strategy has been advocated by writers on organisational change (e.g. Twain, 1983; and Stolz, 1981), reviewing factors influencing the uptake of research findings who concluded that it improved the chances of an innovation taking root in a setting. Similar approaches to the implementation of change in a psychiatric hospital and in a variety of schools have been described by Towell and Harris (1979) and Burden (1981) respectively but the applicability of the strategy to mental handicap services has as yet hardly been explored.

The second area is the role of the "front-line manager" in training initiatives resulting from any such collaborative exercise. The front-line manager is ideally placed to take over the organisational and facilitative role adopted by researchers in most experimental studies of staff training. For supervisory staff to take on this role, they would require training in the following activities.

a) encouraging service consumers, i.e. clients or their families, to collaborate with them in service development;

b) encouraging all care staff to collaborate in this process of service development;

c) monitoring and evaluating their services;

d) identifying priority areas for service development in collaboration with staff and service consumers;

e) drawing up new procedures in collaboration with

staff and service consumers for staff in those areas;

f) providing staff with feedback on their performance of these new procedures;

g) monitoring and evaluating these innovations through a combination of direct observation of staff and client behaviour, examination of service records and regular consultation with both staff and services consumers.

A first step towards such an approach has been made in the form of a manual for front-line managers which describes this process (Porterfield, Evans and Blunden, 1983). The intention is that this manual should be used as a "service development package" and evaluated in a wide range of settings.

The programme of research reported in this chapter has been suggestive rather than conclusive. However, when its findings are considered along with the results of other work in this field, which has examined mental handicap services from the perspective of both behaviouristic and sociological accounts of their functioning, a relatively coherent picture emerges. Organisational behaviour management strategies, such as written procedural guides and feedback on performance, are effective in changing the behaviour of staff in these settings. Ensuring that staff of all levels are involved in taking responsible decisions about their own job functions and the management of clients is associated with a better quality of staff-client interactions. Therefore a strategy has been proposed where the decisions on new procedures and methods of managing them and monitoring their impact are actually formulated between supervisors, direct care staff, clients and their families. Fifteen years of research on producing changes in tightly defined direct care staff behaviours have brought us to the point where the relative impact of different methods is now largely determined.

The challenge now is to discover the best means of involving direct care staff, their supervisors, clients and their families in developing these methods so as to produce appropriate and durable improvements in services for mentally handicapped people.

References

Albuquerque-Williams, L. and Martin, G. (1979) 'Self-recording Training to Improve Effective Use of Temporary Summer Staff Institutions for the Developmentally Disabled: A Demonstration Project', Journal of Practical Approaches to Developmental Handicap, 3, 18-22

Ayllon, T. Layman, D. and Kandel, H.J. (1975) 'A Behavioural-educational Alternative to Drug Control of Hyperactive Children', Journal of Applied Behavior Analysis, 8 137-146

Ayllon, T. and Roberts, M.D. (1974) 'Eliminating Discipline Problems by Strengthening Academic Performance', Journal of Applied Behavior Analysis, 7, 71-76

Ayllon, T. and Wright, P. (1972) 'New Roles for the Paraprofessional' in S. W. Bijou and E. Ribes-Inesta (eds.), Behavior Modification: Issues and Extentions, Academic Press, New York

Blatt, B. (1967) Christmas in Purgatory : A Photographic Essay on Mental Retardation, Allyn and Bacon, Boston

Boles, S.M. and Bible, G.H. (1978) 'The Student Service Index: A Method for Managing Service Delivery in Residential Settings' in M. S. Berkler, G.H. Bible, S.M. Boles, D.E.D. Dietz and A.C. Repp (eds.), Current Trends for the Developmentally Disabled, University Park Press, Baltimore

Bruininks, R.M., Kudla, M.J., Wieck, C. A. and Hauber, F.A. (1981) 'Management Problems in Community Residential Facilities', Mental Retardation, 18, 125-130

Burden, R.L. (1981) 'The Educational Psychologist as Instigator and Agent of Change in Schools: Some Guidelines for Successful Practice' in I. McPherson and A. Sutton (eds.), Reconstructing Psychological Practice, Croom Helm, London

Burg, M.M., Reid, D.H. and Lattimore, J. (1979) 'Use of a Self-recording and Supervision Programme to Change Institutional Staff

Behavior', Journal of Applied Behavior Analysis, 12, 363-375

Burgio, L.D., Whitman, T.L. and Reid, D.H. (1983) 'A Participative Management Approach for Improving Direct Care Staff Performance in an Institutional Setting', Journal of Applied Behavior Analysis, 6, 37-53

Cataldo, M.F. and Risley, T.R. (1974) Evaluation of Living Environments; The MANIFEST Description of Ward Activities' in P.O. Davidson, F.W. Clark and L.A. Hamerlynck (eds.), Evaluation of Behavioural Programs in Community, Residential and School Settings', Research Press, Champaign, Illinois

Cohen, J. (1960) 'A Coefficient of Agreement for Nominal Scales', Educational and Psychological Measurement, 20, 27-46

Coles, E. and Blunden, R. (1979), The Establishment and Maintenance of a Ward-Based Activity Period Within a Mental Handicap Hospital, Mental Handicap in Wales - Applied Research Unit Research Report No. 8, Cardiff

Coles, E. and Blunden, R. (1981) 'Maintaining New Procedures Using Feedback to Staff, a Hierarchical Reporting System, and a Multidisciplinary Management Group', Journal of Organizational Behavior Management, 3, 19-33

Davey, G. (1981) 'Behaviour Modification in Organisations' in G. Davey (eds.), Applications of Conditioning Theory, Methuen, London

Department of Health and Social Security. (1969) Report of the Committee of Inquiry into Allegations of Ill-Treatment of Patients and other Irregularities of the Ely Hospital, Cardiff, Chairman: Mr. Geoffrey Howe Q. C. (Cmnd 3975), HMSO, London

Department of Health and Social Security and Welsh Office. (1971) Better Services for the Mentally Handicapped, (Cmnd, 4683), HMSO, London

Fielding, L.T., Erickson, E. and Bettin, B. (1971) 'Modification of Staff Behavior: A Brief Report',

Behavior Therapy, 2, 550-553

Gardner, J.M. (1971) 'Behavior Modification in Mental Retardation: A Review of Research and Analysis of Trends' in R.D. Rubin, H. Fensterheim, A.A. Lazarus and C.M. Franks (eds.), Advances in Behavior Therapy, Academic Press, New York

Gardner, W.I. (1971) Behavior Modification in Mental Retardation, Aldine, Chicago

Goffman, E. (1961) Asylums: Essays on the Social Situation of Mental Patients and Other Inmates, Doubleday, New York

Greene, B.F. Willis, B.S., Levy R., and Bailey, J. S. (1978) 'Measuring Client Gains from a Staff-implemented Program', Journal of Applied Behavior Analysis, 11, 395-412

Hall, R.H. (1967) 'Some Organizational Considerations in the Professional-organizational Relationship', Administrative Science Quarterly, 12, 461-478

Hart, B.M. and Risley, T.R. (1976) 'Environmental Programming: Implications for the Severely Handicapped' in H.J. Prehm and S.J. Deitz (eds.), Early Intervention for the Severely Handicapped: Programming and Accountability, Severely Handicapped Learner Program Monograph No. 2, University of Oregon

Hemming, H., Lavender, T. and Pill, R. (1981) 'Quality of Life of Mentally Retarded Adults Transferred from Large Institutions to New Small Units', American Journal of Mental Deficiency, 86, 157-169

Hollenbeck, A.R. (1978) 'Problems of Reliability in Observational Research' in G.P. Sackett (ed.), Observing Behavior Vol. 2: Data Collection and Analysis Methods, University Park Press, Baltimore

Hope, R. (1977) Behaviour Assessment Record, Unpublished manuscript, Department of Psychology, Lea Hospital, Bromsgrove, Worcestershire

Horner, R.D. (1980) 'The Effects of an Environmental "Enrichment" Program on the Behavior of Institutionalized Profoundly Retarded Children', Journal of Applied Behavior Analysis, 13, 473-491

Hutchison, J.M., Jarman, P.H. and Bailey, J.S. (1980) 'Public Posting with a Habilitation Team: Effects on Attendance and Performance', Journal of Organizational Behavior Management, 4, 57-70

Iwata, B.A. Dorsey, M.F., Slifer, K.J., Bauman, K.E. and Richman, G.A. (1982) 'Towards a Functional Analysis of Self-injury', Analysis and Intervention in Developmental Disability, 2, 3-20

Jones, A.A., Evans, G. and Blunden, R. (1982) Evaluation of a Method of Encouraging Skill Usage Among Mentally Handicapped People in a Hospital Setting, Mental Handicap in Wales - Applied Research Unit, Research Report No. 14, Cardiff

Jones. A.A., Evans, G. and Blunden, R. (1984) 'Introducing a General Prompting and Recording System: Its Effect on Client and Staff Behavior in an Institutional Ward', Applied Research in Mental Retardation, 5, 125-136

Jones, K., Brown, J., Cunningham W.J., Roberts, J. and Williams, P. (1975) Opening the Door: A Study of New Policies for the Mentally Handicapped, Routledge and Kegan Paul, London

Kazdin, A.E. (1973) 'Issues in Behavior Modification with Mentally Retarded Persons', American Journal of Mental Deficiency, 78, 134-140

King, R.D., Raynes, N.V. and Tizard, J. (1971) Patterns of Residential Care: Sociological Studies in Institutions for Handicapped Children, Routledge and Kegan Paul, London

Kissel, R.C., Whitman, T.L. and Reid, D.H. (1983) 'An Institutional Staff Training and Self-management Program for Developing Multiple-Self-care Skills in Severely/profoundly Retarded Individuals', Journal of Applied Behavior Analysis, 16, 395-415

Kreitner, R., Reif, W.E. and Morris, M. (1977) 'Measuring the Impact of Feedback upon the

Performance of Mental Health Technicians', Journal of Organizational Behavior Management, 1, 105-109

Kushlick, A. (1975) 'Improving the Services for the Mentally Handicapped' in C.C. Kiernan and P. Woodford (eds.), Behaviour Modification with the Severely Retarded, Associated Scientific Publishers, Amsterdam

Kushlick, A., Blunden, R. and Cox, G. (1973) 'A Method of Rating Behaviour Characteristics for Use in Large Scale Surveys of Mental Handicap', Psychological Medicine, 3, 466-478

Matlock, B.L. and Adams, G. (1978) 'A Component Analysis of Staff Training', Boulder Behaviorist, 6, 7-8

McCormick, M., Balla, D. and Zigler, E. (1975) 'Resident-care Practices in Institutions for Retarded Persons: A Cross-Institutional, Cross-cultural Study', American Journal of Mental Deficiency, 80, 1-7

Miller, R. and Lewin, L.M. (1980) 'Training and Management of the Psychiatric Aide: A Critical Review', Journal of Organizational Behavior Management, 2, 295-315

Milne, D. (1982) 'A Comparison of Two Methods of Teaching Behaviour Modification to Mental Handicap Nurses', Behavioural Psychotherapy, 10, 54-64

Morris, P. (1969) Put Away: A Sociological Study of Institutions for the Mentally Retarded, Routedge and Kegan Paul, London

National Development Group for the Mentally Handicapped (1976) Mental Handicap: Planning Together, DHSS, London

National Development Group for the Mentally Handicapped (1978) Helping Mentally Handicapped People in Hospital, DHSS, London

National Development Group for Mentally Handicapped People (1980) Improving the Quality of Services for Mentally Handicapped People, DHSS, London

Nelson, R.O. and Hayes, S.C. (1981) 'Theoretical Explanations of Reactivity in Self-monitoring', Behavior Modification, 5, 3-14

O'Brien M., Porterfield, J., Herbert-Jackson, E. and Risley, T.R. (1979) The Toddler Center: A Practical Guide to Day Care for One- and Two-Year Olds, University Park Press, Baltimore

Page, T.J., Iwata, B.A. and Reid, D.H. (1982) 'Pyramidal Training: A Large Scale Application with Institutional Staff', Journal of Applied Behavior Analysis, 15, 335-351

Panyan, M., Boozer, H. and Morris, M. (1970) 'Feedback to Attendants as a Reinforcer for Applying Operant Techniques', Journal of Applied Behavior Analysis, 3, 1-4

Paulson, S.R. (1974) 'Causal Analysis of Inter-organizational Relations: An Axiomatic Theory Revisited', Administrative Science Quarterly, 19, 319-337

Porterfield, J., Blunden, R. and Blewitt, E. (1980) 'Improving Environments for Mentally Handicapped Adults Using Prompts and Social Attention to Maintain High Group Engagement', Behavior Modification, 4, 225-241

Porterfield, J., Evans, G. and Blunden, R. (1981) The Client Behaviour Measure and Staff Behaviour Measure: Manual for Time-sampling Procedures, Mental Handicap in Wales Research Unit, Cardiff

Porterfield, J., Evans, G. and Blunden, R. (1982) Improving Mental Handicap Services: Involving Clients' Families and Staff in Selecting Areas for Service Development, Mental Handicap in Wales Applied Research Unit, Research Report No. 13, Cardiff

Porterfield, J., Evans, G. and Blunden, R. (1983) Working Together for Change: A Service Manager's Guide to Involving Staff and Families in Service Improvement, Mental Handicap in Wales Applied Research Unit, Cardiff

Pratt, M.W., Luszcz, M.A. and Brown, M.E. (1982) 'Measuring Dimensions of the Quality of Care in

Small Community Residences', American Journal of Mental Deficiency, 85, 188-194

Prue, D.M., Krapfl, J.E., Noah, J.C., Cannon, S. and Maley, R.F. (1980) 'Managing the Treatment Activities of State Hospital Staff', Journal of Organizational Behavior Management, 2, 165-181

Quilitch, H.R. (1975) 'A Comparison of Three Staff-Management Procedures', Journal of Applied Behavior Analysis, 8, 59-66

Raynes, N.V., Pratt, M.W. and Roses, S. (1979). Organisational Structure and the Care of the Mentally Retarded, Croom Helm, London

Repp, A.C., and Dietz, D.E.D. (1979) 'Improving Administrative-related Behaviors at a State Institution', Mental Retardation, 17, 185-192

Risley, T.R. and Cataldo, M.F. (1974) Evaluation of Planned Activities: The PLC-Check Measure of Classroom Participation, Center for Applied Analysis, Kansas

Skinner, B.F. (1953) Science and Human Behavior, The Free Press, New York

Skinner, B.F. (1972) 'Compassion and Ethics in the Care of the Retarded' in B.F. Skinner (eds.), Cumulative Record : A Selection of Papers Appleton-Century-Crofts, New York

Stolz, S.B. (1981) 'Adoptions of Innovations from Applied Behavioural Research: "Does Anybody Care?"', Journal of Applied Behavior Analysis, 14, 491-505

Towell, D. (1982) 'Developing Mental Handicap Services. Part 2 : Generating a County-wide Programme of Informed Change', Hospital and Health Services Review, (February), 40-44

Towell, D. and Harries, C. (1979) Innovation in Patient Care, Croom Helm, London

Twain, D. (1983) Creating Change in Social Settings, Praegar, New York

Tyne A. and Wertheimer, A. (1980) Even Better

Services? Review of mental handicap policies in the 1970s, Campaign for Mentally Handicapped People, London

Wallace, C.J., Davis, J.R., Liberman, R.P. and Baker, V. (1973) 'Modelling and Staff Behavior', *Journal of Consulting and Clinical Psychology*, *41*, 422-425

Welsch, W.V., Ludwig, C., Radiker, J.E. and Krapfl, J.E. (1973) 'Effects of Feedback on Daily Completion of Behavior Modification Projects', *Mental Retardation*, *10*, 24-26

Woods, P. and Cullen, C. (1983) 'Determinants of Staff Behaviour in Long-term Care', *Behavioural Psychotherapy*, *11*, 4-18

PART III: TRAINING IN SPECIFIC SETTINGS

Chapter Seven

TRAINING SOCIAL SERVICE STAFF FOR FIELDWORK SETTINGS INVOLVING PEOPLE WITH MENTAL HANDICAP

Chris Kiernan

Introduction

With the gradual realisation of the ideal of providing care in the community, Social Services Departments in Local Authorities have an increasing role. Their responsibility takes into account the needs of both the individual with mental handicap and also his or her family. The still dominant philosophy of genericism of social work in the U.K. argues powerfully for a range of problems and issues which arise in family units to be dealt with by one social worker, rather than the family being fragmented, each representing a problem which has to be dealt with by a specialist.

In this chapter we will explore some of the issues in training social work staff within the context of a study completed in a London Borough in the late 1970s. Without a doubt some of the problems which emerged in that study have, by now, been ameliorated. In addition some of the emerging problems may have been greater in that Authority than in others. Our purpose is to draw attention to issues rather than to quantify their impact.

The Study

The study was ambitious aiming to survey the needs of families and of children and young people (up to age 20) with handicapping conditions, and then to work with the Local Authority in developing suitable services. The survey covered mental handicap, physical handicap and sensory deficits. The follow-up service developments covered mainly mental handicap in the form of a Home Intervention Scheme

(HINTS) and the development of residential provision for 16 children and young people with mental handicap. In this chapter we will discuss only the results of the studies as they affect provision of services for individuals with mental handicap and their families. This is, however, an artificial distinction for fieldworkers since their responsibilities covered all handicaps, giving them both problems of being aware of a range of needs but of prioritising amongst relevant groups.

The Local Authority in which the study was located was organised in a fairly typical way. The Social Services Department (SSD) was headed by a Director with four divisions, Fieldwork, Residential and Day Care, Central Administration and Research, Development and Training, each being led by an Assistant Director or, in the case of Research, Development and Training, by the Deputy Director. Below the Assistant Director level were principal assistants, heads of homes and area officers and fieldwork teams. These divisions immediately created problems of organisation of services for people with handicaps since the separation in management terms of Residential and Day Care and Fieldwork led to the organisation effecting little collaboration or contact at the grass roots level. Problems of contact were not eased by the fact that the Authorities' policy was to employ as many qualified social workers on the Fieldwork side as possible. This meant that Fieldwork social workers were better qualified and paid than their peers in the Residential and Day Care division. There was no joint training and little opportunity to interact because of physical location and low frequency of formal case conferences or the like.

In 1976, six half-time specialist social workers were appointed to Area teams and, subsequently, half-time specialists were attached to each of the Authority's five special schools. The appointments ran counter to a strong genericist bias in the Authority. The majority of social workers in the Authority were understood to be against a policy of appointing specialists since it was felt that this would lead back to the years before the reorganisation of social work services in the 1970s, when a family could have input from several social workers, each dealing with one aspect of the problems of a family. The generic viewpoint argues, at its extreme, that specialist training is not necessary since social work with people with handicaps requires only the application of social work principles to their cases.

Partly against this background the appointments were of individuals who would be specialist in terms of case load rather than in terms of background training. Of the first ten appointments made, only three had relevant training and three had no prior experience with relevant groups of clients. Specialists were appointment to Area teams at a basic grade but were nonetheless seen as key individuals acting as a resource to teams. In other words, they might have little or no experience with handicapped people, little authority in the team, but be expected to advise and take responsibility if required. The place of specialist social work in special schools was also ambiguous. From interviews with the social workers themselves and heads of schools it emerged that idiosyncratic patterns of working were developed depending on the skills and background of social workers, their perception of their role and the way in which the schools and heads saw their role. One social worker reviewed all children in the school, identified all of the families who had social work input and then ensured that the remainder were allocated such support if necessary. She then liaised across agencies, organising information from several sources, and gathered and disseminated information on services and benefits as well as doing individual and group work with parents. Another construed her role as advising parents on practical and emotional problems. In this case there was an overlap with the head teacher who had previously counselled and guided parents.

Despite these problems the scheme appeared to meet its main aim. In 1974 a survey completed by the Authority development officer showed that, of a sample of 66 families of pupils attending special schools, only 18 (27.3 per cent) had had visits from a social worker in the preceding year. By 1978, when we surveyed families, the proportion had risen to 60.34 per cent. This rise was not accounted for solely by increased visiting by specialist social workers but does suggest a general trend in line with stated aims.

During the period over which the project ran a District Mental Handicap Team was set up. A social worker was appointed to the team but she was not employed through Social Services funding and was, as a consequence, independent of Social Services management. The development of the Team was not helped by a difference between the boundaries of the Local Authority and the Health District.

This account raises a number of critical general issues in training of staff in social service settings. The absence of a common background of training of residential, day care and fieldwork staff was exacerbated in the setting in which the study was done by the emphasis on appointing well qualified staff in Fieldwork. The genericist emphasis in the Authority led to specialist social workers being appointed in terms of case load rather than training. A brief survey of training courses for social workers, done in 1978, showed that there was great variation in input on handicap on courses for the Certificate for Qualification in Social Work. Some courses had units devoted to handicap, others had little or no coverage, arguing the pure genericist position. This, and the emphasis on covering several categories of handicap given to the Area team appointments, would mean that if additional in-service training was seen as desirable it would need to be very extensive in its coverage and available on a modular basis. However, before such training could be justified, the basic genericist argument would need to be overcome.

Other training issues were raised by the study. Specialists were expected to work either as consultants or as change-agents within their area teams or schools. This points to a clear need for training in relevant intervention techniques. In practice, the specialists within the Authority met together regularly as a group to discuss issues of common interest, including difficulties they were experiencing in intervening effectively. However no formal in-service training was provided.

The provision of extensive local in-service training has to be taken in the context of a possibly high turnover of staff. In the area which we investigated the 11 posts were filled by 18 social workers in a three year period. Clearly a heavy investment in in-service training may not be economical if turnover is to be as high as this.

What are the Tasks?

The tasks of social workers in fieldwork settings can

be roughly grouped into those concerned with family support and intervention, including advice on benefits and allowances, and those concerned with helping the family to liaise with other components of social service provision and other agencies.

In our study we placed particular emphasis on the support and intervention role of social workers. During the 1970s there was a great increase in the emphasis on the role of parents as educators of their handicapped offspring. By 1975 there were a substantial number of models available in the research literature but few examples of projects embedded in service settings (Kiernan and Woodford, 1975). The study was informed by this position. It was argued that, since fieldworkers had access to families and broad responsibilities, they were ideally placed to undertake intervention as one aspect of a broader role with the family.

Home Intervention Scheme (HINTS)

The Home Intervention Scheme (HINTS) was set up by the research team as part of the overall study. It was the primary responsibility of two research officers, SD and GH. The basic aim of the scheme was to run a Portage-style intervention with field social workers intervening in families (Shearer and Shearer, 1972). The philosophy adopted was that parent training could provide help through the direct amelioration of problems, for example in assistance with toilet-training and other self-help skills, but that it could also provide indirect help. It was felt that the achievement of such goals as improvement of overall relationships between the handicapped child and parents, acceptance of the child by his parents, and improvement of relationships between the handicapped child and siblings, could also be facilitated by intervention directed at change in the handicapped child's behaviour. In these cases the client to whom the intervention was directed might be the parent or sibling, the achievement of educationally relevant goals being either secondary or immaterial.

The approach represents a shift of emphasis away from the concept of parents as ancillary educators which is often embodied in home teaching programmes (e.g. Cunningham, 1975). This shift is seen as appropriate for a number of reasons. First and foremost, social services personnel are responsible for aspects of counselling and care of families and individuals as clients. The study explored the feasibility of employing child management techniques in the service of social work goals rather than educational goals. Second, it can be argued that the education of the handicapped child and young person is the responsibility of the Education authorities, this responsibility extending to the specification, if necessary with the parents, of overall educational goals. With the improvement in educational provision it may be suggested that the parent role can be described as involvement in the child's education to the extent that the parent is willing and able, rather than as a necessary element. Finally, the concept of parents as ancillary educators, is, in some schemes, taken to imply that parent trainers should confine themselves strictly to advising on educational matters (Smith, Kushlick and Glossop, 1977). Aspects of parent-child interaction, or broader questions concerning family functioning, are seen as irrelevant to the trainer-parent interaction. At the extreme, parents may be 'rewarded' for successful completion of teaching assignments by being allowed to discuss non-educational issues for fixed, brief, periods of time, or trainers are advised to refer all non-educational issues to other agencies. This model is appropriate to settings where it was initially developed in which the trainers had either no professional training or where their training was not relevant to either teaching or social work tasks (Shearer and Shearer, 1972). Strict application of the model with trained social services or health personnel is likely to be professionally unacceptable because such personnel would construe their role as broader than simply parent training. Since training covers several relevant areas of family functioning, restriction would seem to have little justification. In our case, working with such personnel, we were at pains to define the role of the home teacher as integrating educational with other professional skills.

The Home Intervention Scheme Outline

In this section we will outline the development of HINTS from its inception in 1978 to 1980. In subsequent sections we will describe in detail the personnel who participated, the families, the training programmes pursued, with indication of outcome, and the final evaluation.

The Home Intervention Scheme (HINTS) was included as part of the project as a home teaching scheme involving only specialist social workers. The scheme began in September 1978 with three volunteer specialist field social workers. They were given a six session training course in the use of behavioural techniques. The course was integrated with assessment and development of intervention programmes with three families of severely mentally handicapped children. The scheme utilised the Portage project materials (Bluma, Shearer, Frohman and Hilliard, 1976), and followed the Portage pattern in requiring weekly visits to parents and weekly meetings with a research officer, (a clinical psychologist, SD), with whom they discussed the evolution of programmes. Initial assessments and activity charts, recording details of daily sessions, were kept by some parents. Details of weekly meetings reporting progress on target behaviours and events within the families, were recorded at each meeting by the HINTS Organiser.

The initial project ran for a period of nine months. The main project began in September 1979 and ran through until August 1980. Seventeen social services personnel and one specialist health visitor were involved in the main project. The pattern of initial training, integrated with weekly visits to parents of handicapped children, was repeated. Although two patterns of social worker training, one intensive (three or four days), and one extended over six weeks, were offered, none of the personnel trained on the intensive course joined the scheme without requesting further training on the extended course. During the main phase of HINTS five groups were run each week in order to allow adequate consultation. We continued to utilise the Portage materials, but these were complemented by other sources of ideas, advice and guidance in order to offset perceived short-comings. In particular, it was necessary to complement the early stage of the language section and to provide further breakdown and more teaching suggestions, to cope with individual needs. These sources included books from the Human Horizons series and other materials devised for parent use in the U.K. (e.g. Cunningham and Sloper, 1978; Jeffree and McConkey, 1976; Jeffree, McConkey and Hewson, 1979; Kiernan, Jordan and Saunders, 1978). Groups were served by three research officers. One, a trained social worker, attended all meetings. The two others, both psychologists, each attended one or two of the groups each week.

Outcome was assessed through a variety of measures derived from the intervention and from the groups themselves. Initial assessments and activity charts, recording details of daily sessions were kept by some parents. Details of weekly meetings reporting progress on target behaviours and events within the families were recorded by the HINTS organisers. In addition, home teachers and parents of children and young people involved in both the initial and the main schemes were interviewed at the end of the intervention in July and August 1980. The parent interview was a modified version of a Family Interview used at the beginning of the project to assess the individual within the family. Our aims in doing the parent interviews were to assess the degree to which the HINTS children were representative of children and young people with severe mental handicap in the Authority, to gain a picture of the impact of overall changes in the services from the time at which initial interviews were conducted, and to evaluate the impact of the HINTS on the families. All interviews were conducted by research officers who were independent of the HINTS group. Finally, psychological tests were employed with the children and young people in the initial and main study in order to provide additional descriptive information on the sample.

The Training Courses

Analysis of the pattern of qualifications of specialist social workers suggested the need for two in-service training courses.

Course A was entitled 'The Handicapped Person in the Family'. The course began with an introduction to the research project and discussion of the definition of handicap and local statistics on handicap. This session was followed by a discussion of pre-school and school age experiences and problems, with exploration of the implications of these data for counselling and services. The course continued with discussion of methods of intervention, including parent groups, with special reference to mobility, self-help, communication and social behaviour. The views and problems of brothers and sisters of the handicapped siblings were discussed in the context of survey data from the project. Sexual development and post-school occupation and residential provision were covered, with concluding sessions on the welfare rights of families and discussion of the course with the group.

Course A was always provided as an in-service course within a week. From December 1978 courses lasting four days, Monday, Tuesday, Thursday and Friday, each day comprising two sessions, 10.00 am to 1.00 pm, 2.00 to 4.00pm, were offered. This was subsequently reduced to three days, Monday, Tuesday and Wednesday within a week. In all 13 courses were run.

Course size was restricted to eight to ten participants in order to allow for discussion. In practice, non-attendance was common. Of the total of 117 individuals signing up for courses only 73 attended (62.4 per cent). Of these, 26 failed to attend at least one day of the course. The commonest reason given was court attendance, followed by other crisis events. Consultation with Training Officers in the SSD suggested that the high rate of no-show for the courses was comparable with their previous experience. An overall estimate of 40 per cent no-show was made by them. We did not follow up non-attenders systematically, but such follow-up as was made gave staff absences and clients' crises as the main reasons for non-attendance.

On the 73 individuals attending A courses, 29 were field social workers, one, a senior social worker, and one an assistant social worker (42.5 per cent). The largest other groups attending were from residential facilities for the handicapped people (23, 31.5 per cent). Of these, 17 people were from a facility for mentally handicapped children which was linked to the project. The remaining personnel were recruited from day centres for handicapped people, or centres where there were individual handicapped children, (13, 17.8 per cent), and from fostering or medical social work services.

Course B covered discussion of a broadly educational or behavioural approach to mental handicap, means of assessment, intervention in terms of self-help skills, play and communication, and methods of dealing with problem behaviour. Basic behavioural principals of goal setting, establishment of teaching settings, and the use of prompting and reinforcement were illustrated within presentations and in pre-scripted role play settings in which, typically, the course presenters acted as the mentally handicapped individual and the participant as teacher. These examples were video-recorded and the play-back used as a basis for discussion. Course notes were provided to participants. These notes covered the specific topic areas outlined above and also discussions of techniques of behaviour change. In addition the Portage Guide to Home Teaching and the Portage Guide to Early Education Manual and Materials (Bluma, Shearer, Frohman and Hilliard, 1976) were made available along with Human Horizon series texts for parents.

Two types of B course were developed, the Intensive and the Extended. As already indicated, the content of the courses was identical in terms of presentation of concepts, examples and role play. The two forms differed in that the Intensive courses were spread initially over four working days, Monday, Tuesday, Thursday and Friday, with two sessions per day, 10.00 am to 1.00pm and 2.00pm to 4.00pm, and subsequently over three days, Monday to Wednesday, whereas Extended courses were spread over six weekly, three hour sessions.

Participants in Intensive courses had no contact with mentally handicapped individuals during the course. In fact, only 49.4 per cent of the participants had contact with mentally handicapped clients as part of their current work experience. On the other hand, participants in the Extended courses had regular weekly contacts with families. If Extended course participants did not have clients on their case loads, i.e. 55.9 per cent of participants, they were provided with such clients in order to take part in the scheme.

In all, 111 individuals attended the Intensive course and 21 the Extended courses. Of this latter group 11 individuals attended **both** the Intensive and Extensive courses. Overall, 50 (41.2 per cent), of the individuals attending were qualified social workers, four were seniors and ten assistant social workers. The largest other group was employed in residential work with the mentally handicapped people (32, 26.4 per cent). The remaining 25 participants came from day care for the mentally handicapped people, fostering, occupational therapy and medical social work.

The 11 individuals who were involved in the Intensive course and who opted to join the HINTS scheme all requested additional training in the form of the Extended course in the build-up of their HINTS involvement. All expressed the opinion that they would not be able to work with families on the basis of the Intensive course. This view is also reflected by the fact that none of the Intensive course participants who did not switch to HINTS, none reported having adopted techniques described on the course when surveyed in follow-up. We would suggest from these results that the Extended version of the course, with its discussion of interventions which were being developed, is viable as an in-service basis for introduction of the use of behavioural techniques whereas the Intensive course, as presented, does not provide such as basis.

The interpretation of these data needs to be taken in context of the practicalities of the case loads and working situations of participants. As already noted, only around half of the participants in the courses had any current professional contact with mentally handicapped individuals and, of these, a majority of clients were not believed to be in need of intervention.

The Home Teachers

In the two years of the project, 21 personnel joined the HINTS group. In the pilot project all three social workers were specialists. Eighteen people took part in the main study. Of this group three were appointed as specialist social workers for handicapped people, one a specialist social worker for adoption, four field social workers attached to Area teams and one an assistant social worker. In addition, one was a specialist health visitor, one a peripatetic house mother, and one a play organiser for handicapped children. Six participants were residential social workers from the facility for mentally handicapped children. Of these, one worker dropped out of the scheme before becoming involved with a family.

A clear routine was followed prior to recruitment to the HINTS group. After an initial approach from the potential home teacher, the organiser visited the relevant Senior Social Worker within the worker's Area team or the equivalent manager. The purpose, framework, workload and pattern of involvement was described and discussed in these meetings. This contact was necessitated since HINTS organisers were to some degree in a management role which could have conflicted with established frameworks in field and residential work.

In the evaluation interview at the end of the project, the 18 main project Home Teachers were asked to say why they had decided to take part in the scheme. Fifteen of the 18 respondents saw the approach as offering more relevant help to families. Eleven said that they had reasons related to professional development. Four had personal reasons, including a belief that parents should be more involved in their child's education (3), and an interest in behaviourally oriented work (1).

Home teachers were asked whether they had experience with handicapped people before their involvement with HINTS. All 17 respondents to the question reported experience with mentally and physically handicapped children, 15 through their paid employment and eight through voluntary work. Eleven of the home teachers had also had contact with mentally handicapped adults and 11 with physically handicapped adults. Clearly, all the residential social workers had current direct contact with the mentally handicapped people, as did the relevant specialists. The field social workers varied in their case loading of mentally handicapped clients or their families from nil to 21 cases (median 6).

The Children and their Families

The reasons for selection of families for HINTS work were diverse. Only seven of the families were on case loads before the project. Five of the families were referred for HINTS work by other agencies, none being known to Area teams. However a further six families were known. Of these, two requested home teaching and the other three were believed to be interested in participating. In the other case the reason for referral was that a residential placement had broken down and it was believed that the family needed to learn to manage the child at home. A comparison of HINTS families with parallel families from the Family Interview sample will be provided later in this chapter.

The sex, ages, main diagnoses, estimated DQs and secondary problems of HINTS children are shown in Table 1. Thirteen of the children were girls, nine boys. Ages ranged from under a year at the beginning of the intervention to nearly 20 years. Eleven of the children attended school. Of these, nine attended schools for children with severe learning difficulties, one a school for pupils with mild learning difficulties and one a school for physically handicapped children. The remaining children were in contact with an assessment centre for pre-school children. The oldest client attended a social services day centre for mentally handicapped adults.

Table 2 provides further detail about the families of the children in terms of number of siblings, ethnic origin, first language of mother, occupations of fathers and mothers, if the father was living at home, and type of housing. It will be noted that nine of the families were from England, two of West Indian origin, four Asian, two Greek Cypriot, two Irish and one a mixed Spanish-Greek Cypriot and one an Irish-Sri Lankan couple. This high proportion of non-English families reflects the general position in the Local Authority area. This is also reflected by the fact that for seven of the mothers, English was not their first language.

Table 3 lists the number of additional problems experienced by the families and identified by the social workers at the beginning of the main project. The commonest reported were poor health of a family member other than the handicapped child or young person, and relationship problems between parents, for both married and unmarried couples.

The period of involvement with HINTS by home teachers ranged from 15 to 33 weeks (median 23 weeks). During this time they attended between 8 and 24 weekly group meetings (median 17 attendances). None of the home teachers who participated in the main project dropped out once intervention had been established. As already noted, one residential social worker began the scheme but dropped out without establishing contact with a family, withdrawing from the scheme as a result of a change in duties leading to a substantial increase in responsibility.

Table 4 shows the number of successful and

Table 1. Sex, date of birth, main and secondary diagnoses of children and young people in the pilot and main HINTS study.

Child number	Sex	Date of birth	Main diagnosis	Secondary handicap	IQ	Main or pilot study
1	F	22. 4.79	General developmental delay		[illegible]0	Main
2	M	28.11.78	General developmental delay		[illegible]0	Main
3	F	26. 8.78	Downs syndrome		[illegible]0	Main
4	F	4. 1.78	Downs syndrome	Heart and lung malfunction	[illegible]0	Main
5	M	1.12.76	Downs syndrome		53	Main
6	F	18.11.76	Downs syndrome	Myopic	54	Main
7	F	17.11.76	Downs syndrome		[illegible]5	Pilot
8	F	26. 5.76	Downs syndrome		–	Pilot
9	M	1. 9.75	Downs syndrome		–	Pilot
10	M	31. 5.75	Downs syndrome		–	Main
11	F	10.11.74	Brain damage	Epilepsy	[illegible]7	Main
12	F	8. 9.74	Brain damage	Autistic symptoms	[illegible]3	Main
13	M	10. 7.74	Brain damage	Multiple handicap	[illegible]3	Main
14	M	12.10.73	Neuro fibro matosis	Multiple handicap	[illegible]8	Main
15	M	30. 9.73	General developmental delay	Digestive tract	[illegible]7	Main
16	M	28. 8.73	Brain damage	Hyperactivity	–	Pilot
17	F	5. 9.72	Brain damage	Epilespy/hyperactivity	[illegible]5	Main
18	M	15. 7.72	Brain damage	Epilespy	[illegible]6	Main
19	M	8.10.70	Brain damage	Epilespy	[illegible]8	Main
20	F	13. 3.69	Cerebral palsy	ESN (M)	60	Main
21	F	5. 9.67	ESN (S)	Epilepsy	51	Main
22	F	3.11.59	Brain damage	Autistic symptons	50	Main

Table 2. Number of siblings, cultural group, mother's first language, parent occupations, father living at home and housing in pilot and main HINTS study.

Child number	No. of siblings	Cultural group	Mother's first language	Father's occupation	Mother's occupation	Father	Type of housing F-flat H-house	Main/ pilot
1	0	West Indian	English		None	No	F council rented	Main
2	4	West Indian	English		Office cleaner	No	H council rented	Main
3	1	English	English		None	No		Main
4	1	English	English		Waitress	No	F council rented	Main
5	1	Indian	other	Doctor (GP)	Doctor (GP)	Yes	H owner occupied	Main
6	0	Indian	other	Accounts asst.	None	Yes	H owner occupied	Main
7	2	Irish	English	Labourer	Clerk	Yes	H council rented	Pilot
8	2	English	English	GPO tech. Off.	None	Yes	F owner occupied	Pilot
9	2	Irish	English		Waitress	No	H council rented	Pilot
10	1	Greek Cypriot	other		None	No	H owner occupied	Main
11	1	English	English	L. T. cleaner	None	Yes	H council rented	Main
12	1	English	English	Biochemist	None	Yes	H council rented	Main
13	0	Span/GkCyp.	other	Hairdresser	None	Yes	H owner occupied	Main
14	2	English	English	Street cleaner	None	Yes	H council rented	Main
15	1	Indian	other	Shop owner	Shop assistant	Yes	H owner occupied	Main
16	0	English	English	L. T. foreman	None	Yes	F private rented	Pilot
17	2	Irish	English	Painter/Dec.	None	Yes	H council rented	Main
18	1	Greek Cypriot	other	Pasty cook	Dressmaker	Yes	H private rented	Main
19	2	English	English	Club steward	Barstaff	Yes	H private rented	Main
20	1	Indian	other	Ins. agent	None	Yes	H owner occupied	Main
21	4	Irish/SriLanka	English	Factory worker	Schl Meals ass	Yes	H owner occupied	Main
22	4	English	English	Book keeper	None	Yes	H owner occupied	Main

Table 3. Additional problems identified by social workers in HINTS main sample.

Child Number	Poor or unsuitable housing	Low income	Relationship problems between parents	Single parent	Lack of personal resources or knowledge	Lack of local facilities or services	Problems facing minority cultural groups	Poor health of family member other than N	Handicap of family member other than N	Difficulties experienced by other children in the family	Other specified in S.W. interviews.	Totals
1												3
2												5
3												0
4												7
5												3
6												4
10												7
11												4
12												5
13												3
14												2
15												3
17												3
18												4
19												3
20												1
21												7
22												7
Totals	5	8	12	4	8	6	8	10	2	7	3	73

Table 4. Successful and unsuccessful home visits, client discussed in HINTS group, by phone and individually.

Child No.	Home visits Succ	Unsucc.	Clients discussed in group	Consultations Phone	Ind	Total time per case Hrs	Mins
1	6	4	13	0	0	27	00
2	14	1	18	2	0	47	10
3	9	1	13	2	0	32	10
4	14	1	15	3	0	44	30
5	16	1	15	3	0	48	30
6	19	0	18	1	0	56	20
10	13	1	17	1	0	43	50
11	20	3	22	2	0	64	10
12	18	0	8	2	2	48	00
13	12	0	17	2	2	43	40
14	20	0	19	1	0	59	20
15	16*	0	14	0	2	48	00
18	23	0	18	0	1	65	00
19	19	1	18	1	2	58	20
20	12	0	12	2	2	38	40
21	17	1	12	1	0	46	50

*Two 'phone consultations were also made.

Successful home visit Travelling time	90 minutes 30 minutes	120 minutes
Case discussion Travel time	30 minutes 30 minutes	60 minutes
Unsuccessful visit (travel)	30 minutes	
Individual consultations Travel	30 minutes 30 minutes	60 minutes
Telephone	20 minutes	

unsuccessful home visits made by home teachers in the main project. The numbers of successful visits made ranged from 6 to 23 (median 15 visits) and or unsuccessful visits from 0 to 4. Of the 295 visits attempted 280, or 94.9 per cent, were sucessful. In addition to the visits made to family 15, the home teacher had two telephone consultations.

The third column in Table 4 shows the number of occasions on which the client was discussed in HINTS group meetings. Column four shows the number of telephone consultations with the HINTS organisers. Column five shows the number of face to face individual consultations outside HINTS groups. The number of case discussions in groups ranged from 8 to 24 with a median of 15 discussions (88.6 per cent), 24 telephone discussions, and 13 individual discussions.

The duration of visits and discussions was variable but could be estimated as around one and a half hours for a visit and 30 minutes per case discussion. If we assume an additional 30 minutes' travelling time for successful visits, unsuccessful visits, case discussions and individual consultations, and 20 minutes for a telephone consultation, we can compute the time spent per case. These data are given in Table 4 and will be discussed more fully in the results section. For the moment we can point out that the range of working hours involved per case is from 27 to 65 with a median at 47 hours 35 minutes.

In line with the overall approach of integrating HINTS work within a more general framework of social work goals, each home teacher was asked to specify both developmental goals for the child or young person and family goals.

Child related goals can be most conveniently described in the context of the programmes developed.

Several family goals were specified which could be classified under 14 headings. The commonest goal, given for seven of the 18 families, was to help the parent to allow the handicapped child greater independence. Three goals were given by five home teachers. These were to improve specific relationships within the families, to allow the parent to aid in the handicapped child's development, and to help parents to gain a more realistic view of the handicapped child's abilities. Four goals were selected for three families. These were to structure work already done by parents, to encourage more positive interactions between the parent and handicapped child, to relieve tensions caused by the parents' inability to deal with the handicapped child or young person, and to encourage the family as a whole to help the handicapped member rather than leaving the responsibility to the mother. Two goals were selected twice, to increase parental confidence in dealing with the handicapped child and to help focus the needs of the handicapped child in relation to siblings. Four further goals were selected once: a general improvement in parenting skills; an increase in parental enjoyment of the handicapped child; giving the handicapped individual skills necessary for hostel placement; to support and prepare the parent for separation.

On a rough classification, five of these goals may be said to be skill related (i.e. aiding development, increased parenting skills, structuring existing work, allowing the family to help, giving hostel placement skills). These cover 13 of the goals specified. The remaining 31 goals (70.4 per cent) relate to various aspects of the attitudes or beliefs of parents and other family members. These goals are in the main concerned with increasing the parents' confidence in their own abilities, those of the handicapped child, and their enjoyment of interaction with him or her.

Achievement of Goals

Programme success was assessed by the parent and home teacher. Successful completion of a programme was assessed on the home visit through the parent demonstrating new behaviour to the home teacher.

Table 5 shows the total activities set per child in the main programme, the total successful and total unsuccessful teaching programmes, a breakdown of type of task in context of the Portage checklist with behaviour management as an additional category, a listing of the number and percentage of programmes recorded, total and average professional time spent for each client on each successful programme.

Of the 413 tasks set, 359 were completed successfully (86.9 per cent). Percentage programmes completed ranged from 100 per cent (4 children) to 65.5 per

Table 5. Achievement of child-related goals.

Child No.	Total activities set	Total successful	Total unsuccessful	Infant stumulation	Socialisation	language	Self help	Cognitive	Motor	Behaviour management	Recorded	% recorded	Total professional time Hours/minutes	x time per successful programme Hours/minutes
1	2	2	0	-	-	-	1	1	-	-	0	0	[illegible]	[illegible]
2	30	29	1	-	4	9	4	5	8	-	0	0	47.10	1.38
3	22	21	1	-	-	2	7	11	2	-	6	27.3	32.10	1.32
4	6	7	1	-	-	-	5	-	3	-	4	50.0	44.30	6.21
5	27	25	2	-	1	1	14	7	4	-	0	0	48.50	1.56
6	40	37	3	-	4	15	4	4	13	-	11	27.5	56.20	1.31
10	11	11	0	-	-	6	5	-	-	-	0	0	43.50	4.0
11	17	15	2	-	-	2	0	2	-	4	4	23.5	64.10	4.17
12	10	10	0	-	-	1	2	3	3	1	4	40.0	46.40	4.40
13	6	6	0	-	1	-	4	-	1	-	2	33.3	43.30	7.17
14	29	19	10	12	-	-	13	-	4	-	13	44.8	59.20	3.27
15	25	23	2	-	2	7	6	7	2	1	11	440	48.00	2.5
17	27	24	3	-	4	4	1	6	5	7	20	74.0	52.30	2.11
18	44	34	10	7	-	-	36	-	1	-	34	77.3	65.00	1.55
19	32	27	5	4	-	3	18	3	4	-	5	15.6	58.50	2.10
20	20	19	1	-	2	-	8	10	-	-	4	20.0	38.40	2.2
21	44	36	8	-	-	-	14	24	2	4	37	84.1	53.20	1.29
22	19	14	5	-	-	-	10	4	-	5	6	31.6	46.50	3.21
Total	413	359	54	23	18	50	161	87	52	22	161	-	-	-
Median	23.5	19.0												
Mean	22.9	19.9												

cent, with a median percentage completed at just over 92 per cent.

Data on the mean amount of professional time spent per successful programme ranges between 78.9 and 115.8 hours (median 97.4 hours).

These two dependent variables, number of successfully completed programmes and professional time per successful programme, will be used as reference points for the remainder of this analysis. In addition, number of programmes attempted will be used as a dependent variable in some cases.

The commonest type of programme was in the self-help skill area (39.0 per cent of all programmes), followed by 'cognitive programmes' which included play activities (21.1 per cent). Motor and language programmes were employed in 12.6 and 12.1 per cent of cases. Programmes suitable for less able children, those in infant stimulation, were used for three children (5.6 per cent of all programmes). Programmes classed in the socialisation section were employed in only 18 instances (4.4 per cent). Finally, behaviour management programmes were employed with six of the children and in a total of 5.3 per cent of programmes. These programmes all dealt with relatively mild problem behaviours. In three instances they dealt with 'hyperactive' behaviour, the child being taught to remain on task, in two cases with toleration of having hair brushed and one of having hair washed. Two more substantial problems were approached. One, open masturbation, was dealt with in the home. The other, an incontinence problem, was tackled in the short-term care unit of the residential care facility.

All of the children and young people in the scheme were involved in at least one self-help skill programme. Thirteen children were involved in at least one cognitive programme and the same number of children in motor programmes. Ten were involved in language programmes.

Only 39 per cent of programmes were recorded by parents (161 of 413). Parents ranged in their recording from nil to 37 per cent to 84.1 per cent of all programmes attempted (median 29.6 per cent).

In several cases the requirement to record was not

pressed by home teachers. This was an agreed policy for three families where one aim of intervention was to encourage the family to play with their child in a more relaxed way than initially observed; two families in which parents could not be convinced of the value of recording, and one family in which the mother was very hostile to recording on the grounds that it was 'like filling in a form for the Town Hall'. In addition one family was judged to be too hard-pressed to warrant insistence on recording, and three families did not record consistently for reasons which were unclear. One mother in this group agreed to record with reluctance but then did not complete charts or lost them. For three further families, parents were working with children whose progress was slow and unreliable. Parents tended to be depressed by what they perceived as failures revealed by recording and, consequently, home teachers did not insist that records be kept.

This left a core of five families for whom recording presented no problems and who recorded regularly. It was reported that one family enjoyed keeping records.

The influence of recording on performance was explored through several questions in the HINTS interview evaluation. Home teachers reported that, for those families where recording was encouraged, they had simplified recording by providing charts with simple instructions (13 instances) and provided drawings or other aids (two instances each). Eleven home teachers reported using demonstration and explanation of recording and four explanation and discussion. The remaining three reported that special explanations of recording were not necessary. There were no differences in number or proportion of programmes recorded relating to these reported strategies.

Comparison of the number of programmes attempted by the group who recorded (29.0 per cent) and the remaining families (20.9 per cent) does not reveal a significant effect of recording. Similarly, comparison of the mean percentage of programmes completed by the group who recorded (88.2 per cent) and the group who did not (89.1 per cent) does not reveal a significant effect.

In practice the group for whom recording was no apparent problem recorded an average of only 62.5 per cent of their programmes as opposed to the remaining families who recorded an average of 21.6 per cent ($U=5.5$, $n_1=5$, $n_2=13$, p 0.05). There are no clear relations between the numbers of programmes recorded and number of activities attempted in the group as a whole nor between percentage of programmes recorded and percentage of programmes successfully completed. The relationship here is negative, although the correlation is not statistically significant.

These findings suggest that recording does not clearly relate to performance and that initiation and successful completion of programmes was dependent on factors other than recording in the situations studied in this report.

As already noted, the number of successfully completed programmes and the professional time involved in each successful programme appear to provide valuable indices against which to evaluate the effect of other variables. The last statistic is of particular relevance in terms of service significance. In our analysis these statistics reflect two sets of variables, home teacher variables and client variables. The latter set comprises both parent and offspring variables.

Correlations between the number of successfully completed programmes and professional time involved per successful programme were computed with a range of variables. With others, where dichotomous or tricotomous classification was appropriate, t-tests or median tests using chi squared or Fisher Exact Test were employed. The following variables were investigated, age: cultural group, English as a first language, social class, type of housing, number of other children, quality of housing, income, relationship with father, personal resources, local facilities, health of other children, total additional problems, child's developmental level and type of employment of home teacher.

Three variables, poor housing, low income and type of employment of home teacher, were related to outcome. Parents rated as having problems with low income **and/or** poor housing were found to take more time per successful programme, an average of over 4 hours 30 minutes, than did families without such problems, who averaged 1 hour 53 minutes ($t=3.48$, $df=16$, p 0.01). Separately, the two variables did not relate to outcome at acceptable levels of statistical significance. The group of Residential Social Workers took significantly less time per successful programme than the combined group of field, specialist and other personnel. The mean time per programme for the Residential group was around 2 hours 11 minutes, for the other home teachers 4 hours 34 minutes ($t=4$, $df=16$, p 0.01). However, further analyses indicated that less problematic cases had been allocated to the residential social work group. The effect of income or housing problems were nonetheless significant.

The failure to reveal any substantial correlations among the variables selected may reflect a number of problems. We have already noted that outcome variables reflect both home teacher and client variables and that client variables comprise parent, or in practicc, family, and offspring variables. This complexity may well have prevented the effects of some variables of interest from emerging.

Second, it may well be that the relatively obvious variables described and the relatively crude level of measurement, were insensitive to effects. This explanation is quite feasible. Further studies may well examine more subtle variables, especially those concerned with parental perceptions of the handicapped child and difficulty of modifying behaviour. Some method of rating the parents 'readiness' for intervention, which could reflect notions derived from psychodynamic literature, would assess the influence of these variables. What the current study suggests is that a variety of obvious variables do not relate strongly and simply to outcome.

Of the 35 social work goals established, 25 were rated by the home teacher and HINTS organisers to have been achieved (71.4 per cent); eight were partly achieved (22.8 per cent) and the remaining two were not. The most commonly set goals related to encouraging the parents to set appropriate goals and/or to interact more positively with the child. These were most commonly achieved (15 goals, 13 achieved, one partial, one failed). Other goals commonly achieved included allowing the child more independence (three), and relief of anxieties about development (two) full, (one) partial. Of the four goals related to improving child-family interactions in general, two were judged to have been achieved fully (broadening contacts between the child and his father and brother, and encouraging family participation with the child thereby relieving the child's boredom and reducing family tension). Two others were only partially achieved (to adjust the child's behaviour to fit into the family, and to involve the child with other family members). Other goals achieved included increasing awareness of the child's needs and preparation for separation.

The relatively small number of failed social work goals and the task-oriented nature of most of the goals make examination of the inter-relations with other variables problematic. In practice, correlations with the child and staff related variables described above reveal little of interest. In particular there is no evidence of an influence of type of employment on outcome.

Home Teachers' Evaluations of HINTS

The replies to several questions on this interview have already been noted. Other questions clustered round several themes including development of interaction with the family, perceived success, the HINTS group and the impact of HINTS work on other responsibilities. Eighteen home teachers were interviewed.

A marked improvement in the level of confidence shown by parents in relating to their children was reported for eight families and some improvement for a further five. In only three cases was no change reported. Home teachers did not rate any family as showing loss of confidence.

As we have seen, home teachers rated the majority of families as having problems other than those directly related to the handicapped child. Nine of the home teachers suggested that the intervention had helped families tackle other problems. In seven cases no differences were noticed and in two cases changes were noticed but were not thought to be related to home teaching. Consistent with this trend, five of the seven home teachers who had had previous experience of their family suggested that important family issues had been discussed for the first time as a result of home teaching. Five of the six residential staff reported that matters other than those directly related to home teaching were raised during the intervention. Issues included general family and marital problems, problems concerning the acceptance of the handicapped child by the father or siblings and, in one case, the question of adoption of the handicapped child. These data are consistent with reports of 11 home teachers who felt that their relationship within the family had changed, and nine of the 17 relationships between the family and the community had changed.

Changes in the social worker relationship to the family were not always felt to be beneficial. Three social workers found conflict between their social work and home teaching because of their perceived relative importance, and parental concern with social work matters as opposed to home teaching.

Home teachers saw the most useful aspect of the HINTS approach as working jointly on a task with the family, followed by the fact that the work was focused and structured. Weekly visiting and the opportunity to observe the child closely in the family were less highly rated aspects of the approach. The relatively low rating of weekly visiting is somewhat surprising.

There were no clear potential problems of time commitment arising from a model of intervention which requires daily parent work and weekly or fortnightly visits and meetings. However, nine of the home teachers rated the model as very flexible and providing no problems in adaptation to individual family style. A further seven found some difficulties and one reported substantial difficulties.

Of 17 respondents 13 felt that there had been significant advantages for the child and 12 for the parents. None of the six residential social workers saw advantages for the family as a whole, although nine of the 11 other home teachers did. Two home teachers reported problems resulting from home teaching. These were sibling jealousy, which was felt to have been present prior to HINTS work but aggravated by it, and difficulties which the parents experienced with recording.

A possible area of potential professional difficulty concerns the integration of HINTS work into a normal case load. The responses to questions about difficulties as a result of time spent on home teaching showed that, out of 11 respondents, one found great difficulty because of ability to take on new cases at allocation, and one because of being unable to spend enough time with the HINTS family.

It will be recalled that build-up of HINTS work involved the organiser in approaching the relevant senior social workers in Area teams, in company with the field worker, and explaining and negotiating the contact. A parallel procedure was followed for residential social workers. These arrangements apparently worked satisfactorily. None of the home teachers reported problems in relationships with seniors or equivalents. Only two home teachers, both residential personnel, reported problems with colleagues.

The final section of the HINTS evaluation interview dealt with the weekly group meetings. All respondents felt that they had benefited from discussing their child with the organisers. Of 16 respondents, 15 reported that they were happy to share discussion with other home teachers, and all respondents felt that the opportunity to discuss their case with the group was beneficial. Fifteen of the 18 home teachers said that they found the possibility for sharing ideas beneficial and 12 that they found it beneficial to share difficulties. All bar two of the respondents felt that the format could be improved. Ten home teachers felt that the addition of individual sessions to group meetings would be beneficial, although it is worth noting that **none** of the respondents favoured exclusively individual sessions. Fourteen home teachers out of 16 felt that the need for weekly meetings declined after the 'initial period' and favoured fortnightly or even monthly meetings with added telephone conversations. Two respondents suggested that group meetings were time consuming and sometimes time wasting.

Parents' Experience of HINTS

As part of a broader evaluation parents were asked for their views on the scheme. One section of the Family Interview administered after the HINTS intervention was inserted as related specifically to HINTS or other interventions. Several of the questions provided simple confirmation of the HINTS evaluation completed with home teachers. Parents confirmed that home teaching had been provided in the parental home on a weekly basis in the case of 16 of the 18 respondents and fortnightly for the remaining two.

Parents reported spending various amounts of time on teaching. One parent reported spending 10 minutes per day, and two others, two hours in two one-hour blocks. The median total time spent teaching was between 30 and 45 minutes (mean=46.4 minutes per day).

Parents said that they favoured self-help skills in their choice of area of work. Nine parents opted for this area as opposed to five for motor development, defined as sensorimotor-play; five for tasks involved in cognitive development within the Portage checklist, two each for language development and remediation of over-activity; and one for remediation of temper tantrums. Three parents said that they did not have perferences so the home teacher had suggested areas.

Only 11 parents reported that advice was easy to put into practice and eight said there were some difficulties. In general these problems were not related to the manner of giving advice. For instance, one parent said that it was difficult to do programmes because the child was sick from time to time, another because the child 'liked an audience' and, from time-to-time, would not cooperate when she was alone with him.

Advice was consistently rated as helpful to both parents and handicapped child or young person. Three parents said that the practical help was mostly of value to them as parents and one that it was mostly of help to the handicapped child. Reassurance and confidence building were seen as mainly helpful to the parents, although one mother also said that it was helpful to siblings.

A more mixed picture emerged in response to enquiries concerning advantages or disadvantages to the family as a whole. Ten parents reported only advantages, including one parent who reported that, as a result of home teaching, the child's brother did puzzles with him. Five parents saw both advantages and disadvantages. One parent reported that, as a result of being taught to play with soap suds, the child had developed an irritating interest in the sink plug. In other cases home teaching had created problems within the family, partly through focusing on the child's difficulties and partly because of the mother giving extra time to the handicapped child.

One normal sibling remarked: "You're always doing things with A, and you don't do things with me". These problems need to be taken in the context of the fact that all bar three families contained siblings and of the occasional reports in other protocols of siblings benefiting through being involved with the handicapped child.

The Representativeness of the HINTS Families

The type of intervention employed in the HINTS scheme is becoming increasingly common as the Portage model is adopted more widely. If this model is to be seen as a crucial component of provision it is important to establish its value in dealing with the range of problems emerging in a Local Authority. This could be done in the current project since we had data on a random sample of children and young people with severe learning difficulties in the Authority.

Comparison of the individuals in the HINTS group with the sample suggested that they were of equivalent ability in mobility, sensory functioning and sensory-motor coordination. The HINTS group was rather less able in the understanding and use of speech but equivalent on other measures of communication. Rather more HINTS group children were said to have problems than the comparison group.

These data are suggestive of the success of the HINTS programme in catering for a cross-section of children and young people whose parents are able to work with them on broadly educational programmes. However, none of the parents worked with offspring who showed substantial behaviour problems. These were, in general, avoided by the HINTS organisers on the grounds that they required specialist input.

Conclusions

The evaluation of the HINTS programme suggested overall success. Training was feasible, the format of management meetings was acceptable and could be integrated into normal day-to-day work, as could home visiting. Targets were achieved and rated well by home teachers and parents. The scheme overall suggests that home teaching can be undertaken by social service personnel. The particular contributions which social workers could make to home and teaching and which home teaching may make to achievement of social work goals was less clear. Home teachers felt that such goals could be achieved more readily because home teaching provided a rapid way of building up contact. However the scheme did provide an opportunity for more frequent visiting than may otherwise be normal. The hypothesis that involvement with the parent in a child-oriented activity which the parent sees as relevant, helps to establish a valuable relationship which can be used to further social work goals, has high face-value but remains to be tested.

The HINTS programme was considered sufficiently successful by the SSD for it to be continued as part of normal service provision, eventually under the management of a senior social worker. Within the pattern of provision HINTS represented a parallel component to other social work activities. In other words, the only way in which it could be fitted into the organisation of service and in-service training was to use it, as needs were felt to arise, with individual social services personnel as a complement to their normal practice. There was no policy commitment to the scheme and no guarantee that children and young people with mental handicap would have social services input which would ensure that, if they or their families could benefit, they would be involved in the scheme. Because of the organisational climate of the service it was up to the individual social worker to opt for the HINTS programme. Attempts to coerce on the grounds of perceived need would almost certainly have been resented and resisted.

The dominant impression emerging from the experience of the HINTS programme was that the high degree of autonomy given to individual social services personnel in respect of their methods of working was both a strength within the system and a weakness. It was a strength because it allowed new methods of working to be rapidly introduced and exploited by interested individuals. It was a weakness because it appeared to reduce the likelihood that new methods of working could be introduced as a matter of agreed policy. 'Policy' would have had to be 'agreed' with all personnel rather than a policy decision being made and implemented in a top-down manner. Although there are clear problems with top-down decision-making, the extreme opposite of individual autonomy of practice is the rule.

These complications, and others following from the emphasis on genericism and the equivocal status of specialists in our case study, produced a programme which was in many ways grafted onto a service rather than being an inherent part of it. It is possible that given time and continued success, such a programme could become an integral part of the service. The likelihood of this would seem to be increased if it were to be an aspect of the work of, for example, a Community Mental Handicap Team which had a broader perspective.

The HINTS Programme has been offered as an example of in-service training within an SSD. The intervention was, we believe, relatively successful both in exploiting the strengths of SSDs, in allowing change and in revealing the way in which such organisations limit and contain change.

The research described in this paper was completed with the assistance of funding from the Department of Health and Social Security

References

Bluma, A., Shearer, J., Frohman, A. and Hilliard, J. (1976) Portage Guide to Early Education, Cooperative Educational Service Agency 12, Portage, Wisc

Cunningham, C. (1975) 'Parents as Therapists and Educators' in C. C. Kiernan and F. P. Woodford (eds.), Behaviour Modification with the Severely Retarded, Associated Scientific Publishers, Amsterdam

Cunningham, C. and Sloper, P. (1979) Helping Your Handicapped Baby, Souvenir Press, London

Jeffree, D. and McConkey, R. (1976) Let Me Speak, Souvenir Press, London

Jeffree, D. M., McConkey, R. and Hewson, S. (1979) Let Me Play, Souvenir Press, London

Kiernan, C. C., Jordan, R. R. and Saunders, C. A. (1978) *Starting Off*, Souvenir Press, London

Kiernan, C. C. and Woodford, F. P. (1975) 'Training and Reorganisation for Behaviour Modification in Hospital and Community Settings', *British Association of Behavioural Psychotherapy Bulletin*, *3*, 31-34

Shearer, M. S. and Shearer, D. E. (1982) The Portage Project: A Model for Early Childhood Education', *Exceptional Children*, *39*, 210-217

Smith, J., Kushlick, A. and Glossop, C. (1977) *The Wessex Portage Project: A Home Teaching Service for Families with a Pre-school Mentally Handicapped Child*, Research Report No. 125, Health Care Evaluation Research Team, Wessex R.H.A.: Winchester

Chapter 8

NURSE TRAINING AND INSTITUTIONAL CONSTRAINTS

C. Cullen

It is not always necessary to employ others to help mentally handicapped people. They may have family and friends who are happy to take that role, or they may be sufficiently independent to be able to live with minimal support. Where it is necessary to have paid staff, the issue arises of what **kind** of staff. In the United Kingdom there are two main statutory agencies which currently have responsibilities for providing residential services for mentally handicapped people: the Health Service and the Local Authority. It is with the former group that this chapter is concerned, although many of the issues raised are relevant to all varieties of residential service.

The care staff employed in the National Health Service are **nurses** and **nursing assistants**. During the past decade there has been a shift to the view that the Health Service is an inappropriate agency for providing residential services to mentally handicapped people. In 1979 a Committee of Enquiry into Mental Handicap Nursing and Care, the Jay Report (DHSS, 1979), recommended that a new caring profession should emerge, and that nurses, as the term is presently understood, should cease to have responsibility for providing services to mentally handicapped people. This endorsed the earlier recommendation of the Briggs Report (DHSS, 1972) which was looking at the future of nursing in general. The new profession, according to the Jay Report, should have a common training so that there would be no distinction between Health and Local Authority care as there is at present. Half the workforce would have a new qualification and half would receive in-service training, maintaining the current pattern of having a mix of both qualified and unqualified carers. Unfortunately, though, there has been very little progress in implementing the recommendations of either the Briggs or the Jay Reports. Services are still divided between the two statutory authorities, albeit with a slow shift away from the Health Service. There is still, then, a need for nurse training, at least in the near future.

One of the distinctions between the Health and Local Authorities is that, in general, the formal care for people with more severe handicaps while the latter tend to provide services for people with lower levels of handicap. It might reasonably be supposed, therefore, that there is more of a need for training for nurses and that, once trained, nurses should be in a good position to help a wide range of mentally handicapped clients. A corollary of this argument is that lessons learnt from attempts to train nurses should be valuable in designing training programmes for all staff working with mentally handicapped people.

The body which has had responsibility since 1983 for monitoring the standards of training for nurses is the English National Board for Nursing, Midwifery and Health Visiting. There are also Welsh and Scottish Boards. Before 1983 there was the General Nursing Council. A Register of nurses is maintained and nurses have to undergo a course of training which is approved by the Board in order to be entered on the Register. The syllabus of training is determined by the Board who are advised by multi-disciplinary panels; new syllabi are prepared every ten years or so in response to changing service demands. The latest revision was in 1982 and nurse training schools henceforth must operate the new syllabus if they wish to remain accredited.

The content of the 1982 syllabus are impressive. Its main sections are

1. The nursing process
2.a The skills of communication
  b Alternative methods of communication
3. Education and mentally handicapped people
4. The sociology of organisations
5. Normalisation and human rights
6. Management
7. Principles of development

8. Causation, nature and effects of mental handicap
9. Partnership with families

The exact mode of teaching each of these sections is determined by each nurse-training school, taking into account local service provisions and the availability of practical placements, but there is a national final examination which all students undergo. Consequently, there ought to be a reasonably sophisticated group of nurses, spread throughout the country, working in residential services for mentally handicapped people.

The underlying philosophy of the course is stated in the preface to the syllabus, and is adapted from Henderson (1961):

> "The function of the nurse for people with mental handicap is directly and skilfully to assist the individual and his family, whatever the handicap, in the acquisition, development and maintenance of those skills that, given the necessary ability, would be performed unaided: and to do this in such a way as to enable independence to be gained as rapidly and fully as possible, in an environment that maintains a quality of life that would be acceptable to fellow citizens of the same age."
>
> (ENB,1982)

On the face of it, a person having successfully undertaken a course of training such as this would be in an ideal position to serve mentally handicapped people in a residential setting. However, nurses who were trained under the previous syllabus (GNC, 1970) also had what was, then, a progressive and comprehensive training. As Williams and Jackson (1975) state "...the 1970 GNC syllabus includes sufficient material to form an excellent training in the care of the mentally handicapped" (p. 242). But the history of hospital-based residential services for mentally handicapped people shows clearly that nurse-training has **not** resulted in a high quality of life. There has been a steady stream of inquiries into conditions in mental handicap hospitals, starting with Ely Hospital in 1969 and continuing to the present day (Beardshaw, 1981). Most mental handicap hospitals are not the subject of allegations of cruelty and malpractice, but there is still reason to believe that the service they provide is of a lower quality then we would like.

Consider, for example, the nature of the interactions between nurses and residents. As part of the Resident's Development Project (aspects of which are described below) an analysis of the relationship between residents' behaviour and nurses' behaviour was carried out. (This is described fully in Cullen, Burton, Watts and Thomas, 1984.) Ten mentally handicapped male residents of a small hospital were observed continuously for ten minutes at a time, five times each day. Two of the times, mid-morning and mid-afternoon, were while the people were in a recreation hall. The remaining three periods, before breakfast, after lunch and before the evening meal, were on the ward.

The data were collected using a portable keyboard linked to a memory, each key corresponding to a specific behaviour category. An observational period was started by the observer recording on the keyboard the following information: number of residents present, number of staff present, date, time, location, session length, coder and coding system. To start the session clock, the observer made a judgement about the resident's behaviour and about the reactions of staff or other residents to that behaviour (see below) and depressed the two relevant keys in the order: resident behaviour - reaction of staff or other resident.

If the resident changed his behaviour, or if there was a change in the reaction to that behaviour, then the two appropriate keys would be depressed. When this happened, the duration of the two previous behaviours were stored in the memory and timing of the two new behaviours was started. At the end of ten minutes there was a visual signal, and the session would be terminated.

Resident behaviour was categorised as **appropriate**, **inappropriate** or **neutral**; nurse reactions as **positive** or **negative**; and the reactions of other residents as either **positive** or **negative** if there was no reaction from nurses. When there was no reaction from anybody, this was recorded as **no attention**. A full description of the definitions of these categories is given in Cullen et al (1984).

Resident Behaviours	Reaction						
	Unobserved	Other residents Positive	Other residents Negative	Staff Positive	Staff Negative	Staff No attention	Total
Unobserved	0.01	0	0	0	0	0	0.01
Appropriate	0	0.01	0	0.01	0	0.06	0.08
Neutral	0	0	0	0.01	0	0.61	0.62
Inappropriate	0	0.01	0	0.01	0.01	0.25	0.28
Total	0.01	0.02	0	0.03	0.01	0.92	

Table 1: Relative proportion of time spent in each behaviour category (averaged across two settings).

Table 1 shows the relative proportion of time spent in each behaviour category by the residents and their reaction to that behaviour. Data are presented averaged across the two settings because there was very little difference between them (cf Cullen et al., 1984). It is clear that the overwhelming effect of the residents' behaviour was little attention from nurses and virtually no attention from other residents. Regardless of what they were doing, residents received no attention for 92 per cent of the time. Most of the time (62 per cent) was spent in neutral behaviours and when they were not 'doing anything' they were much more likely to be engaging in inappropriate behaviour (28 per cent of the time) than in appropriate behaviour (8 per cent of the time).

Table 2 shows the frequency and mean duration of the different combinations of resident behaviour and staff or resident reaction.

The total time spent observing was 30,475 seconds. When all entries coded as **no attention** (0) are excluded, since they cannot count as interactions, the following information may be derived. During the observation periods, there were an average of 0.4 interactions per minute, each with a mean duration of 9.1 seconds. Since we were observing ten people, this means that each person could expect to have some reaction to his behaviour on the average once every 25 minutes and that interaction is likely to last for less than 10 seconds. Grant (1974) compared the levels of interactions in two hospitals and obtained broadly similar results. He found that 42.8 per cent and 63 per cent of the interactions were less than 10 seconds in duration and that there was a mean of 26.5 minutes and 20.1 minutes between interactions in the two settings.

Clearly, then, hospitals staffed by nurses and nursing assistants, some of them trained according to a syllabus with many fine characteristics, still have major problems in providing an environment in which mentally handicapped people lead purposive and fulfilling lives, interacting with those around them in meaningful and useful ways. There are variables at work which negate the hoped-for effects of nurse training. Brown and Walton (1984) have investigated some of the factors which influence mental handicap nurse training. They conducted a nation-wide survey of nurse-training schools and identified several

Observational category	Frequency	Mean duration (seconds)	SD
U	13	12.8	11.0
A + *	25	9.0	7.5
A +	42	10.1	10.5
A O	68	26.9	42.3
A -	7	8.3	4.9
N + *	13	7.1	6.5
N -	2	4.0	0
N +	26	11.4	10.6
N O	322	58.0	106.6
N -	2	4.0	0
I + *	25	13.8	17.0
I - *	11	5.1	3.7
I +	19	18.5	31.2
I O	207	37.4	50.9
I -	20	9.0	8.9

Table 2: Frequency and mean duration (in seconds) of each combination of resident behaviour and reaction to it. Resident behaviour is coded as appropriate (A), neutral (N) or negative (-). No reaction is designated as 0, and reactions by other residents are marked by *. Occasions on which behaviour was incompletely observed or recorded are denoted at U.

factors associated with dissatisfaction with nurse training. These included poor relations between the service and the training school, inappropriately trained tutors, low staffing levels, outdated attitudes of some service staff and tension between the move towards community services and the existence of the present hospital 'power base'. While there is little doubt that many of these issues are important, the research project did not identify **causal** factors and it is left open to supposition whether or not changing any of them will result in a significant change within the residential services.

It could be that, even though nurse training might be suitable for preparing care staff, hospitals employ so few appropriately qualified nurses that any benefits are lost. In 1979 the Committee of Enquiry into Mental Handicap Nursing and Care (DHSS, 1979) found that less than 45 per cent of nursing staff in hospitals were qualified and this figure **includes** a grade of nurse not on the Register referred to above, but on a Roll (enrolled nurse) and therefore having a less extensive training than that of the registered nurse. This is a national picture, the exact situation varying from hospital to hospital. In 1981, in one medium sized hospital with 130 residents, only 9 per cent of the staff were on the Professional Register (Cullen, 1981), while in the writer's present hospital, housing around 50 residents, 11 per cent of the nursing staff are appropriately qualified. There seems to be, therefore, a **prima facie** case for providing in-service training for those nurses who do not have a mental handicap qualification and for those who trained many years ago. This has been one of the main planks of service plans for the past decade and was one of the main recommendations of the Brown and Walton (1984) study.

Does in-service training have the desired effect? Exactly what "the desired effect" might be is open to interpretation, but one widely accepted aim would be that the staff would, after such training, interact with mentally handicapped people in such a way that the behavioural repertoires of the residents would be positively increased. Watson and Uzzell (1980), for example, found that they were able to teach aides an important behaviour modification procedure (backward chaining) on a practical basis and that such training resulted in the staff then being able to teach self-care skills to multi-handicapped clients. These training skills were maintained at a high level over at least 22 weeks. However, academic instruction in the principles of backward chaining was found to have little effect on practical skills. It seems as though this is an example of in-service training being effective. However, one reads in Watson and Uzell's report that "maintenance of training skills at a high level was probably due to the supervisory procedure and certification requirements employed" (p.50). Obviously, there are additional variables present which are having an important effect over and above any effect which the in-service training **might** be having.

Milne (1985) reviewed seventeen studies of in-service training of nurses in terms of their specification of the independent variable (cf Peterson, Homer and Wonderlitch, 1982). He found that the exact nature of the in-service training given was rarely specified, so that it would be difficult to replicate procedures, and that it was equally difficult to compare studies. He echoed the sentiments of Bernstein (1982) who provided a conceptual review of training evaluation and said that "most behavioural research on effective training procedures is not nearly as sophisticated as behavioural research on other topics" (p.1).

Many other authors, having surveyed the literature on nurse training, have arrived at a similar conclusion. Ziarnik and Bernstein (1982) put it this way:

> "The issue is whether staff training works. An in-depth review of the literature on staff training would have to result in an answer of **sometimes**. As with most outcome evaluation problems, the answer partially depends on who and how you ask".
> (p.10)

Quilitch (1975) was equally pessimistic after comparing three staff training procedures:

> "It is generally assumed ... that in-service training leads to improved staff performance and, finally, more effective service programs ... workshops are frequently used to deliver this training and generally consist of prepared talks ... audio-visual aids ... case presentations and live demonstrations ... discussion groups ... handbooks and texts ... specially prepared

> instructional materials ... refreshments ... and questionnaires allowing participants to evaluate the workshop ... Available research does not bear out the optimistic assumptions made about services provided by six institutions for the retarded (it has been) found that the least effective of the six had the strongest in-service training program and ... that, overall, there was simply no relationship between institutional effectiveness and in-service training."
>
> (p.64)

It behoves us now to move in search of factors in addition to training which might influence the way in which staff interact with handicapped people. This does not mean that training is unimportant, because it is clearly impossible for a nurse to perform a task he or she has not been taught to do. Rather, it means that training is only one factor which operates in the complex world of residential care. Ziarnik and Bernstein (1982) assert:

> "It is our contention that the effectiveness of staff training has yet to be demonstrated because it is often incorrectly applied. That is, the assumption underlying the decision to provide staff training is that staff cannot perform the needed skills. The assumption is not always correct. Poor performance may be related to a variety of factors, only one of which is skill deficiency."
>
> (p.111)

The Resident's Development Project

In 1981, the Department of Health and Social Security funded a research project which was originally to apply some of the lessons learnt from an earlier project on the in-service training of teachers (cf McBrien and Foxen, this volume). This project in its turn had been a development (see Hogg, Foxen and McBrian, 1981) from a study of the in-service training of nurses in a mental handicap hospital (Kiernan and Riddick, 1973). The circle had apparently turned full circle, and, taking seriously the doubts about the value of in-service training referred to above, it was more appropriate to investigate factors other than nurse training.

Around this time, nursing within the United Kingdom

was undergoing a shift in emphasis and was moving towards developing a distinct professional identity. Following trends in the United States, British nurses were turning towards the **Nursing Process** as a definition of the nursing role. The nursing literature of the late 1970s onward was dominated by descriptions of the Nursing Process in the various branches of the profession. In 1977 the General Nursing Council issued a policy statement which asserted that:

> "The concept of the Nursing Process provides a uniform thread for the study of patient care and a helpful framework of nursing practice."

In June 1981 the Chief Nursing Officer sent a letter to Area Nursing Officers and others describing the Process " ... to stimulate discussion and initiative at local level" and named a link-person at the Department of Health and Society Security to co-ordinate new developments in the field. The 1982 syllabus for training nurses in the field of mental handicap is based on the concept of the Nursing Process. Clearly, here was a contextual factor which had to be taken into account in any research into nurse training or practice.

It is difficult to arrive at a succinct description of the Nursing Process. Kratz (1977) describes it as "...a kind of prescription of how nurses do, or ought to do, their work". Other writers describe it as an "attitude". Its two characteristics which everyone agrees on are:

* it is a client-centred rather than task-centred approach to nursing

* it is a problem-solving or goal-planning approach

There are four 'steps' in implementing the Nursing Process:

1 assessment of the client's needs
2 determination of a (nursing) plan of action
3 implementation of the plan
4 evaluation of the success of the plan

This 'prescription for practice' obviously fits very well with the behaviour modification approach which had been important in mental handicap nurse training throughout the 1970s (cf Berni and Fordyce, 1977). The important question, though, concerns whether nurses will adopt the Nursing Process as anything more than a verbal exercise. What would be the consequences for the profession of working within the framework of the Nursing Process? A search of the literature reveals several potential good reasons why the framework should be adopted:

a Since the Process demands a high degress of specificity, the nurse is forced to define that elusive concept 'quality of care' (Altschul, 1977; Hegvary, 1979). Defining a target is the first stage in achieving this.

b The status and identity of the profession would be enhanced by a clear delineation of the nursing role (Crow, 1977; Kratz, 1977; Davis, 1978). This is important in attracting high quality people into the service, which, in turn, should lead to an improved service for mentally handicapped clients.

c The process emphasises a non-medical view of the client, directing the nurse towards activities of daily living rather than disease processes (Luker, 1977). Within mental handicap nursing this is particularly relevant, as one of the main reasons for moving towards community care and away from hospital care has been to eliminate the view held by some that mental handicap is an "illness" and can be "treated" by medical personnel.

d Increased communication and understanding between nurses and relatives, between nurses and other professional staff, and between nurses on different shifts has been noted (Ashworth, Castledine and McFarlane, 1978; Clark, 1978).

e Increased job satisfaction has been reported after implementation of the Nursing Process (Ashworth, Castledine and McFarlane, 1978).

f A formal system for daily working allows job specification in sufficient detail to predict realistic staffing levels (Ashworth, 1980; Clark, 1978).

g With increasing public accountability for service provision, Neilson (1978) has suggested that there are compelling legal reasons for implementing the

Nursing Process. It is important to be able to identify actors, actions, and the determinants of those actions as a means of safeguarding nurses against charges of malpractice and as a means of monitoring the standard of nursing care.

With such an array of supporting reasons, the case for changing nursing practice and training away from the conventional mode to the Nursing Process seems unassailable. Unfortunately, though, 'right' has rarely been a factor in implementing models of practice within the mental health field. Asserting that a particular approach is likely to result in a better level and quality of service rarely leads to the adoption of that approach. In an important review of the adoption of innovations, Stolz (1981) tried to identify 'possible key variables' which could influence whether a programme was implemented on a wide scale. Of the ten she describes, one stands out as absent from the Nursing Process literature: research data showing that the innovation is effective. For all the hundreds of thousands of words written on the subject, there is virtually nothing to show that adopting a Nursing Process format leads to a measurably better service for the client. It seemed reasonable, therefore, for the Resident's Development Project to turn its attention to this problem.

Any evaluation of a programme implementation has to have a set of criteria in terms of which the effectiveness of the programme can be measured (Morris and Fitz-Gibbon, 1978). These ought to reflect the ultimate goal of the programme. The majority of studies which have evaluated staff training and practice systems have measured change in **staff**. Such measures have included the attitudes of staff, their ability to perform in role-plays or with mentally handicapped clients, their knowledge of concepts and procedures and their skill in describing and understanding situations involving mentally handicapped people (cf Milne, 1985; Sebba, 1985). Such measures are necessary for a complete understanding of the requirements of the users. We wanted an instrument which would take into account the nature of the environment in which the handicapped individuals were living. It was important to be able to assess what residents were actually doing rather than what it was thought they might be capable of doing. Also, if the assessment was to be of help in identifying reasonable targets for future training, there must be some indication of which skills would be likely to be maintained and be of use to the person after training. Since commonly available checklists did not appear to satisfy these criteria, we developed the **Offerton Self-Care Checklist** (Burton, Thomas and Cullen, 1981). This is an acceptably reliable instrument which incorporated one device generally missing from other similar checklists. If a maximum score was not achieved for any particular skill, a reason had to be given. The analysis of these reasons proved to be extremely informative and opened potentially important areas for research into the context within which staff training and management takes place.

The checklist was completed by a **rater**, who interviewed an **informant**, usually the nurse in charge, who knew the resident. In addition to the checklist, there was a series of supplementary questions which formed the basis for a structured interview with the informant. These questions related to the self-care routines on the ward and followed the checklist in overall structure. The checklist and questionnaire were administered for all 130 residents of the hospital.

The data collected were qualitative, although certain quantitative statements can be derived. Analysis proceeded as follows:

(i) a sample of checklists and questionnaires were examined by three team members who then agreed a set of categories for the different types of constraints identified.

(ii) the categories were then tried out with data from one ward, the information from questionnaires and checklists being sorted into the agreed categories as appropriate.

(iii) having ascertained that the method was feasible and that the categories were meaningful in relation to the actual constraints identified, the information from the other five wards was also sorted into these categories.

The method used is equivalent to that termed "hunting" by Selvin and Stuart (1966) in their classic paper on data-dredging procedures. Since our categories could only be derived from the data and hence were not independent of them, we could not formally use stage (iii) of our analysis to check the validity of the categories. Our choice of categories was influenced by the data themselves and by our observations of the setting. This is a limitation to the analysis. The ultimate utility of the categories can only be determined by further independent studies. In practice, nobody who has looked at the analysis and its results has expressed any reservations, so at least they have high face validity.

Explanations of why a resident did not obtain the maximum score on an aspect of self-proficiency tended to refer to some aspect of the environment as well as, or rather than, a lack of ability on the part of the resident. For example, if the question was about the ability to pour hot liquids such as tea, it was found that very few residents were given an opportunity to do so. It was the custom for staff always to do this. Many of the residents were reported as not using toilet paper - because there was actually none available in the toilet area. Apparently toilet paper was kept in the ward office because when it was freely available a small number of residents were likely to flush large amounts down the toilet bowl thereby blocking the hospital's ancient sewers. Since the analysis was carried out, describing these and similar factors at numerous conferences and seminars and publishing an abbreviated description in the nursing press (Cullen, 1984; Thomas, Burton and Cullen, 1982) has increased my confidence that they are common in mental handicap hospitals in the United Kingdom.

The constraints were categorised as follows:

a Resident's (physical characteristics): some physical quality of a person which prevents her/him from carrying out a particular task, such as a severe physical handicap.

b Resident's (behaviour): an aspect of a person's behaviour which prevents them or others from behaving adaptively. For example, someone who throws cups might be denied the opportunity to pour tea for themselves.

c Staff (rules): refers to the formal regulations of

an institution, such as a policy which states that there must always be more than one staff member present with a resident who is being bathed. This effectively prevents the mentally handicapped person bathing with due regard to privacy.

d Staff (routines): those aspects of staff behaviour which, although not the subject of formal hospital policies nevertheless become the standard mode of operating. Tea may be served from a large jug, with milk and sugar added, by the staff, so preventing the resident from deciding how much, if any, sugar to add, and whether tea will be taken black or white.

e Environment (high cost): most hospitals have buildings which are unsuited to normal living. For example, people cannot care for their own clothes if proper cupboards and wardrobes are not provided, but to provide them might require major expenditure.

f Environment (low cost): some changes to the fabric or fittings of a hospital may cost relatively little, yet their absence can mean an important opportunity is denied. For example, if salt and pepper pots are not provided, a person cannot be expected to know how much of each to put on food.

There is an illusory simplicity in categorising constraints with the consequent danger of underestimating the complexity of the underlying causes. There is a relation between the categories; they are not necessarily discrete entities. For example, if there is no toilet paper in the toilet area because one of the residents habitually puts whole rolls down the bowl, this may be categorised as **resident's (behaviour)**. However, there is probably also a **policy** in operation because of the **high cost** of building problems (old-fashioned sewers which easily become blocked).

Some constraints could not be easily categorised. Approximately 30 per cent of the residents had no teeth or dentures. Some had them but did not use them, or had them in the past and they had been 'lost' because they were never used. Others had no teeth but had never been offered dentures. It was occasionally difficult to assign a case to a category because we had to guess at likely determinants. The only completely reliable way to overcome this problem would be to carry out an experimental analysis and this was impractical under the circumstances.

However, the reliability of categorisation was surprisingly good. A rater independent of the project team re-categorised the data and percentage agreements between her and the team rater were computed. Each source of constraint was treated as separate and distinct, with no attempt made to give weight to disagreements, even though, in practice, certain disagreements are less serious than others. For example, disagreeing over whether to place an item in **environment (high cost)** or **environment (low cost)** is less serious than a disagreement over whether to place an item in **environment (low cost)** or **staff (rules)**. Two slightly different measures of agreement were calculated:

1 Percentage agreement on responses to all items was 84 per cent
2 Percentage agreement on actual constraints identified was 84 per cent

Since the independent rater knew little about the hospital, it could be expected that she lacked certain contextual information which was available to the other rater. Even so, the acceptably high level of agreement allows some confidence in the value of the exercise.

Table 3 shows the total number of constraints and the number expressed as a percentage of the total, for each category. We were also looking at care practices in a local authority hostel so we carried out the same exercise there. These data are also presented in Table 3. A comparision of the hostel, with its relatively more able and independent residents, with the hospital, which had a very wide range of levels of dependency, would be unfair, so the data for one ward are also presented separately. This ward was the home of a group of relatively able men who were ready to be discharged to a hostel and, thus, can be considered as equivalent in many respects to the hostel residents.

There are many constraints in the hospital when compared with the hostel, but when the hostel is compared with the pre-discharge ward, there is much closer correspondence. The overall number of different constraints is about the same, and staff

Source of constraint			Hospital	Pre-discharge	Local
Residents	-	Physical characteristics	1 (2.0)	2 (10.5)	0 (0)
	-	behaviour	3 (6.1)	5 (26.3)	2 (11.1)
Staff	-	rules	3 (6.1)	1 (5.3)	2 (11.1)
	-	routines	22 (44.9)	6 (31.6)	7 (38.9)
Environment	-	high cost	8 (16.3)	C (0)	4 (22.2)
	-	low cost	12 (24.5)	5 (26.3)	3 (16.7)
TOTAL			49	19	18

Table 3: The constraints in three settings. The number of constraints in the TOTAL column for the hospital as a whole represents each constraint only once, thus there were 49 different constraints identified in the whole hospital. Percentage of the total is in parentheses.

behaviour, which accounts for the largest proportion of constraints within the hospital, is similar. As we might expect, there are no reported constraints due to high cost buildings or equipment in the purpose-built hostel, but there were four on the pre-discharge ward.

From these figures we can reach certain unequivocal conclusions. The single biggest contributor to the constraints on the residents' performance of self-care behaviour is **staff routine.** Specific rules of the hospital or hostel are only a small influence. Staff routines are ways of behaving which could be changed easily, without recourse to hospital management. The next biggest contributor is **low cost physical environment**, i.e., items of equipment or facilities which are relatively easy to obtain or change and which should certainly be within the capabilities of the nursing or hostel management to change.

This supports the view of many practitioners and researchers involved in mental handicap residences - it is the **little** things which, probably because they ought to be easy to change, are so frustrating and which seem to form the major hinderance to improving the service. The whole is greater than the sum of the parts, with the aggregate effect being disproportionate to the relatively minor effects of the individual components. When constraints such as routines are ignored in attempts to improve services, the results are generally disappointing. For example, it is relatively straightforward to demonstrate an immediate improvement for residents when moving them from a large institution to much smaller community residences (cf Birenbaum and Seiffer, 1976; Felce, Kushlick and Smith, 1983). However, when the same population is examined after there has been time for any re-location effects to have dissipated, the results may be disappointing:

> "...for these mentally retarded people who had left large and isolated state schools and had lived at a community residence for almost 4 years, a career-like sequence in the direction of moving from dependency to greater self-reliance was not found. The period of personal exploration and the acquisition of new experiences that initially accompanied resettlement had given way to a prosaic routine of sleep, work, and at-home recreation of

a passive nature; weekends were often reserved for visiting family or receiving visits. This picture of living is not too different from that of those who are not retarded, but are marginally employed or mostly unemployed."

(Birenabaum and Re, 1979 p. 329)

It is not unreasonable to suppose that routines and minor environmental factors can operate in any residence, regardless of its size or location. One of my clients, for example, is a 27 year old man who was always met by his mother as he alighted from the 'bus which brought him from the training centre where he spent his day. He then walked home, a distance of around 300 metres, holding his mother's hand. Since we were trying to work towards greater independence, we discussed the possiblility of the young man walking alone from the 'bus to home. It transpired that the main reason for his being met was that it was a well established routine and he did not have his own door key in case his mother was out. It was not surprising that the first day he was given a key and allowed to walk home alone he did so with no trouble, even opening the door himself.

Since such a large proportion of the factors which inhibit the development of mentally handicapped people lie within the practical remit of nurses and others to change. The question to answer is "why don't they do so? Why persist with practices which are not in the best interests of mentally handicapped people?" I have already argued that it is **not** only because the staff are inadequately trained. One argument often heard is that staff must have "the wrong attitude" if they allow themselves to develop such damaging and inhibiting routines. We examined the attitudes of the nursing staff as our next step.

Moores and Grant (1976, 1977a, b) conducted an extensive study into the pattern of care delivered by nurses in mental handicap hospitals, a significant part of which was a study of the attitudes, expectations and perceptions of the nurses. We took this as our starting point, using items from their scale and from those of Butterfield, Barnett and Bensberg (1968) who investigated the attitudes of attendants in several institutions.

Certain systematic alterations to the existing scales were made. We replaced the word 'patient' with 'resident' and substituted 'severely mentally handicapped', for low grade: Items concerned with the employment potential of mentally handicapped people were excluded because, in the current economic climate, the nurses' views could be determined by factors other than their views of the residents' potential. Moores and Grant had also used items from earlier questionnaires aimed at identifying authoritarian attitudes and we excluded these because they appeared to contribute very little to the analysis by Moores and Grant and because Ajzen and Fishbein (1977), in their review of the field, had concluded that attitude-behaviour relations are only seen when there is a reasonable correspondence between the question and the subject of the enquiry.

Some items were included in our scale because they related to matters of current interest within the hospital.

The resulting 48-item questionnaire was presented in a Likert-type format with a 5-point scale from Disagree Strongly to Agree Strongly. The questionnaire was distributed to all ward staff. A total of 84 were distributed, with 51 being returned, a response rate of 61 per cent. It was not possible to increase the response rate because anonymity had been guaranteed to respondents as a way of increasing the likelihood of honest answers, so we did not know who had not responded.

Responses were analysed with the aid of a CDC 7,000 computer using the Statistical Package for the Social Sciences. Factor analyses of these data were performed and a two-factor solution was chosen as most meaningful. Factor I accounted for 65.2 per cent of the total variance and Factor II accounted for 34.8 per cent. The items in Factor I, together with the number of staff who felt strongly, are shown in Table 4. The items in this first factor correspond closely to the factor labelled 'staff expectations' by Moores and Grant. Nurses scoring **high** on this were **pessimistic** about the potential of residents in their care. High scores also indicated an element of social restrictiveness in matters such as allowing mentally handicapped people to marry and the need for hospitalisation. Table 6 shows the mean score obtained by four different types of nurse. Qualified staff have a more optimistic view than do unqualified staff, but qualified staff who work at night have the

Agree or Strongly Agree	Disagree or Strongly Disagree	Statement
14	29	Becoming involved in the social life of residents at weekends is stretching the role of the nurse too far.
33	6	Nurses should treat residents as equals.
18	26	Given the current shortage of money, it would be shortsighted to provide residents with more personal possessions as they would not look after them properly.
29	18	Despite the social and economic problems that could arise the mentally handicapped should still be allowed the opportunity of marriage.
25	25	On wards where residents are severely mentally handicapped, all one can do effectively is look after the residents' basic physical needs - such as toileting, feeding and dressing.
25	17	Kindness is more important than any therapeutic programme for the severely handicapped.
34	14	It is part of nursing staff's responsibility to ensure that epileptic residents do not have any access to dangerous items, e.g. kettles.
5	31	The provision of training programmes having any real value for residents is just too expensive for mental handicap hospitals.
12	33	Residents without behaviour problems should take precedence when choosing residents to go on holidays and outings.
40	7	There will always be a number of mentally handicapped people for whom hospitalisation is the only solution.
9	33	In the residents' interests, staff and residents should have their meals together.

Table 4: Pattern of responses to items included in Factor 1.

Agree or Strongly Agree	Disagree or Strongly Disagree	Statement
28	16	Doctors in this hospital rarely ask for information about particular residents from nursing staff.
41	7	In this hospital the opinions of nurses who work alongside residents are rarely sought when decisions are made to transfer residents to other departments.
41	7	There are too many hospital bosses here telling you what to do and not enough people to do the work.
23	22	Untrained nursing staff have too many menial tasks to perform in this hospital.
25	17	Nurses are expected to do too much house-keeping on the wards.
39	8	Most ward staff feel that they are not included enough when plans for the residents are being made.

Table 5: Pattern of responses to items included in Factor 2.

	Qualified	Unqualified
Day staff (N = 43)	26.2	35.0
Night staff (N = 8)	42.6	34.3

Table 6: Mean scale score on Factor 1.

	Qualified	Unqualified
Day staff (N = 43)	20.7	23.1
Night staff (N = 8)	22.2	18.3

Table 7: Mean scale score on Factor 2.

most pessimistic view. Being untrained in itself is not, therefore, sufficient to account for low expectations of mentally handicapped people. It is at least in part a function of working conditions. At night time there being a very different 'sub-culture' in hospitals. Figure 1 shows the distribution of scores across the hospital as a whole. The pattern is towards generally low expectations.

The second factor we identified was related to the nurses' feeling of satisfaction with their role. People scoring high on this factor could be said to feel alienated, uninvolved and under-valued by the system. Table 5 shows the items included in this factor, together with the number of those who felt strongly. Table 7 shows the mean scores obtained by three different types of nurse. There is no real difference here among the staff. Figure 2 shows the distribution of scores, with a strong trend towards feelings of alienation and dissatisfaction.

Reviews of attitude studies are split on the value of this kind of research. Some maintain that there is no reliable relation between a person's attitudes and what they do, while others assert that behaviours may actually determine attitudes rather than attitudes influencing behaviour. However, Ajzen and Fishbein (1977), in reviewing the literature, argue that there can be a strong link between what a person says about a situation and what they do in that situation, especially when the questions asked are closely related to actual behaviour. If we take this view, then the findings of our study are worrying. There is a generally low level of expectation of the potential of mentally handicapped people, and the nurses felt alienated and dissatisfied with their role. It is hard to imagine how such staff can be expected to change the routines and practices which, it was argued earlier, have inhibiting effects on the residents. Attitudes can be setting events (cf Wahler and Fox, 1981) in the same way as routines and environmental factors. They may be important for that reason.

The management of nurses' behaviour

The pattern of institutional care is obviously complex. The research literature on staff training gives us little confidence that basic or in-service

SCORES

10 - 15	0
16 - 20	2
21 - 25	5
26 - 30	14
31 - 35	11
36 - 40	10
41 - 45	3
46 - 50	5
51 - 55	1

Figure 1: Distribution of expectation scores. Possible range is 11 (high expectations) to 55 (low expectations).

SCORES

5 - 7	0
8 - 10	0
11 - 13	3
14 - 16	4
17 - 19	9
20 - 22	8
23 - 25	14
26 - 28	11
29 - 31	2

Figure 2: Distribution of involvement scores. Possible range is 6 (involved) to 30 (alienated).

training will have much lasting effect on nurses or other care staff, yet it is their behaviour with mentally handicapped people which is partly the key to the problem. There is little research evidence to support the view that factors such as the location of a residence or even its size will have an influence on the nature of service provision **divorced from** the behaviour of the carer. What seems to be needed is to train nurses and other staff at the same time as changing the organisations in which they work. This is going to be a more difficult task than simply setting up training courses or altering the location and size of residences.

Even if nurses had the skills to help mentally handicapped people why should they? What is likely to maintain the behaviour of care staff? Activities which they already carry out regularly and reasonably efficiently include ensuring that residents are clean, have food and receive medication. They also tidy linen cupboards, make beds and other similar domestic activities. Why do they do this? Murphy (1983) investigated this by issuing a questionnaire to nurses at a large mental handicap hospital. He asked staff to rank their various duties in order of importance according to the criteria of:

a consequences for not performing the task

b the importance of that duty for career prospects

c the importance for job satisfaction

d the importance to the resident

They were also asked in open-ended questions why they performed each of their duties and what would be the specific consequences for failure to perform them. A content analysis was carried out on the answers.

Twenty one qualified nurses completed the exercise. The results of the study indicated that, in general, activities such as running individual training programmes, arranging leisure activities and talking to residents were ranked as less important than administrative duties and carrying out basic nursing procedures in terms of the severity of consequences for not carrying them out and in terms of prospects for career development. Such activities were ranked highest in terms of job satisfaction and importance to residents. Moreover, content analysis of answers to the question "What would be the consequences to you for not running individual training programmes or leisure activities" suggested little outcome. For not attending to administrative duties and nursing procedures, however, disciplinary action was predicted. This study was essentially exploratory, so too much emphasis cannot be placed on its findings, but it seems that daily contingencies are probably an important avenue to explore if we want to change staff behaviour. A survey of contingencies which are used by supervisors indicates that they are overwhelmingly punitive (Mayhew, Enyart and Cone, 1979) and it seems sensible to explore other possibilities.

Researchers on the field of organisational behaviour management have examined the effectiveness of several variables on the therapeutic behaviour of direct care staff. These have included public posting of treatment activity information, public and private feedback on client improvement, praise from supervisors for treatment occurrence, eligibility for a weekly lottery as a consequence of treatment occurrence, monetary or other tangible rewards and so on. (See Jones et al. this volume) The effect of such procedures has sometimes been good, with some long-lasting and socially valid changes in staff behaviour. Many of them, though, are expensive in financial or resource terms and are thus unlikely to be adopted on a large scale in mental handicap services. Some of the procedures - such as the public posting of the results of treatment procedures carried out by particular nurses - would not be adopted on a large scale in work places in Britain because they would be culturally inappropriate (cf Guthrie, Guthrie, Fernandez and Estrera, 1982; Goldstein, 1974).

Reid and Whitman (1983) have reviewed procedures which aim to establish and maintain therapeutic staff behaviour in institutions. Methods which manipulate the antecedents of staff behaviour are **instructional manipulations**, both general and specific, in which staff are told what their job entails and **modelling**, where staff are shown how to do a job. The conclusion they reach is that the effectiveness of such procedures has yet to be conclusively demonstrated, although there is a good case for supposing that antecedent manipulations can set the occasion for other staff management procedures to be effective. Although it is not noted as such by Reid and Whitman (1983), nurse training might be viewed as a setting condition and might therefore be a **necessary** condition for other procedures to have an effect. As discussed earlier in this chapter, nurse training does not seem to be a **sufficient** condition.

Reid and Whitman (1983) also describe contingency management procedures where the consequences for staff behaviour are manipulated. Again, they are forced to conclude from the studies they review that convincing evidence of efficacy is still lacking, although there are promising trends. A similar picture emerges from their review of self-control procedures, in which care staff are taught to monitor their own behaviour.

The staff-management programmes which show the most promise are those that are multi-faceted, where a number of procedures are combined. An example of such a programme would be that reported by Kissel, Whitman and Reid (1983). Direct care staff were trained to teach mentally handicapped people to brush their teeth. They were trained using written instructions, both videotaped and live modelling, rehearsal and videotaped feedback. To maintain their skills, staff were taught to record, graph and evaluate their own behaviour and the resident's behaviour. Results were very encouraging, with significant gains in the resident's self-care skills of tooth brushing haircombing and handwashing; the latter two skill areas showing that the staff training had generalised to untrained tasks. Because of the complexity of the 'package', it was not possible to isolate the effects of individual components.

This study may be compared with the procedure reported by Page, Iwata and Reid (1982) which had fewer componments. They used a pyramidal training model, with three supervisors taught to train forty-five direct care staff. Daily feedback was provided to the supervisors on the performance of the care staff. Although there were increases in the supervisors on the performance of the care staff, in this case teaching communication skills, there was no generalisation to a different area, teaching gross-motor skills. Improvements in the residents' skills were "small but noticeable".

Because of the difference in the nature of the staff management procedures and the tasks being taught in these two studies, it is not possible to draw any firm conclusions, but it is worth considering the possibility that procedures which are simpler are less likely to achieve lasting significant effects. It is clearly necessary, as Reid and Whitman (1983) argue, to identify the potent components of staff training and management 'packages' but we must be careful to avoid searching for the holy grail of staff management - the single procedure which will be the key to the problem. That mistake has already been made by those who have advocated staff training in the absence of other important organisational changes as a way of improving mental handicap services.

Conclusion

Mental handicap services, in common with all care-systems for disadvantaged people, are changing rapidly. Although it is asserted by some that the emphasis is changing from institutional to community care, a more jaundiced but probably realistic view is that the change is from living in institutions to living in smaller residences. If the process of **care** is to improve, then there must be serious attempts to change care practices before mentally handicapped people leave the institutions, since there is little evidence to support the view that they will alter simply as a result of changing location. Whether or not **nurses** will be carers in the future is not an issue. The same problems will arise whatever the carers are called. Slama and Bannerman (1983) describe the issue vividly:

> "Implementation of behavioural treatment in an institutional setting with unmotivated staff who lack behavioural sophistication, a low staff to client ratio, and a poor physical and management environment is usually a difficult process. It is even more challenging when the clients are severely and profoundly retarded adults who show aggressive and problem behaviours"
>
> (p. 171)

Not all staff have to face such a difficult situation, but the quotation outlines some aspects of the predicament which faces service providers today. Staff have to be **motivated**, which means paying attention to the contingencies under which they operate and the attitudes they bring to the job. They have to become **sophisticated**, which means that training procedures need to be correspondingly sophisticated. The **environment** in which they work has to be conducive to helping mentally handicapped people with conditions such as appropriate staff-client ratios, a minimum of inhibiting routines and a facilitative management structure. Further, in order to help the more difficult of our mentally handicapped clients, all these factors will have to operate together and in the same direction. The challenge of nurse training is not simply how to do it more effectively, but how to do it effectively and alter the ecosystem of a mental handicap residence at the same time.

References

Ajzen, I. and Fishbein, M. (1977) 'Attitude-behavior Relations: A Theoretical Analysis and Review of Empirical Research', Psychological Bulletin, 84, 888-918

Altschul, A. T. (1977) 'Use of the Nursing Process in Psychiatric Care', Nursing Times, Sept 8, 1412-1413

Ashworth, P. (1980) 'A Way to Better Care', Nursing Mirror, August 28, 26-27

Ashworth, P., Castledine, G. and McFarlane, J. K. (1978) 'The Process in Practice', Nursing Times Supplement, Nov 30, 3-4

Beardshaw, V. (1981) Conscientious Objectors at Work, Social Audit, London

Berni, R. and Fordyce, W. E. (1977) Behavior Modification and the Nursing Process, Mosby, St Louis, CV

Bernstein, G. S. (1982) 'Training Behaviour Change Agents: A Conceptual Review', Behaviour Therapy, 13, 1-23

Birenbaum, A. and Re, M. A. (1979) 'Resettling Mentally Retarded Adults in the Community - Almost 4 Years Later', American Journal of Mental Deficiency, 83, 323-329

Birenbaum, A. and Seiffer, S. (1976) Resettling

Retarded Adults in a Managed Community, Praeger Special Studies, New York

Brown, J. and Walton, I. (1984) How nurses learn: A national study of the training of nurses in mental handicap, Final Report. University of York, Department of Social Policy and Social Work

Burton, M., Thomas, M. and Cullen, C. (1981) Offerton self-care checklist, Hester Adrian Research Centre, University of Manchester

Butterfield, E. C., Barnett, C. D. and Bensberg, G. J. (1968) 'A Measure of Attitude which Differentiates Attendants from Separate Institutions', American Journal of Mental Deficiency, 72, 890-899

Clark, M. O. (1978) 'Why We need the Nursing Process? - For Practical Reasons', Nursing Times, Nov 30, 21-24

Crow, J. (1977) 'The Nursing Process - Theoretical Background', Nursing Times, June 16, 892-896

Cullen, C. (1981) Residents' Development Project - Annual report to the Department of Health and Social Security. Hester Adrian Research Centre, University of Manchester

Cullen, C (1984) '"But we've always done it that way": Obstacles to Implementing the Nursing Process in Mental Handicap Settings', Senior Nurse, 1(24), 10-11

Cullen, C., Burton, M, S., Watts, S. and Thomas, M. (1984) 'A Preliminary Report on the Nature of Interactions in a Mental Handicap Institution', Behaviour Research and Therapy, 21 579-583

Davis, B. D. (1978) 'Why Do We Need the Nursing Process? - For Professional Reasons', Nursing Times, Nov 30, 1986-1987

Department of Health and Social Security, Scottish Home and Health Department and Welsh Office, (1972) Report of the Committee on Nursing. Chairman: Professor Asa Briggs. Cmnd 5115, HMSO, London

Department of Health and Social Security (1979) Report of the Committee of Enquiry into Mental Handicap Nursing and Care, Chairman: Mrs Peggy Jay. Cmnd 7468-I HMSO, London

ENB (1982) Syllabus of Training: Professional Register (part 5) (Registered Nurse for the Mentally Handicapped), English and Welsh National Boards for Nursing, Midwifery and Health Visiting, London

Felce, D., Kushlick, A. and Smith, J. (1983) 'The Planning and Evaluation of a Programme of Community-based Residences for Severely Mentally Handicapped People' in S. E. Breuning, J. L. Matson and R. P. Barrett (eds.), Advances in Mental Retardation and Developmental Disabilities, JAI Press, Greenwich

GNC (1970) Syllabus of subjects for examination for the certificate of the nursing of the mentally subnormal, General Nursing Council, London

Goldstein, G. S. (1974) 'Behaviour Modification: Some Cultural Factors', Psychological Record, 24, 89-91

Grant, G. W. B. (1974) An examination of care patterns in subnormality hospitals with differing resource levels, Unpublished doctoral dissertation, Department of Management Science, University of Manchester Institute of Science and Technology

Gutherie. M, Guthrie, H. A., Fernandez, T. L. and Estrera, N.O. (1982) 'Cultural Influences and Reinforcement Strategies', Behavior Therapy, 13, 624-637

Henderson, V. (1961) The Nature of Nursing, Collier Macmillan, London

Hegvary, S. T. (1979) 'Nursing Process: The Basis for Evaluating the Quality of Nursing Carers', International Nursing Review, 26, 113-116

Hogg, J., Foxen, T. and McBrien, J. (1981) 'Issues in the Training and Evaluation of Behaviour Modification Skills for Staff Working with Profoundly Retarded Multiply Handicapped Children, Behavioural Psychotherapy, 9, 345-357

Kiernan, C. C. and Riddick, B. (1973) A draft programme for training in operant techniques, Institute of Education, University of London, London

Kissel, R. C., Whitman, T. L. and Reid, D. H. (1983) 'An Institutional Staff Training and Self-management Programme for Developing Multiple Self-care Skills in Severely/Profoundly Retarded Individuals', Journal of Applied Behavior Analysis, 16, 395-415

Kratz, C. (1977) 'The Nursing Process', Nursing Times, June 9, 854-855

Luker, K. A. (1977) 'A Framework for the Nursing Process: Problem Oriented Recordings', Nursing Times, August 30, 1488-1490

Mayhew, G. L., Enyart, P. and Cone, J. D. (1979) 'Approaches to Employee Management: Policies and Preferences', Journal of Organizational Behavior Management, 2, 103-111

Milne, D. (1985) 'A Review of the In-service Training of Nurses in Behaviour Therapy', American Journal of Mental Deficiency, 80, 644-649

Moores, R. and Grant, G. W. B. (1976) 'Nurses' Expectations for Accomplishment of Mentally Retarded Patients', American Journal of Mental Deficiency, 80, 644-649

Moores, R. and Grant, G. W. B. (1977a) 'Feelings of Alienation among Nursing Staff in Hospitals for the Mentally Handicapped', International Journal of Nursing Studies, 14, 5-12

Moores, R. and Grant, G. W. B. (1977b) 'Optimists and Pessimists: Attitudes of Nursing Staff toward the Development Potential of Mentally Handicapped Patients in their Charge', International Journal of Nursing Studies, 14, 13-18

Morris, L. L. and Fitz-Gibbon, C. (1978) Evaluator's Handbook, Sage, Beverly Hills

Murphy, R. J. (1983) An investigation into the determinants of nursing staff behaviour in the long term care of the mentally handicapped, unpublished manuscript, Calderstones Hospital,

Blackburn

Neilson, A. F., (1978) 'Why Do We Need the Nursing Process? - For Legal Reasons', Nursing Times, Nov 30, 1984-1985

Page, T. J., Iwata, B. A. and Reid, D. H. (1982) 'Pyramidal Training: A Large Scale Application with Institutional Staff', Journal of Applied Behavior Analysis, 15, 335-351

Peterson, L., Homer, A. L. and Wonderlich, S. A. (1982) 'The Integrity of Independent Variables in Behavior Analysis', Journal of Applied Behavior Analysis, 15, 477-492

Quilitch, H. R. (1975) 'A Comparison of Three Staff-management procedures', Journal of Applied Behavior Analysis, 8, 59-66

Reid, D. H. and Whitman, T. L. (1983) 'Behavioral Staff Management in Institutions: A Critical Review of Effectiveness and Acceptability', Analysis and Intervention in Developmental Disabilities, 3, 131-149

Sebba, J. (1985) 'Evaluating the Effectiveness of Teaching Behavioral Methods to Staff Training in Mental Handicap', Behavioral Psychotherapy, 13, 101-109

Selvin, H. C. and Stuart, A. (1966) 'Data Dredging Procedures in Survey Analysis', American Statistician, 20, 20-23

Slama, K.M. and Bannerman, D. J. (1983) 'Implementing and Maintaining a Behavioural Treatment System in an Institutional Setting', Analysis and Intervention in Developmental Disabilities, 3, 177-191

Stolz, S. B. (1981) 'Adoption of Innovations from Applied Behavioral Research: "Does Anybody Care?"', Journal of Applied Behavior Analysis, 14, 491-505

Thomas, M. Burton, M. and Cullen, C. (1982) 'Take a New Look at Your Ward: Increasing Opportunities for Learning on Wards with Mentally Handicapped Residents', Nursing Times, 78, 1068-1070

Wahler, R. G. and Fox, J. J. (1981) 'Setting Events in Applied Behavior Analysis: Towards a Conceptual and Methodological Expansion', Journal of Applied Behavior Analysis, 14, 327-338

Watson, L. S. and Uzell, R. (1980), 'A Programme for Teaching Behavior Modification Skills to Institutional Staff', Applied Research in Mental Retardation, 1, 41-53

Williams, C. and Jackson, M. (1975) 'Nurse Training in Behaviour Modification' in C. C. Kiernan and F. P. Woodward (eds.), Behaviour Modification with the Severely Retarded, Associated Scientific Publishers, Amsterdam

Ziarnik, J. P. and Bernstein, G. S. (1982) 'A Critical Examination of the Effect of Inservice Training on Staff Performance', Mental Retardations, 20, 109-114

PART IV: METHODS OF DISSEMINATION

Chapter 9

A PYRAMID MODEL OF STAFF TRAINING IN BEHAVIOURAL METHODS: THE E.D.Y. PROJECT

J.A. McBrien and T.H. Foxen

Introduction

In 1976 the Department of Education and Science began funding a four year research project at the Hester Adrian Research Centre, University of Manchester entitled 'Education of the Developmentally Young Mentally Handicapped Child: A Programme of Evaluated Dissemination and Research', known as the E.D.Y. Project. The need for this research had emerged from a body of work carried out over the previous three years at H.A.R.C. (Hogg, 1975; Hogg, Foxen and McBrien, 1979).

The aim of the Project was to develop and disseminate a method of training staff working with severely mentally handicapped children to use a behavioural approach to teaching. Over the four years, a model of staff training was developed and researched on two levels. First, a training course in behaviour modification for 'hands on' staff was developed, consisting of an initial training in basic skills followed by training for generalisation of these skills - the in-service course for staff. Second, a training course for key personnel in education was developed, based on workshops, to teach these professionals to run and evaluate the staff training course in their own Local Education Authorities (L.E.A.). It is the purpose of this chapter to report in detail on the E.D.Y. Project.

The E.D.Y course is essentially a training to use an individual teaching strategy. It can only be effective when organisational changes are made and management support is forthcoming to ensure that individual teaching time is available. The realisation of this led the project team to a consideration of room management as a technique for providing such changes. This aspect of the research will be referred to in the conclusions but not dealt with in detail.

E.D.Y. Project

The In-Service Course for Staff

The course consists of three training phases by the end of which staff should be competent to devise, execute and evaluate individual training programmes with children in their classroom. The course is concerned with teaching method and not with content. Decisions as to curriculum are not addressed by the course except as they arise in choosing a task to teach within the training sessions. An outline of each of the three phases will be given, followed by detailed description of the materials and methods used in each.

Phase I consists of the bulk of the training in the form of ten one hour training sessions per member of staff. Variations on the 'pure' model of one trainee per one instructor are common and will be discussed later but for the purposes of describing the course, it will be assumed that sessions are conducted on a one to one basis as originally intended. The ten sessions of Phase I cover ten content areas of behaviour modification, the trainee receiving instruction through written material, role play and practice with children. Practical skills are evaluated throughout, and theoretical knowledge before and after the course. At the successful completion of Phase I, trainees received a certificate from the University of Manchester and proceed to Phase II. A trainee may be any member of staff, e.g., qualified teacher, nursery nurse, classroom assistant.

Phase II is a period of generalisation and consolidation of skills learned during Phase I. While Phase I sessions concentrate on the sequential acquisition of techniques, practising with a different child in each session, in Phase II the trainee selects one child and one task and works intensively with the child in the classroom over approximately a ten week period with close supervision from the instructor. Practical skills and child progress are continually monitored.

Phase III is a repeat of Phase II with a different child and task but with support for the trainee systematically faded. Once again, child progress and trainee performance are monitored.

Course Materials

The written materials for the trainee are contained in self-instructional form in the Trainee Workbook (Foxen and McBrien, 1981). These have undergone a considerable evolution, generally in the direction of making them shorter and simpler in theoretical content and more explicit and detailed in terms of preparing the trainee for the practical sessions. The first (pilot) version of the course used Kiernan and Riddick's (1973) 'Programme for Training in Operant Techniques' (see Hogg, Foxen and McBrien, 1979). This was substantially revised and rewritten by Foxen (1978b) and again by Foxen and McBrien (1981) which is the present version. This is currently undergoing further revisions in the light of national feedback. The present version contains ten units covering Operant Behaviour, Reward Assessment, Reward Training, Prompting, Generalisation and Discrimination. A short discussion of each of these is given, followed by programmed questions to aid comprehension. This is followed by a detailed breakdown of the content of the practical session, including a description of the videotape demonstration to be shown and recording sheets to be used. At the end of the workbook are recording sheets for Phases II and III. Trainees retain the workbook after the course as a permanent record and as a reference source.

The course materials also include a one hour demonstration videotape and an Instructor's Handbook (McBrien and Foxen, 1981a).

Pedagogic devices

Behaviour modification is a set of practical skills, albeit derived initially from experimental studies of learning. The emphasis of the course is more on the acquisition of these skills than on gains in theoretical understanding. It is important to note that behaviour modifiers have been using different techniques to teach staff from those which the staff are being taught to use with their clients. In developing the course, therefore, it was necessary to consider which pedagogic devices should be used, their sequencing and time allocation. The time allocation would need to reflect the effectiveness of the different pedagogic devices. Some consideration was therefore given to instruction theory.

One such theory (Bruner, 1966) has suggested three levels for the representation of knowledge: the symbolic (or cognitive) level; the iconic (or perceptual) level; and the enactive (or behavioural) level. Bruner (1964) suggests that these three modes of representation form a developmental sequence in order of difficulty: enactive, iconic, symbolic. The overall question to be asked of each part of the training is 'what level of representation by the trainee is required to understand the knowledge content being taught?'. A second, related question is 'which pedagogic devices are available which demand a low representational level for understanding, e.g., iconic or enactive, but which effectively teach the skills to be learned by the trainee?' The major pedagogic devices available are discussed below in relation to these two questions.

The Socratic technique

This is the traditional inductive or question and answer method. The technique is based on the belief that the student 'knows' the answer and it is the function of the teacher to 'bring it out' by skilful questioning. Much of traditional teaching involves this method, but it is of doubtful generality because it only works with the 'best' students. The technique depends heavily on the symbolic level of representation. Watson and Bassinger (1974), for example, have shown that academic knowledge (symbolic level) does not necessarily correlate with practical skills (enactive level). It was felt that the poor educational background of some trainees often promoted the learning task to an academic (symbolic) level beyond that required to learn the behavioural (enactive) skills being taught. The high level of representation which written and spoken information demands suggests that these should only occupy a small part of the course. Revisions of the course have reduced the amount of time spent on questioning the trainee about the reading material from one hour to none at all, trainees merely being asked at the end of the session if they have any questions about what they have read.

Social modelling and audio-visual demonstration

It is generally accepted that much learning occurs as a result of imitation of others (Bandura and Walters, 1963; Piaget, 1951). It would appear that social modelling exploits the iconic level of representation. As such, this pedagogic device should be able to transmit knowledge not understandable at the symbolic level. Teaching through modelling has been shown to be highly successful (Lange, 1971). It has also been shown that film or video models have a similar effect to live models and on this basis a course demonstration videotape was produced showing trainers using the various techniques with children.

The limitations of social modelling suggest that while it is an essential pedagogic device, it should only occupy a small part of the practical session. In the workbook, following the programmed questions is a short description of the video model. This is accompanied by a recording sheet with relevant headings (such as reward, prompt, target behaviour) to cue the trainee. Recording the child's and teacher's behaviour is an integral part of the whole course. The recording sheet to be used throughout the course for child behaviour is introduced in Unit 3 and is practised on each video demonstration as well as in other parts of each session. Each practical session starts with 15 minutes watching and rating the demonstration video.

Educational role play

Role play is now a familiar technique in many fields in which training in practical skills is required. Its importance seems to lie in its provision of relevant practice (enactive level) without the aversive consequences of error responses in the natural situation. Gagne (1962), for example, discusses the use of flight simulators for rapid training of war-time personnel. The equivalent method for the teaching situation is to provide a child simulator for the trainee to practise with (Corsini and Cardone, 1966).

It is interesting to note that the Stanford University

team which developed the micro-teaching approach (Allen and Ryan, 1969) originally tried role playing techniques using student-teacher peers as pupils. They apparently rejected role play because the students found it unrealistic. It is possible that the feeling of unreality in the students was due to their unfamiliarity with the children being role played. To achieve verisimilitude, the person role playing the child must be very familiar with the child. This means the technique is applicable to all 'hands on' staff but would suggest caution when applying it to pre-service teachers in college or to pupil nurses. Our experience is that staff who are familiar with their clients are adept at role playing, needing only a little modelling and encouragement to try it for the first time.

Role play has the benefit of removing the need for new understanding by the trainee at the academic or cognitive level before attempting the role play. This is usually in the form of written or spoken instruction given before the trainee has the opportunity to accommodate at the enactive level.

Finally, role reversal maximally exploits the established pedagogic device of social modelling. In the role reversal situation, with the trainee enacting the child, the instructor is in a position to model the technique he or she wishes the trainee to learn. After the role reversal, the trainee reverts to his or her normal social role. The instructor who has just witnessed the model of the child is then in a position to provide a child simulator for the trainee to practise with. In this natural role play situation, the trainee can practise using the new technique without the threat of real failure. The potential advantage of role play over shaping techniques based on operant principles is that it can exploit the more advanced levels of representation available to the trainee. If these views are correct, then role play would appear to be an ideal instructional strategy. In the course, twenty minutes of each practical session is devoted to role play, ten minutes in which the trainee takes the part of the child and receives a life model of the technique and ten minutes in which the trainee practises the technique using the instructor as a simulated child.

Simulated practice with a child

The natural follow-on from the role play is simulated practice with a real child. It is equivalent in some ways to micro-teaching which involves a short lesson in a highly structured but simplified situation. The difference is that whereas in micro-teaching feedback is delayed until the end of the short teaching period and followed by a reteach, in the E.D.Y. course feedback is given trial by trial so that trainees have an opportunity to correct their own behaviour immediately and be reinforced for correct responding. Although trainees can experience the consequences of their behaviour, overall responsibility is taken by the instructor.

The emphasis on all three levels of representation, particularly the enactive, which is involved in role play and simulated practice suggests that these two pedagogic devices should constitute the major part of the practical session. Thus, following the twenty minutes spent on role play, twenty minutes is spent on practice with a child with trial-by-trial feedback from the instructor. A task will have been selected beforehand by the instructor in consultation with the trainee (as will rewards) and these will have been used in the role play.

Shaping and feedback

For shaping to take place, a response must be emitted in order to provide an opportunity for reinforcement. This has been called the problem of 'the first instance' (Skinner, 1968). The video model can serve to sensitise the trainee but its effect will again depend on the present skill repertoire of the trainee. The first role play sequence further primes the required response, but it is not until the second role play with the trainee practising his or her own role as teacher, that the instructor can start to shape her behaviour. The teaching role of the instructor can then be seen as giving positive feedback to the trainee for approximations to target behaviour and appropriate prompting (i.e., shaping). In this context, role play sets the occasion for the occurrence of new trainee behaviour which can then be reinforced.

It is essential that the instructor be prepared to give positive reinforcement for approximations rather than no feedback or negative feedback for 'inadequate' performance. Watson (1972) has suggested that a ratio of four positive to one negative comments should be aimed for. It is our experience that trainee errors which are not corrected in the role play are repeated unmodified in the simulated practice with the child. It is possible to use negative feedback in the role play since in this pretend situation the trainee is more prepared to accept critical guidance.

In the simulated practice, however, the trainee's behaviour becomes more realistic. Negative comments tend to have the predictable emotional concomitants which are associated with punishment and which interfere with learning. In the simulated practice, therefore, it is essential to follow Watson's dictum. This bias towards positive feedback is not a typical teaching style and instructors need to learn to use it. The typical situation is one where the instructor ignores errors but does not see opportunities for reward, thus conducting the simulated practice in silence and leaving the trainee no wiser. The course recommends that feedback is given positively and frequently during practical sessions. Negative comments are rephrased in the form of single, unambiguous instructions (verbal prompts) preceded by a positive comment. In this way the feedback necessary to shape up behaviour is given during the session and not delayed until the end. Given the limitations of delayed feedback, in that it gives no immediate opportunity for self correction, the course has not used delayed video feedback to trainees on their own performance. Early experience with this demonstrated that it added nothing to what had already been said and possibly only accentuated to the trainee examples of incorrect responding.

The session finishes with some remarks about the child's behaviour and arrangements for the next session. The reading material may be discussed briefly at this stage if trainees have any questions. The reason for keeping any discussion of the reading material until this point is that trainees have by that time received instruction on the enactive and iconic levels concerning what they have read, which should have reduced some of the difficulties in understanding.

Implications

The course uses the pedagogic devices as described to maximise learning at all three levels of representation. Two thirds of staff training time is spent in a simulated teaching situation utilising the two major pedagogic devices of role play and practice with a child. If the trainee can achieve success at this level, generalisation to the classroom is more likely. The temporal sequence of the practical session includes two important features. First, there is a progression from symbolic through iconic to enactive levels. Second, there is a progressive reality content from the anonymity of the videtape model, to the very real demands of working with a child from one's own classroom. Figure 1 depicts the use of the various pedagogic devices and their temporal sequence in the standard one hour training session.

Evaluation methods used in Phase I

Methods of evaluating staff training courses in behaviour modification have been reviewed elsewhere (for example, Mazza and Pumroy, 1975; Carr, 1980) and will not be reviewed in detail here. Questionnaires on course content and opinions of course members are popular and simple. Typically, participants evaluate courses positively and there are dangers in using these as the only method of evaluation. Questionnaires were used extensively in the development of the E.D.Y. course but not to evaluate trainee progress. Trainees completing the course were asked to complete comments sheets concerning what had been most useful on the course and asking for suggestions for improvements. Although comments did tend to be largely positive, analysis of large numbers of comments sheets provided valuable data for the revision of parts of the course. Trainees were also asked to complete ratings of the pedagogic devices using seven point rating scales on a number of attributes of each pedagogic device, e.g., useful/not useful. Data on these and on the comments sheets are reported by McBrien and Thomas (1981).

Quizzes and tests of behaviour modification are another popular method of evaluation and several are reported in the literature (Gardner, Brust and Watson, 1970; Carr, 1980; Kiernan and Riddick, 1973). On the E.D.Y. course a pre-post course quiz is given to

Figure 1. E.D.Y. One Hour Training Session (Phase 1).

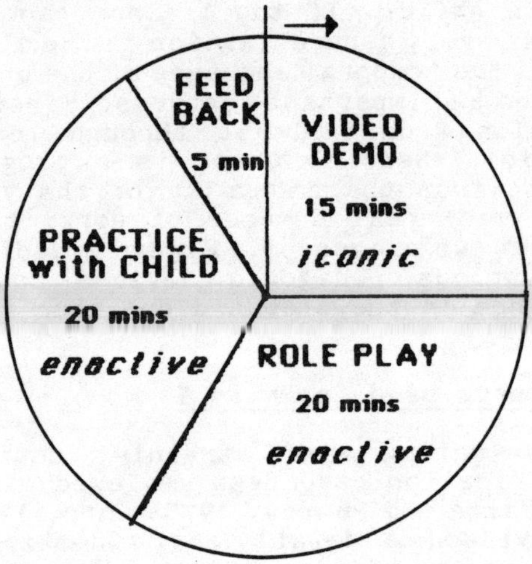

trainees to test knowledge of the terminology and principles of behaviour modification as described in the Trainee Workbook. To pass the course, trainees must score 50 per cent or over at the post test. It was felt important that staff should have a grasp of the terminology of behaviour modification so that a common language could exist between members of staff to facilitate discussion of programmes.

The most common method of assessing the effectiveness of behaviour modification training has been to determine whether or not the trainee has changed the behaviour of the client. This is used as an indirect measure of trainer effectiveness. O'Dell (1974) and Griffin (1979) criticised the tendency for most studies at that time to rely on changes in the mentally handicapped person's target behaviour as the only outcome measure of training efficacy. The rating scale used on the E.D.Y. course includes a rating of child behaviour.

Assessment of changes in the trainee's behaviour is essential. Techniques to do this vary from global subjective ratings to detailed analysis of practical skills and complex observational schedules. Typically, the trainee is assessed on a rating scale while teaching a particular skill or dealing with a problem selected by the experimenter - the critical incident technique. Most studies make ratings on role played sessions. However, there are no studies comparing trainees' performance in role played situations with real life interaction with a mentally handicapped person. There are very few studies in which real clients have been used in the evaluation of trainees. Kiernan and Riddick (1973) used a 30 item scale to evaluate their trainees on a pre-post test basis. Trainees were videotaped before and after the course. Hogg, Foxen and McBrien (1981) used a modified form of this scale to evaluate application of Kiernan and Riddick's course with profoundly retarded multiply handicapped children.

The critical incident technique is a potentially reliable and objective method of assessing performance skills, although several pitfalls need to be avoided (Carr, 1980). Gardner and Giampa (1971) highlight the point that the critical incident technique involves only a limited amount of trainee behaviour and thus lacks comprehensiveness and possibly representativeness. It is important to remember why one is making such evaluations. If the aim of training is to train staff to use certain techniques in specified circumstances, e.g. training teachers to use behaviour modification techniques when working on programmes with individual children for short periods each day, then the critical incident technique would seem to be entirely appropriate.

On the E.D.Y. course the assessment of practical skills was seen as the most important part of the evaluation. Practical skills were identified as those described in the Trainee Workbook. In earlier work, the rating scale developed by Kiernan and Riddick (1973) was used but found to be unwieldy in developing an exportable staff training course. It required videotaping facilities and each ten minute pre-, and posttest took up to two hours to rate. It also yielded a large amount of redundant data (see Hogg et al. 1981 for details). In developing an exportable course, a method was needed for assessing a trainee's skills in a live teaching session which had good reliability and which could be taught to course instructors during a workshop. Accordingly, the Kiernan and Riddick scale was drastically revised and shortened to form a new scale - the Trainee Assessment Form (T.A.F.).

The T.A.F. has five categories, four relating to the trainee's behaviour and one to the child's. These are: 'prepares child for task', 'presents tasks', 'prompts', 'child's response', and 'rewards'. The scoring system allows for three types of correct response ranging from excellent to poor approximation, two types of incorrect response, failure to respond and incorrect response, and an "irrelevant" score. Good reliabilities exist for all categories of the T.A.F., less satisfactory ones having been dropped during the research (see Foxen, 1978a). Trainees are rated on the T.A.F. for units 3 - 10 of the course while they are working with a child. Unit 3 is then used as a pretest measure and Unit 10 as a posttest. Trainees must score 65 per cent or over on the posttest to pass the course.

Generalisation of skills - Phase II

The project team was well aware that a major and valid criticism of all training courses is their failure to generalise to the work setting of the trainees. Kiernan (1975) has called this the 'circus effect'.

A team of experts arrives with a package of new techniques, passes them on to 'hands-on' staff using a variety of methods for doing so and then 'the circus leaves town'. Staff are left with a few practical hints, on rare occasions some practical experience and often a handbook of some sort describing the theory of a behavioural approach. They are left without structured programmes and without support or feedback on their attempts to put the new approach into practice. The finding that generalisation will not take place unless programmed has often been stressed in the literature (Watson, 1975; Hart and Risley, 1976; Stokes and Baer, 1977). The E.D.Y. project was faced with the question of how best to induce generalisation. In a sense, this inducement begins in Phase I, since this extends from simulation, through practice, to direct teaching. Phase II forms the next logical step of providing staff with practice in using the techniques in the less sheltered setting of the classroom.

Phase II consists of individual child training programmes run by staff who have successfully completed Phase I. The programmes are jointly set up by the newly qualified trainer and instructor and although the trainer carries out the programme from day to day in the classroom, it is closely monitored by the instructor who has overall responsibility for its success. The main aim of Phase II is to ensure that the trainer experiences success with the techniques and that by its completion will be able to use the skills of behaviour modification and programme planning in the work setting. Two major functions of Phase II were envisaged. First, it would be a period of consolidation in which the trainer rehearsed the newly learned skills in a task seen as relevant to the child's development, over an extended period of time. Second, it would be a period of generalisation in which the trainer was expected to practise the skills in a new, unshelterd setting, e.g. the classroom or toilets and to incorporate the practice periods into the normal working day.

The project team felt strongly that a structured approach to programme planning was vital. Programmes which were ill-thought out usually failed early on. Accordingly, a Phase II programme is set up through a series of six meetings between trainer and instructor, timed to suit both with at least one meeting held weekly. Programme sheets are included in the workbook for each meeting. In these meetings, trainers select three children with whom they would like to work and a tentative task area for each. All three are assessed on one or more developmental scales or checklists relevant to the selected task area, including any already available in the school, e.g. a Portage checklist. With advice from the instructor, the trainer then chooses one of these three, a tractable child to work with on a task regarded as relevant to the child's educational or social needs. In the third meeting the child is observed on the task and a preliminary task analysis is made with full assistance from the instructor. The trainer takes several baselines on these steps. The task analysis is then refined and decisions are made on the steps to teach, rewards, methods of prompting, time out, etc. and on the training schedule, e.g. ten minutes from 1.30 - 1.40, Monday - Thursday. The trainer decides on the type of recording sheet to use for recording child behaviour, usually the sheet used throughout Phase I.

The instructor's role throughout centres on giving full support to the trainer in meeting the objectives. The sixth meeting constitutes the first training session with the child and from then on the trainer carries out the programme alone three to five times a week according to the agreed timetable. The instructor monitors once a week. At the monitoring session, the instructor's task is to review the records of child progress for that week, observe the session for that day, record the trainer's use of the techniques on T.A.F. and give reinforcement. When the pre-arranged termination criteria have been reached, instructor and trainer hold a review meeting to decide on continuation, maintenance and generalisation of the programme. A follow-up meeting takes place about three months later. The child is observed on the targeted behaviour and records reviewed. In this way Phase II provides a detailed and permanent record of individual child progress which can be incorporated into the school record keeping system. Data on Phase II are available from a variety of sources. The T.A.F. analyses reveal utilisation of Phase I skills by the trainer. Child progress data are available in the form of the trainer's own records of each trial of each training session and there is a reliability check on this in the form of the instructor's weekly recording. The programme summary sheets reveal the number of trials and sessions taken for the child to reach criterion on each step and the frequency with which trainers managed to carry out sessions.

Phase III

This is a repeat of Phase II with systematically faded support from the instructor. The six programme planning meetings are collapsed into three. Trainers are given a freer choice in child and task selection and are not discouraged from selecting a child with special problems or a more complex task. The third meeting, observation of the child, is still crucial in so far as the instructor must decide at this point if the programme is likely to work or not. The trainer is then left to make a task analysis, take baselines and draw up programme details with minimal support. The instructor attends the first training session and thereafter monitors fortnightly still completing T.A.F. assessments and giving feedback. Detailed results of Phase II and III programmes run by the project team are reported in McBrien and Foxen (1981b).

Evaluations of the in-service course

The three phases of the course have been described above in terms of their content, pedagogic devices used and methods of evaluation. Following the development period, the course materials were made self instructional and published by Manchester University Press. Figures on the number and type of staff trained are given in a later section. We are concerned in this section with formal evaluations of the course. The research team evaluated the trainees trained by them during the funded period of the research using pre- and posttest measures on the T.A.F. and the quiz for Phase I, and repeated T.A.F. measures during Phases II and III. Information was also sought through questionnaires. Subsequently, more detailed evaluations have been undertaken on Phase I and recently on Phase II. Three of the studies which examine the internal validity of Phase I will be briefly reported here but the reader is referred to the studies themselves for further information.

Farrell (1982) made an evaluation of an E.D.Y. course run for five teachers and five classroom assistants from the same school for children with severe learning difficulties. Each trainee was videotaped at pretest, posttest and at a seven week follow up and the videotapes were rated blind by two independent raters. Farrell's results show a significant improvement for teachers at posttest and at follow up over pretest scores and a difference between teachers and assistants in favour of teachers. These results formed the first attempt to make an independent evaluation of the course. They suggest that the course may be better suited to qualified teachers than to untrained assistants.

This latter finding was further explored by Farrell and Sugden (1984) in an evaluation of a Phase I E.D.Y. course for eight classroom assistants. All eight were trained nursery nurses, in contrast to other classroom assistants in the school who had no qualifications. The trainees were videotaped on four occasions - two pretests, an immediate posttest and a ten week follow up. The main conclusion was that the assistants made significant gains in their total T.A.F. scores for all teaching techniques taken together immediately after training and that these improvements were maintained at follow up. However, analysis of individual rating categories showed that improvements had only been made on two categories (rewards and task analysis) and no improvement was shown on presents task or prompts. (The authors used a modified form of T.A.F. which dropped 'prepares child' and included a rating of task analysis.) Individual results were also reported and these showed considerable variation between trainees. These results contradict the earlier findings of Farrell and suggest that non-teaching assistants can benefit from the course. It must also be remembered that these assistants were trained nursery nurses. These studies represent an advance on previous work in the evaluation of behaviour modification courses in that they used videotapes of live teaching sessions, rather than role play, and the tapes were rated independently by trained raters who were not involved in the training course and who were blind to occasion (see also Barrowclough, 1981). However, with the possible exception of Farrell and Sugden, they do not control for a possible practice effect from pretest to posttest, a very real danger as pointed out by Carr (1980). The studies use a one group pretest-posttest design, the limitations of which have been pointed out by Cook and Campbell (1979).

The third study is that by McBrien and Edmonds (1985)

which used a non-equivalent control group design (Cook and Campbell, 1979) to examine immediate effects of Phase I training on teacher behaviour and generalisation of any behaviour change. The experimental and control groups each consisted of four teachers from each of two E.S.N.(S) schools. The experimental group received a standard E.D.Y. course and the control group no training. Each trainee from each group was tested on three occasions: at pretest, posttest and at a fourteen month follow up. No further training took place between the posttest and follow up. Sessions were videotaped and rated independently by two trained raters, blind to condition and occasion. Results showed that the experimental group improved its scores significantly on posttest compared to pretest and maintained this improvement at the fourteen month follow up. The experimental group score was above the pass mark for the course on posttest and follow up. The control group did not change their scores from one occasion to another and remained well below the pass mark on all occasions. There was a significant difference between groups in the expected direction. Analysis of individual results showed considerable variation between teachers. These studies give some support to the internal validity of the course and to the long term maintenance of skills. Controlled studies remain to be reported on the effects of Phase II training and on the effects on children taught by trained staff. Research is underway in this area through Project Impact at the Hester Adrian Research Centre.

THE NATIONAL DISSEMINATION EXERCISE

National coverage

It was the brief of the project to establish a method of disseminating the in-service course described above on a national basis. The project was to select key Local Education Authority personnel who were in a position to organise and run in-service training in the special schools. The project team selected Educational Psychologists and Advisers for Special Education as the professionals most likely to be able to influence teaching in the schools. It was decided that each of the 104 L.E.A.s in England and Wales would be asked to identify one representative, either an Educational Psychologist or an Adviser, who would undergo training to run the E.D.Y. course and who would subsequently run the course in that L.E.A. It was also decided that each representative would need to be given practical experience of running the course if dissemination was to be effective. The method selected to identify representatives was to write to the Chief Education Officer in each Authority explaining the aims of the research and asking him or her to select a suitable candidate. The difficulties to which this method led will be discussed later.

A workshop method of training was selected whereby representatives came to Manchester for five days to receive practical training in running the course. It was decided that twenty workshops, each lasting five days, would be run with five instructors attending each workshop. In this way 100 instructors could be given practical training over a period of four school terms, five workshops per term between September 1977 and December 1978. This provision was thought to be more than adequate since a maximum of 25 per cent representation from the Authorities was expected. As will be shown, this was not to be the case.

Workshop location

In order to run the workshops, direct access to children and staff of special schools was required. Facilities were made available to the research team in a new special school in Manchester (Melland School). The training course was set up in the school with school staff as trainees. Instructor workshops took place in the school at the same time. In basing the workshops in a school, instructors could participate in actual staff training courses in a setting not dissimilar to that which they would encounter in their own Authorities. This arrangement had the added benefit of creating a strong link between a research project and an applied educational facility.

Workshop model

It should be made clear that the functions of the course and workshop were different. The function of the staff training course (Phases I, II and III) is to teach behaviour modification skills to staff working in special school classrooms, referred to as course trainees. The function of the E.D.Y. one week workshops was to teach L.E.A. representatives how to put on such a course in their own Authority. These representatives were referred to as course instructors. The workshop was not designed to provide a training in behaviour modification for instructors, although it could serve this purpose to some extent.

In order to provide practical experience for instructors, it was necessary to set up a ten unit course in microcosm, so that instructors could gain experience of the whole Phase I course which they were expected to run on return to their L.E.A. By doubling up the number of sessions for trainees, it was possible to train five to seven trainees over a period of five workshops, two units per trainee per workshop. At the same time, 25 instructors (five x five) could learn how to run the course. The workshop model therefore provided a very efficient dissemination procedure.

Regarding the use of pedagogic devices, it was decided that role play and simulated practice were likely to be relevant for use with instructors in the same way as they were being used with trainees. The main pedagogic devices will be described in detail below, but there were several additional teaching aspects included in workshops which are worth mentioning. Instructors were given the opportunity to use a developmental scale - the Object Schemas Scale - derived from Uzgiris and Hunt (1975). Seminars were given during each workshop at the end of the day. These were designed to broaden the scope of the workshop and to provide a forum for discussion of practical issues relevant to teaching in E.S.N.(S) schools.

Pedagogic devices used with instructors

The major pedagogic devices used with instructors during workshops were reading materials, social modelling, role play, simulated practice with trainee and child, shaping, delayed verbal feedback, problem setting and goal planning. These are briefly discussed below and fuller details are available in Foxen (1978a).

Reading material

Instructors were sent the written materials for trainees before a workshop and needed to become familiar with their content. Unlike trainees, all instructors had an advanced educational background, including in most cases, some training and/or experience in behaviour modification. Although reading material relies on the symbolic level, the instructors' professional backgrounds made this device very important. The theoretical units served as academic content revision, while the description of the practical sessions served as a written course guide. The written materials, however, did not serve to give the instructor practical skill in running a course at the enactive level. After the end of the funding period, instructional methods used on workshops were distilled into an Instructor's Handbook. Clearly this made a significant difference to the nature of the course removing all opportunity for practical training of instructors and relying on a self-instructional model. The implications of this will be discussed in a later section.

Social modelling

As well as the models provided by the course demonstration tape, a sequence of live models was provided by the research team (Foxen and McBrien) acting as coordinators and by other instructors as they ran staff training sessions during workshops. During the workshop week, each instructor ran two and observed eight of the ten units. They therefore had a live social model of the whole course. Since real trainees and children took part in the practicals, the modelled sessions had high verisimilitude.

The limitation of this modelling was that instructors were in a learning situation themselves and therefore unlikely to provide high standard models. Although this device was at the iconic level, the high verisimilitude of simulated practice models, combined with instructors' expertise suggest that social modelling was a critical workshop pedagogic device. The live modelling of each unit should have given the instructor a model of Phase I in its entirety, requiring only practical experience in their own setting to consolidate understanding.

Role play and simulated practice

As noted earlier, the critical feature of role play is familiarity with the child. To overcome the difficulty of instructors being unfamiliar with the children, they were first introduced to the children in the classroom and then the following sequence of role plays was used before the training session with a member of staff began:

1. Coordinator models as trainer and child.
2. Instructor role plays child, while coordinator role plays trainer.
3. Instructor role plays trainer, while coordinator or another instructor role plays child. When the member of staff came into the session, the role play sequences took their usual form between instructor and trainee.

Shaping and prompting

This pedagogic device is an art which the instructors had to learn, as did the coordinators. The role play and simulated practice for the instructor provided the context in which instructor skills could be shaped up by the coordinators. The role of the coordinator was to use positive and negative feedback during role play when the trainee was absent. During simulated practice with the trainee, it was essential for the coordinator to adopt Watson's dictum of a feedback ratio of four positive to one negative comment to the instructor. The scope for this depended on the prior role play preparation of the instructor and at times proved problematic. There was rarely sufficient time for the pre-session role plays and these were particularly necessary for instructors whose knowledge of behavioural techniques was slight.

Delayed verbal and audio-visual feedback

Time was allocated for verbal feedback to instructors in a group setting after sessions. Although video feedback was not presented during the workshop, unless there was extreme disagreement about what had happened, the instructors and coordinators had written records of the session to which they could refer. This was especially true of the T.A.F. which gives a trial by trial account of the trainee and child's behaviour. It was also possible to code on the T.A.F. the feedback given by the instructor to the trainee. The delayed and hence post hoc nature of this verbal feedback may have served to consolidate understanding at the most advanced (symbolic) level.

Problem setting for discovery learning

For discovery learning (insight) to occur, successful problem solving had to be engineered. The effectiveness of this device was dependent on the preparation of instructors for the two sessions for which each was responsible. The scope for role play preparation before a session was limited both by time and motivation, since instructors and coordinators already needed to prepare and run four one hour sessions per day. In both respects, a longer workshop was needed. Despite these limitations, each instructor was presented with two sessions which he or she had to learn to run however well prepared or otherwise. Problem setting with practical assignments was seen as an essential feature of the workshop model being used.

Goal planning

Goal planning (Houts and Scott, 1975) is a procedure which, like problem solving, was a general pedagogic feature of the workshop. Goal planning is based on the assumption that achievement or success is the motivating feature of human behaviour (see McClelland, Atkinson, Clark and Lowell, 1953). It is reasonable to assume that instructors arrived at a workshop with varying levels of aspiration. Most would not have run a course in behaviour modification, so that task demand was a challenge. The aim of the workshop was to provide the skills and the motivation necessary to run a training course. Throughout the workshop week, instructors were responsible for instructing trainees on a course set up by the coordinators. As the workshop proceeded, coordinator support was faded so that, by its completion, instructors should have had sufficient knowledge and expertise to run and evaluate the training sessions. The instructors saw a course in microcosm, but did not see the preparation and organisation required to set the course up. Much of the last day was spent in dealing with this aspect.

Each instructor was asked to write out a goal plan for setting up and running an E.D.Y. course in their own Authority. Instructors were asked to specify the strengths and needs which would determine the sort of course they might run, for example, training two staff, training a whole school, running a residential course. As with trainees in Phase II, it was critical that instructors be guided to choose an approach consonant with their strengths and needs list. Having selected one approach, the instructor analysed it into sequential steps, specifying method and target dates for each. The instructor was required to revise and expand the goal plan and return it to the project centre within one week of their return to their own Authority. This marked the beginning of the external evaluation of the workshops.

Rehearsal for setting up a course

A vital first step in setting up a course is to 'sell' the idea to the headteacher of a school. Using role play, instructors were asked to sell the course to a sceptical headteacher role played by the head of Melland School. He asked a series of pre-prepared questions about the course. The role play was seen as a dress rehearsal for the meeting which instructors would later have with the head of a facility in their own Authority. It had the added advantage of allowing instructors to discover what they did know about the content and organisation of the course.

Instructors were also given information on Phases II and III during the workshop but perhaps not in sufficient detail as many appeared not to proceed beyond Phase I in their own courses.

Evaluation of the national dissemination exercise

Evaluation fell into two parts - an internal evaluation of each workshop and an external evaluation of each instructor's activity post workshop.

In all, 22 standard E.D.Y. workshops were run for a total of 101 instructors, representing 73 of the 104 L.E.A.s in England and Wales. Some Authorities sent more than one instructor and the rest consisted of five Manchester University staff, six community mental handicap nurses and three teachers from Melland School. Although not invited to be part of the original sample, Eire and Scotland each sent two instructors to workshops. Three other workshops were held for a further 19 individuals but because these did not follow the usual workshop format, data are not included in the summary results. It will be clear from these figures that the response from the L.E.A.s was far greater than had been anticipated - 70 per cent as compared with the expected 25 per cent. This single factor led the project into several difficulties. The sheer volume of work entailed for a team of two coordinators and one secretary in providing the promised support to each instructor and in following up each in detail meant that some of the research objectives were dropped. In retrospect, it might have been advisable to reduce the number of workshops run.

Internal evaluation of workshops

Evaluation of each instructor during a workshop took a number of forms, only two of which will be commented on here. Instructors were required to answer questions on operant behaviour before attending a workshop. Analysis of their answers suggested that most instructors were familiar with the distinction between operants and respondents and the concept of reinforcement. However, few were familiar with the terms 'controlling stimulus' or 'setting conditions', an understanding of which is important for a functional analysis of behaviour.

An important activity in each workshop was training instructors to use the T.A.F. reliably, as this was to be their main evaluation tool. Pre-training was given on the first day of each workshop with videotaped session, using a backward chaining procedure. Instructors were then given a pretest on a standard session, the same on each workshop. Thereafter they practised using the scale in every session and reliabilities between them and the course co-ordinators were calculated and discussed daily. On the last day, instructors were posttested on the standard tape and informed of their results. As with all aspects of the training, an instructor who failed to learn the T.A.F. coding could not be prevented from running training courses. Those who found difficulty with it were strongly encouraged to practise it further before attempting to use it.

Pretest percentage agreement for five instructors across all T.A.F. categories was 49 per cent, rising to 73 per cent on the posttest.

Instructors were asked to assess different aspects of the workshop. The two highest rated pedagogic devices were consistently 'practice with child' and 'role play'. This gave some support for the emphasis placed on these two enactive modes of learning. The three most frequently occurring aspects which were most liked were 'practical work with children', 'the school based nature of the course' and 'role play', in that order. Suggestions for improvements centred on having more practice on the T.A.F., more feedback after sessions and generally more time for discussion. Interestingly, 15 per cent asked for more role play and only one instructor asked for less.

External evaluation of the workshops

As the number of individuals running courses rose, the project was increasingly occupied with providing instructors with materials which were not, at that time, published and were restricted to members of the sample, answering queries and analysing data returned to the project. Data tracking systems were developed for monitoring the courses being run so that data were available on the activity of each instructor, the use of the E.D.Y. model in each L.E.A., the staff involved and other relevant variables.

A number of record forms were devised for return by instructors giving details of courses run for the purposes of issuing course certificates. These included a data sheet per member of staff trained and a summary sheet per course run. These continue to be collected. The data sheet on each trainee gave results for the pre- and posttest quiz and T.A.F. These data, while providing interesting information on courses run, did not help in establishing the reasons why some instructors had not run courses, the difficulties encountered in setting up a course, or the modifications made by some instructors to be the standard version of the course. To gather information on these aspects, two questionnaires were used, the first addressed to those instructors who had run a course and returned data and the second addressed to those who had not to our knowledge run a course. Additionally, a total of 22 visits were made to courses while they were running, selected on a random basis, mainly but not exclusively in the North West. These were an excellent source of data on the type of course being run.

Data on the reactions of trainees trained by members of the sample were available in the form of comments sheets and ratings of pedagogic devices sent in by instructors. At the end of the funding period a questionnaire was sent to a random sample of trainees trained by a range of instructors asking for detailed information on the course they had received.

Results of the national dissemination exercise

Results are presented to provide information on L.E.A. representation, numbers of courses run and staff trained, the reasons why some instructors did not run a course, and the nature of the courses run.

L.E.A. representation, courses run and staff trained

The pyramid model of dissemination was concerned with the spread of courses through the L.E.A.s. Table 1 gives summary figures on the L.E.A.s in England and Wales in which E.D.Y. courses had and had not been run between December 1978 (the end of the workshops) and December 1984. Of the 101 instructors in the original sample, it was known that by the end of 1980, 58 (57 per cent) had run one or more E.D.Y. courses, although not necessarily in their original L.E.A. In addition, courses have been run in five areas of Eire, in three Scottish Authorities and in the Isle of Man. Courses have also been run in 13 different Health Authorities in England and Wales for nursing staff. It is certain that over 2,500 course certificates had been issued to successful trainees between 1978 and 1984. These figures all refer to courses which have returned data and to trainees who have received certificates and are therefore a conservative estimate of E.D.Y. activity across the country. For example, at the end of the funding period, it was known that 18 of the original sample had run or helped to run versions of the E.D.Y. course for which data have not been returned. These would increase the overall percentage of the original sample who had made use of the workshops to 75 per cent.

The relative activity of Educational Psychologists (E.P.s) and Advisers is shown in Table 2, from which it can be seen that the former were by far the most successful as a target group for dissemination.

Instructors who did not run a course

In April 1980 records showed that 45 of the original sample, representing 32 of the L.E.A.s, had not run a course. These consisted of 34 per cent Educational Psychologists, 65 per cent Advisers and 1 per cent others. Clearly the reasons why these representatives

Table 1: Number of L.E.A.s in England and Wales in which E.D.Y courses were run 1978-1984

	N.	No. known to have run courses	%
No. of L.E.A.s represented on Workshops	73	46	63
No. of non-represented L.E.A.s	31	11	36
Total L.E.A.s	104	57	55

Table 2: Profession of Instructor and Number of E.D.Y. courses run by April 1980.

Profession of Instructor	N	Percentage Running 1 + courses
Educational Psychologists	62	47
Advisers in Special Education	20	10

had not run a course were of interest, given that this was an explicit goal for each workshop attender. Questionnaires were sent out, to which 22 instructors replied (49 per cent). This was an encouraging return rate given that these were instructors who had apparently failed to fulfil their commitment to the project. Some had attended a workshop over two and a half years previously while several had moved areas, retired or left the country.

The 22 returned questionnaires revealed that eight of the respondents considered that they had run some kind of an E.D.Y. course following the workshop, either starting a course and not finishing it, or using some of the materials for various other training purposes. To summarise the replies of these eight, six were from Educational Psychologists and two from teachers.

The six Educational Psychologists: Two had altered the course structure; three had run a course in their original L.E.A. but did not return data and had subsequently changed profession (two of these had subsequently run several E.D.Y. courses). The sixth E.P. had encountered opposition from both the school and from an E.P. colleague and subsequently moved to another L.E.A. where he ran several successful courses.

The two teachers: It is interesting to note that one was a headteacher and the other a class teacher. The headteacher had decided to raise funds for the purchase of video equipment in order to run the course and was currently engaged in this. The class teacher, who had been sent to the workshop as the representative for the L.E.A. by the Adviser in Special Education, reported that she started an E.D.Y. course in her school but had to abandon it:

'I was forced into it by the head making it impossible to carry on. Her line was that a re-organisation of the school structure took priority and she wasn't going to let us have time out of her Friday afternoon music session with the school...'

This reply underlines the importance of pre-selection of representatives from the L.E.A.s.

The remaining 14 questionnaires came from six Advisers and eight E.P.s.

The Advisers: Of the six Advisers who replied to the questionnaire, three cited a change in their job description or role as the major reason for not having run an E.D.Y. course which led to lack of time as a secondary reason. Two of these gave the major reason as a commitment to other in-service courses in their L.E.A. One Adviser selected another in-service course to concentrate on. One moved to another L.E.A. where another Adviser had already attended a workshop and was running a course and it was decided that only one of them should pursue E.D.Y. The sixth Adviser cited no less than nine other in-service courses in which he was regularly involved. For him, E.D.Y. was too intense to be manageable. Nevertheless, this same Adviser wrote on his questionnaire:

'I a) enjoyed and b) learned more from my workshop than from any other course/conference that I have attended'.

Two Advisers owned to being in need of more training in basic behavioural skills before feeling confident to run a course themselves. Many Advisers did not seem to have the background in terms of scientific method or psychological theory to allow them to absorb easily the course philosophy or structure, particularly the evaluation methods. We gained the general impression that Advisers are excessively overworked (four of our small sample suffered physical or mental breakdowns during the course of the research). Despite their role being to organise in-service training, most do not have the pre requisite skills or the time needed to set up and run an E.D.Y. course.

An exception to this is the Teacher-Adviser who, in a humbler position, is also expected to run in-service training. Teacher-Advisers are in an excellent position to run these intensive courses and to follow them up in terms of doing Phases II and III. These people are very experienced with severely mentally handicapped children, experience which Advisers do not necessarily have and it is fully within their professional role to concentrate on staff training. Indeed, one Teacher-Adviser has trained every member of staff in all the E.S.N.(S) schools in a large county L.E.A.

The Educational Psychologists: Five of the E.P.s who replied gave 'lack of time to run a course/work load too great' as the main reason for not having run a course. One gave 'lack of interest from school' as the main reason, although four cited this as a contributing factor. One gave the reason that the school concerned had embarked on a different project. One basically disagreed with the emphasis of the E.D.Y. model on teaching technique and was concerned to develop the curriculum in her school. Of the four mentioning lack of interest from schools, two said this revolved around internal difficulties within the school such as lack of communication between the head and staff. Two said it was because the school had decided on different priorities.

All the respondents, bar the one already mentioned, were positive about the use of a behavioural approach for teaching severely mentally handicapped children and the E.D.Y. workshop they had attended as well as the E.D.Y. course materials themselves. Instructors were also asked why they had attended the workshop in the first place. Answers to this question varied, most saying they wished to learn to run the course, the 'right' answer. Others, however, had attended in order to learn about behaviour modification or about working with E.S.N.(S) children, both inappropriate reasons. Some indicated that they had been sent.

We finish this section with just one quotation from an instructor (E.P.) who did not run a course:

'Parts of the course were like blood transfusions for me and the effects took weeks to wear off. It still annoys me greatly to think that all that mental energy which was plugged into me didn't spread any further when I came back to X.'

The courses run by the sample

A different questionnaire was sent to all the instructors (51) who had run an E.D.Y. course by April 1980, following attendance at a workshop. Of the 39 which were returned, 29 had been completed in sufficient detail giving a return rate of 57 per cent. These 29 consisted of 25 E.P.s, two Advisers and two teachers. They had run between them a total of 98 E.D.Y. courses for 437 trainees. This in itself reveals that many instructors did not stop after running one course but went on to incorporate it as part of their regular work. Questions were asked on

16 separate aspects of the course, not all of which can be dealt with here (see McBrien and Thomas 1980).

Instructors reported that it took anything between two hours and a week's full time work to organise a course. Seventeen of the 29 had trained colleagues as co-instructors and three had set up courses specifically for trainee Educational Psychologists. The number of trainees taken on a course varied from one per instructor to an extreme of 15. The majority felt that two trainees per instructor was the optimal number, whereas the original E.D.Y. model had suggested one trainee per instructor. There are several advantages in taking two trainees together, provided the length of each session is extended to about one and a half hours in order to ensure that each has the required amount of role play and practice with a child. The majority held sessions once a week for ten weeks during Phase I. A few held twice weekly sessions, thus completing Phase I in half a term, and some had held more intensive courses.

The structure of the sessions run is of interest with regard to the proportion of time allotted to each pedagogic device. All but one instructor spent over 50 per cent of each session on the enactive level, i.e. role play and practice with child. The E.D.Y. model taught on the workshops for these instructors suggested 66.6 per cent of each session should be spent in the enactive mode. This figure of 50 per cent obscures the fact that, where there were several trainees in each session, one may have spent 100 per cent of the time merely observing colleagues. Sixteen of the 29 claimed that every trainee had the opportunity for role play and practice with a child on every session.

Role play did not seem to receive the amount of attention suggested by the original model, although only three instructors omitted it altogether. Some trainees never role played at all because of the number of trainees in each session and some role played either the child or the teacher but not both on any one session. Role play generally took up less than 30 per cent of a session (33.3 per cent recommended). This was unfortunate as it is felt to be an essential part of the course, allowing for structured practice without the demands placed on the situation by the presence of a child. It relies on familiarity with the child and on careful planning of each session in advance.

Seventeen of the respondents used the E.D.Y. demonstration video tape and a further three used parts of it. Of the nine who did not use it, some did not have access to video equipment and many found the technical quality to be too poor. This was indeed a valid criticism which was overcome at the end of the funding period when a new tape was made professionally. Those who did not use video spread the time saved fairly evenly over the other parts of the session. One used role play between two instructors as a substitute. The difficulties experienced with the tape make it difficult to draw any conclusions about the value of the demonstration videotape as a pedagogic device.

The percentage of time devoted to the symbolic level ranged from the 16.6 per cent as suggested to those instructors during their workshops to a high figure of 42 per cent. Subsequent revisions of the course have reduced the recommended input at the symbolic level to 8 per cent of a session. All but one instructor allocated time for verbal feedback at the end of each session, although this was not part of the model. This feature must be linked with their responses to questions on the use of the T.A.F. - only 24 per cent used it to help structure feedback during the practical work. The true percentage of the overall course given to the symbolic level is increased by the tendency of instructors to give 'homework' and additional handouts to supplement the course materials. It seems that course tutors cannot easily give up their familiar role as pedagogue, relying on written and spoken information.

Modifications were made by some to the presentation of the units, four omitting the unit on overcorrection, one omitting time out, four presenting the ten units in a different order and two re-writing all the units to make them simpler.

Selection of staff for a course was always made by the head teacher or head of the unit, usually in consultation with the instructor. Several stressed the importance of having motivated volunteer rather than press-ganged candidates. Opinions varied widely as to which grades of staff were most suited to the course, some finding it suited all, others finding it more appropriate for qualified staff. Many found that less qualified staff needed more explanation and encouragement but found them easier to handle and often more receptive than teachers.

Information was also solicited on Phases II and III. Only half the respondents answered this part of the questionnaire (14/29). All of these had carried out Phase II training with all or some of their trainees. Instructors who had done this, clearly found it valuable but organisationally difficult. This was also the experience of the research team at Melland School. Subsequent experience has suggested that the most efficient method of running Phase II is to train the deputy head of the school as the course instructor. The position of the deputy head is such that she or he is likely to be available on a regular basis to organise and monitor sessions.

In conclusion, the dissemination of the course at this stage was encouraging. The pyramid training model appeared to have been successful in terms of the number of staff trained and the number of new instructors trained by the original sample. The quality of the courses being run, as determined by questionnaire, and more convincingly by visits, was good though with some appalling exceptions. The training given to instructors was short. They returned to their Authority armed with only a week's intensive experience of the E.D.Y. course. During the workshop they had been required to instruct unfamiliar trainees in a strange school on two of the course units each, to learn to use the T.A.F. and to absorb the whole structure of the course. In setting up courses at Melland School, the research team had the benefits of working as a team and of being present in the school daily. We were aware that Educational Psychologists are doing well if they are visiting one E.S.N.(S) school once a week. If this is the case, the time allotted to E.D.Y. work in one school has to be tightly scheduled. There is unlikely to be time to meet staff between sessions. Therefore all planning of tasks and children to work with must take place within specified times. Thorough preparation can overcome these difficulties and instructors appeared to gain in competence on their second and subsequent courses.

Data on trainees

As noted earlier, by December 1984 just over 2,500

certificates had been issued to successful trainees. Table 3 give the quiz and T.A.F. scores for a random sample of teachers and nurses (these professions forming the bulk of trainees).

Table 3: Average pre- and post- course scores for trainees by profession*

		QUIZ		TAF	
	N	Pre	Post	Pre	Post
Teachers	40	37	82	82	92
Nursery Nurses	10	17	78	80	93
Classroom Assists	22	26	75	78	94
Nurses (RNMS)	9	32	85	70	92
Nurses (SENS)	3	8	71	65	87
Nursing Assistants	8	7	76	84	92
Other	8	-	-	-	-

* Based on data from the last 100 certificates issued (Oct 1984).

Extensions of the model

Although the course was designed for use in special schools with mentally handicapped children, it has been tried in a variety of different settings with both children and adults. In so far as the course concerns method and not content, it should be applicable to any age group. Its specificity lies in the examples used in the written materials and on the videotape to illustrate what are general principles of behavioural teaching. The use of the course with National Health Service staff has been the most extensive outside the educational field. Detailed descriptions of its use in two Health Authorities are given by Knight, Gale and Pickerill (1985) and by McBrien (1985). The course has been found successful with nursing staff working with mentally handicapped adults. The difficulties are reported to lie in the increased organisational problems of needing to train a large core of staff to influence a small number of clients. These problems are due in part to complex shift systems and high staff turnover.

An interesting project undertaken by Phillips and Sapsford (1985) in the Leicestershire School Psychological Service is the integration of the E.D.Y. course with the Portage scheme. In this, groups of parents and teachers of pre-school mentally handicapped children are jointly trained in the use of the Portage curriculum and the E.D.Y. techniques with the aim of ensuring continuity between pre-school provision and entry into special school.

There have been many adaptations, formal and informal, of the E.D.Y. materials and methods for use in schools. For example, Cotterhill and Leadbetter (1984) of the Birmingham Education Department have re-written the E.D.Y. Workbook in a simplified form entitled 'E.D.Y. Bare' for special school assistants and non-teaching staff. Educational Psychologists in Fife have produced 'McEDY' - a different version of the demonstration videotape. The proceedings of the second E.D.Y. user's conference (Farrell, 1985a) contain sixteen papers on applications of the E.D.Y. course throughout the U.K.

These and other developments have revealed a need for the E.D.Y. materials to be substantially revised and rewritten. At present this is underway with the aim of making the course applicable to a range of staff working with a variety of mentally handicapped clients.

CONCLUSIONS

Selection of a target group for dissemination

The selection of representatives from L.E.A.s was of critical importance for the success or failure of the dissemination. In selecting Educational

Psychologists as the main target group the project was largely successful, some 60 per cent of them having run a course by the end of the funding period. The selection of Advisers met with markedly less success for reasons already discussed. By writing to Chief Education Officers in the first instance, we left the selection of representatives largely to chance. Hindsight suggests it would have been preferable to have contacted Principal Educational Psychologists and to have had a contractual arrangement between the L.E.A. and H.A.R.C. It should have been made clear to each L.E.A. that whoever was sent should a) have been committed to running staff training courses, b) have been guaranteed time, resources and support from within the School Psychological Service to do this and c) have been likely to remain in that Authority for long enough to run at least one course. These precautions would have avoided instructors who were sent on workshops against their wishes, those who came to learn about behaviour modification or about mental handicap, and those who were already planning to leave their post and hence would not be a resource for that Authority. A further contract with the local E.S.N.(S) school might have gone even further in ensuring dissemination.

The importance of pre-selection of candidates is endorsed by our experience of the 'second generation' instructors who were a self-selected group trained by the end of the funding period and all had run at least one course and were among the most enthusiastic and energetic of all the instructors.

The role of the Educational Psychologist

Anecdotal reports from Educational Psychologists suggest that the course gave them, often for the first time, a role in their local E.S.N.(S) school. Where previously they might have had contact only for statutory placements of children, for testing and for crisis intervention, they could now offer a longer term involvement on a structured and regular basis. The running of the course introduces the instructor to the staff and children and provides a sound basis for continued intervention and support. Crisis intervention may assist with the problems of one child for a short period but is likely at the same time to undermine the confidence of the teaching staff in their own ability to deal with problems. Ways are needed to provide 'hands on' staff with the expertise to meet difficulties as they arise. The Educational Psychologist's skills are well employed when applied to staff training and backing this up with regular support and feedback. A quotation from one instructor may support this view:

'General overspill from E.D.Y. has been interesting. There is increased involvement by E.D.Y. instructors in curriculum and assessment in E.S.N.(S) schools. The schools themselves have become quite excited about the techniques and have welcomed the practical basis of the course. The Ed. Psych./E.S.N.(S) school relationship is much enhanced.'

Some of the most successful courses have been those in which the Educational Psychologist has trained the deputy head as a second instructor who between them have then trained the whole school. The deputy head is in an excellent position to monitor Phase II programmes which need intensive input at the start and weekly monitoring. Educational Psychologists, whose workloads take them elsewhere at this point, can continue to provide support for the deputy head in their role as staff trainers. Educational Psychologists should also be in a position to evaluate staff training and child training programmes in the school.

The recipients of the course

The success met with by the instructors serves to underline yet again the overwhelming need for staff training in the special schools. Only two points will be discussed here: the applicability of the course to trained and untrained staff and the degree to which the course fits into the organisation of a school.

It was the finding of the E.D.Y. team that both qualified and unqualified staff could be equally successful on the E.D.Y. course. As we have seen, Farrell (1982) cast some doubt on its applicability to untrained assistants, whereas the more recent findings of Farrell and Sugden (1984) suggest that assistants, at least nursery nurses, can benefit from the course. As the course is largely practical, there is no need for trainees to have an academic background or indeed to be able to read to benefit from the practical aspects of the training. Our own data suggest that Phase II is particularly welcomed by classroom assistants although difficulties may arise. Phase II is naturally construed as a teaching activity which is not the recognised role of ancillary staff (though this is not so in all schools). Trained teachers may feel that this is their preserve. However, this leaves the untrained assistant in charge of the majority of the children while the teacher works on individual programmes. If the assistant stays with her traditional role of mopping up and bottom wiping, then most of the children are not being taught at all. In some classes, the teacher sees her role as organising the class as a group while freeing her assistant to carry out Phase II programmes with individual children. This seems to provide both members of staff with activities suited to their training, expertise and disparate financial status.

Research has demonstrated that severely mentally handicapped children learn most efficiently from individualised instruction tailored to their needs. The more handicapped the child, the less is learnt from mere exposure to educational stimuli of the kind provided in, say, music or story time. Teaching in schools for children with severe learning difficulties aims to provide a balance of individual and group teaching, but in reality the individual contact time for any particular child is often low. A course such as E.D.Y. places a high priority on providing short one-to-one teaching sessions. Phase II, for example, suggests ten minutes per day with one child. It has been our experience and that of the trainers that this ten minutes per day is an extremely difficult goal to achieve in most classrooms. Clearly those who are particularly keen and dedicated will achieve this through elaborate contingency planning, but in so far as it is recommended as a routine undertaking, it is proving difficult to achieve. The room management approach to using behavioural methods with groups of children while freeing a member of staff for individual work seems very promising (see for example Porterfield, Blunden and Blewitt, 1977; McBrien and Weightman, 1980, and Jones et al., this volume). There is a definite role here for instructors in instituting change in teaching patterns.

Quality control

The drawback to making the course materials self-instructional in 1981 lay in the loss of control over the standard of courses run. This was already a problem within the sample trained by the research team as shown by the variation in the courses run. It is of particular concern in the area of evaluation of trainee progress. The two key areas of evaluation are a pre-post course quiz for Phase I and the rating of trainee behaviour with a child throughout all three Phases. Bar deliberate cheating, the quiz remains unproblematic - the scores for pre- and posttests are added up by the instructor and sent to the Hester Adrian Research Centre. The T.A.F. presents far more difficulties. Our concern was to equip instructors with a useable evaluation tool for measuring trainee progress. All instructors in the original sample were taught to use T.A.F. during a workshop and most reached a high level of reliability in scoring by the end of the training. However, there was a disappointing return of adequately completed T.A.F.s as part of the data collection. There could have been a number of reasons for this. First, instructors may not have been adequately trained to use it. Questionnaire responses suggested this was the case for the first time, when, often single-handed, instructors may have felt overwhelmed. The tightly structured sessions require organisation and discipline. The T.A.F., unless well practised, requires a level of concentration difficult to achieve when other constraints are operating. Some instructors reported that they found the T.A.F. distracted them from other aspects of running a session. This is extremely unfortunate as it is the only objective measure of skill acquisition. As instructors became more practised in running sessions, they reported finding the T.A.F. more manageable and more valuable.

Although high reliability between instructors and the research team was reached during workshops, there is bound to be a drift as each instructor continues to use T.A.F. in isolation. Many instructors trained colleagues to use the rating scale and there was no check on their reliability. These problems are much more acute for those instructors who have used the self-instructional package. Users have been encouraged at least to reach reliability amongst themselves when co-instructing and to practise rating on the demonstration videotape for which specimen recordings are provided in the Instructor's Handbook. A solution under consideration is the provision of regular workshops to train new instructors.

Generalisation and maintenance of skills

Much has been written on the generalisation and maintenance of staff training. 'Generalisation' as an end result has been variously defined and past research critically examined in the light of the resulting criteria (see for example Robinson and Swanton, 1980). Clearly it is essential to demonstrate generalisation and maintenance of the skills taught on the E.D.Y. course. Generalisation is typically looked for in terms of time, place, children and tasks.

Phase I teaches the basic techniques of behaviour modification sequentially over ten sessions. In so far as on each occasion the trainee works with a different child and task, generalisation across children and tasks is built in from the beginning. Generalisation beyond the training sessions is not at stake at this stage. At the completion of Phase I, trainees are expected to be able to exhibit a behavioural teaching strategy as defined on the E.D.Y. course and when presented with any child and any task in a pre-prepared, one-to-one training setting. These behaviours should be maintained over time as a well-rehearsed repertoire. The research has demonstrated that upon completion of Phase I, trainees can exhibit these behaviours in one-to-one training sessions when primed to do so, i.e. provided with a distraction-free setting and time to plan the session. The recent research of McBrien and Edmonds (1985) suggests that teachers can maintain these skills without further input for a period of 14 months, although this study was conducted on a very small sample and needs further verification.

Phases II and III are concerned with the consolidation of skills learned on Phase I which should assist maintenance across time, generalisation across children and tasks, and generalisation of skills to settings beyond the training condition. The essential differences between the training condition in Phase I and those in Phases II and III are, first, the trainee has to make a task analysis and create a timetable for training, with considerably less assistance from the instructor. Second, the trainee has to conduct the sessions within the confines of her classroom duties; and third, the trainee must carry out these sessions independently of the instructor several times a week. The regular T.A.F. ratings made by the instructor during these phases allows for an evaluation of generalisation across time and place, or training versus non-training conditions. This should fulfil the criteria of generalisation defined by Robinson and Swanton, i.e. 'similar effects are demonstrated in a non-training condition where the events scheduled are i) less costly than the training events and ii) not similar to those scheduled in the training condition'. Success in this type of generalisation has been demonstrated by the E.D.Y. team for their trainees at Melland School (McBrien and Foxen, 1981b). However, an evaluation of the trainees trained by the instructors with respect to this type of evaluation was not undertaken. This would be fairly straightforward to examine given the large numbers of already trained staff in different parts of the country. If generalisation could be demonstrated for Phase I skills across time and place for staff trained by a wide variety of instructors, it would provide powerful support for the E.D.Y. model of staff training and dissemination. Indeed, without this information it is difficult to promote this model as more effective than any other.

Although an outcome measure of child behaviour change was never an aim of the E.D.Y. project, data on Phase II programmes would easily provide such a measure as these programmes involve minute attention to the rcording of child behaviour on specified targets. It would be feasible to use control groups of both Educational Psychologists and schools not so far exposed to the course in a generalisation evaluation study.

"The Myth of the Hero Innovator"

The paper of the above title by Georgiades and Phillimore was published in 1975. The authors raise some fundamental questions concerning the value of staff training, putting forward the case that innovation and change in schools is slow. In 1960 it was estimated that it takes seven years for 11 per cent of schools to adopt an innovation (Georgiades and Phillimore, 1975). This slow rate of change, the authors propose, is due primarily to a continued emphasis upon training as the predominant change strategy. They cite evidence to suggest that it is a psychological fallacy to assume that work organisations can be changed by changing the behaviour of individual members:

'This then is the myth of the hero-innovator: the idea that you can produce, by training, a knight in shining armour who, loins girded with new technology and beliefs, will assault his organisational fortress and institute changes both in himself and others at a stroke. Such a view is ingenuous. The fact of the matter is that organisations such as schools and hospitals will, like dragons, eat hero-innovators for breakfast.' (Georgiades and Phillimore, 1975).

Georgiades and Phillimore go on to give six guidelines for those intent upon staff training. These guidelines are examined below in relation to three distinct client groups in the E.D.Y. project: the research team, the instructors, the trainees.

Guideline 1: Work with members of the organisation who are supportive of change and improvement. Do not attempt large scale, across the board activity. Do not attempt mass training or large public relations exercises.

The Research Team: The research team needed to select a local E.S.N.(S) school which would be 100 per cent accommodating of the workshops and courses to be held there. A newly opened school - Melland School, Manchester - was selected for a number of reasons. The head teacher had expressed an interest in having a research input from the Hester Adrian Research Centre, was in sympathy with a behavioural approach and was able to hand-pick his own staff. Although there were then five E.S.N.(S) schools in Manchester, the research team chose to concentrate on just one.

The Instructors: In the selection of personnel to become course Instructors, the research team did not entirely follow this guideline, as has already been discussed. It is probably true to say that most of the psychologists and advisers were keen to attend workshops although a few were 'sent' by their Authority. Keeness to attend a workshop was, however, no guarantee of keeness to institute change in the schools - many and varied are the reasons for professionals spending a week away from work.

The Trainees: At the end of a workshop, instructors

were given sessions on role play and goal planning to aid in setting up their own course in a local school. Instructors were encouraged to select keen volunteers from amongst the staff. This strategy has been endorsed by many instructors in their feedback to the project. It was certainly our experience at Melland that, once the keen staff had been trained and we took on new members of staff who were not volunteers, this made for difficulties in the training.

Guideline 2: Develop a 'critical mass'; i.e. a self-sustaining team within the organisation which is self-motivated and powered from within. Do not leave people working in isolation to promote change.

The Research Team: The research team was in itself a self-sustaining team, but this was extended to include the headteacher of Melland School. He became closely involved in the organisation and development of the research in his school. The amount of time which this took should not be underestimated. Over a year was spent in the development of and planning by this team before the first workshop was held. Without the support of the headteacher from this early stage, later difficulties could not have been overcome.

The Instructors: Here again the rules were broken. In taking one instructor from each L.E.A. we were condemning this individual to working in isolation in their own Authority. Many instructors overcame this by developing their own 'critical mass' in their L.E.A. by training colleagues and heads and deputies of schools as co-instructors. A solution which was not thought of at the time would have been to have invited one E.P. and the deputy head from one of his/her local E.S.N.(S) schools to attend the workshop together. In this way the school and the School Psychological Service would have been in agreement in running courses for staff. The skills of teachers in curriculum development and their familiarity with staff and children would have complemented those of the E.P. in knowledge of behavioural techniques, programme planning and evaluation.

The Trainees: The project gave no specific advice as to the selection of trainees except that they should be volunteers and that wherever possible either the head or deputy should be one of the first to be trained in a school. Many instructors and trainees have suggested that pairs of staff from the same class should be trained together in order to provide mutual support following the course. It seems particularly important at this level to ensure the development of a 'critical mass'. Schools are slow to change and newly trained staff do meet with resistance and opposition from those members of staff who have not been through the course.

Guideline 3: Work in 'healthy' parts of the organisation which have the will and resources to improve. Change requires additional energy and talent, especially in the early stages.

The Research Team: The research team made an early decision to develop staff training in the educational setting rather than in the health service. Staff in schools naturally see their role as one of fostering the educational and social development of their mentally handicapped students. There is therefore an already established 'culture' into which to inject new methods. In tackling staff training in hospitals and community settings, much more work would have to have been concentrated on developing in the staff a 'need' for this kind of approach. This may be less true today than it was in 1976.

The Instructors: Guideline 3 seems close to Guideline 1. The E.P. service is keen to develop staff training. E.P.s are generally energetic people who are actively seeking a better defined role, especially in the field of Special Education. They have a training which particularly fits them to carry out behavioural skills training in schools. The Advisory service on the other hand is made up of individuals with more diverse backgrounds and often less formal training. They provide a wide ranging service making it difficult for them to implement change in one specific area.

The Trainees: Choice of schools in which to run the course was left entirely to the instructor. It is abundantly clear that selecting a school which is functioning well, has a cohesive group of staff, reasonable facilities and most importantly a well worked out curriculum, is a great advantage both for the running of the course and for subsequent training activity by trainees. Many comments from instructors reveal that courses which were planned and then abandoned failed because of poor relationships within the school, or because schools were selected which could be considered problematical, e.g. staff undecided on priorities, schools with an almost entirely special needs population, schools undergoing major internal re-organisation, etc.

Guideline 4: Work with those who have as much freedom and discretion in managing their own operations and resources as possible.

The Research Team: In selecting Melland School as the site for the development of the course and workshops, we were working with a school which, because it was newly built and newly staffed, was enjoying a great deal of autonomy and resources. The research team itself, by the nature of its funding, also enjoyed a fair amount of autonomy and the resources of the purpose-built research accommodation within the school.

The Instructors: In selecting Advisers as course disseminators, it might have been thought that these were people with more autonomy and resources than most. However, it seems that despite a brief to develop in-service work, the role of the Adviser is such that they have neither the time nor the availability of colleagues to enable them to undertake this type of course. It should be said that there are some notable exceptions in that some Advisers made considerable alterations in the organisation of their time and have successfully run many E.D.Y. courses. E.P.s seem to have the necessary autonomy and can command sufficient resources such as video equipment and money for materials to put on the course. Paradoxically, the more junior the E.P. the more likely he/she was to run a course. Those of senior grade and below are in an ideal position to organise their time to run courses and to follow them up. Principal E.P.s, in the same way as Advisers, have too many competing commitments. At the other end of the scale, those instructors who were regular class teachers had nothing like the autonomy or resources required.

The Trainees: So far as the trainees are concerned, this guideline again emphasises the need to select senior teachers, especially the head or deputy, as the first trainees on the course. Once these are 'won over' they can create the necessary conditions to allow the less senior staff to undertake the course and subsequently carry out training programmes in the classroom.

<u>Guideline 5: Involve the top management at the appropriate level. Top level management are often too personally identified with the 'status quo' to become totally involved, although their permission for a new project needs to be sought. The best supporters are among the ranks just below the top.</u>

<u>The Research Team</u>: We were slow to take the headteacher at Melland through the course and eventually took him through as an instructor. Although he was not expected to act subsequently as such, his close involvement during the week he attended a workshop was of inestimable value in the future smooth running of both the workshops and child training programmes in the classroom. It may also be of note that once the research team had invited their own top management to participate in the person of the Director of the Hester Adrian Research Centre, this noticeably increased the attention given to the project staff and hence their resources.

<u>The Instructors</u>: One of the basic mistakes made by the research team was in the initial approach made to the L.E.A.s. As had been mentioned under Guideline 1, it might have been better to have written to the Chief Education Officers to ask for their permission and support for the project, but to have sent the invitations directly to the Principal Educational Psychologists asking them to select a suitable E.P. as the representative. The ultimate in top management for this project was of course the D.E.S. who were asked to endorse the letter to Chief Education Officers stressing the implied commitment that representatives would implement the course in their own Authority following attendance at a workshop. While prepared to fund the research for four years, the D.E.S. was not prepared to say anything to the Authorities which might lead to extra expenditure. If such an exercise were undertaken again, we would now feel it essential to have a contractual arrangement with the organisations responsible for dissemination.

<u>The Trainees</u>: While we found it advisable to take the headteacher as one of the first trainees, this should be seen largely as an exercise to gain support for future courses in the school. It allows the head to understand fully the commitment required of his/her staff. It is however the deputy head who can play a key role in developing and maintaining staff training and hence child training in the school.

Guideline 6: Protect the training team from pressure by working in small groups or pairs. Do not attempt to evaluate the training team too early. Reinforce them with specially built-in incentives.

The Research Team: It must be said that the research team felt under tremendous pressure most of the time and did not succeed in finding any source of relief from this. An extra research worker or alternatively limiting the scope of the research from the beginning would have been advisable.

The Instructors: Although the project kept in close contact with instructors which was possibly a source of comfort to them, we could not ensure their protection from hostile colleagues or schools. Again, when instructors have trained colleagues as instructors this has assisted them in combating pressure in the system. As regards reinforcement, E.D.Y. Users' conferences were held in 1979 and 1983 (Farrell, 1985a,b) which provided opportunities for instructors to describe to an interested audience the work which they are doing and to exchange ideas with people in a similar position from different parts of the country.

The Trainees: The same applies to the trainees as to the instructors. Where trainees are taken in pairs, or where the entire staff of a school are trained, they can provide support for one another. Where the head or deputy is in favour of the course, trainees are protected from resistant members of staff. It is an important role for the instructor to provide continued monitoring and support in school following the initial course. The trainee certificate was seen as a reinforcement and incentive for staff and has proved very successful. The project did produce a certificate for instructors but remained undecided as to whether or not this was desirable.

Bearing in mind the sixth guideline, which stresses the importance of not evaluating attempts at change and innovation too early, the time has perhaps now been reached to make a wider ranging evaluation of the course and its dissemination than was possible during the funding period. This is no easy task, but recent developments in research methodology for large scale programme evaluation (Hall, 1983) are showing the way for this to be done. The D.E.S. awarded a new grant to Manchester University which commenced in October 1983 for research to be undertaken into the impact of in-service training in Special Education. As part of this work, a detailed evaluation of the E.D.Y. course is being made, including its impact in different schools, the long term maintenance and implementation of skills by staff and the progress of individual children taught by the trained staff.

Given the extent to which the E.D.Y. course has now been run in E.S.N.(S) schools throughout the U.K., it would seem that the hero-innovators in the form of several hundred instructors and some two and a half thousand trainees have not so far been eaten for breakfast.

Acknowledgements

We would like to acknowledge and to thank the following for their significant contributions to the E.D.Y Project. Mr Mike Gore, headteacher of Melland School, Manchester and his staff and pupils; Dr James Hogg, originator of the research proposals and project consultant; Ms Maria Thomas, research assistant 1979 - 1980; Ms Jane Weightman, temporary director of the project for three months; Ms Irene Jones, secretary for the first three years; Ms Sheila Watt, secretary for the final year; and by no means least Professor Peter Mittler for his continued interest, enthusiasm and support over the years.

References

Allen, D. W. and Ryan, J. A. (1969) Microteaching, Addison Wesley, Reading

Bandura, A. and Walters, R. H. (1963) Social Learning and Personality Development, Holt, Rinehart and Winston, New York

Barrowclough, C. (1981) An Evaluation of a staff

training course in behaviour modification techniques with the severely mentally handicapped, Unpublished M.Sc. Thesis, University of Manchester

Bruner, J. S. (1964) 'The Course of Cognitive Growth', American Psychologist, 19, 1-15

Bruner, J. S. (1966) Toward a Theory of Instruction, Norton, New York

Carr, J. (1980) 'The Organisation of Short Courses' in W. Yule and J. Carr (eds.), Behaviour Modification for the Mentally Handicapped, Croom Helm, London

Cook, T. D. and Campbell, D. T. (1979) Quasi -experimentation Design and Analysis Issues for Field Settings, Rand McNally, Chicago

Corsini, R. J. and Cardone, S. (1966) Roleplaying in Psychotherapy, Aldine, Chicago

Cotterhill, J. and Leadbetter, P. (1984) E.D.Y. Bare, School Psychological Service, Birmingham

Farrell, P. T. (1982) 'An Evaluation of an E.D.Y. Course in Behaviour Modification Techniques for Teachers and Care Staff in an E.S.N.(S) School', Special Education Forward Trends, 9, 21-25

Farrell, P. T. (ed.), (1985a) E.D.Y.: Its Impact on Staff Training in Mental Handicap, Manchester University Press, Manchester

Farrell, P. T. (1985b) 'An Account of the E.D.Y. Project' in D. Milne (ed.), Training Therapists: Methods, Evaluation and Implementation with Parents, Nurses and Teachers, Croom Helm, London

Farrell, P. T. and Sugden, M. (1984) 'An Evaluation of an E.D.Y. Course in Behavioural Techniques for Classroom Assistants in a School for Children with Severe Learning Difficulties', Educational Psychology, 4, 185-198

Foxen, T. H. (1978a) Second Annual Report on the E.D.Y. Project to the D.E.S., Hester Adrian Research Centre, University of Manchester

Foxen, T. H. (1978b) Trainee Manual, Hester Adrian Research Centre, Manchester University

Foxen, T. H. and McBrien, J. A. (1981) The E.D.Y. Course for Mental Handicap Practitioners: Trainee Workbook, Manchester University Press, Manchester

Gagne, R. M. (1962) 'Simulators' in R. Glasser (ed.), Training, Research and Education, University of Pittsburgh Press, Pittsburgh

Gardner, J. M., Brust, D. J. and Watson, L. S. (1970) 'A Scale to Measure Skills in Applying Behaviour Modification Techniques to the Mentally Retarded', American Journal of Mental Deficiency, 74, 633-636

Gardner, J. M. and Giampa, F. (1971) 'The Attendant Behavior Checklist: Measuring On-ward Behavior of Institutional Personnel', American Journal of Mental Deficiency, 75, 617-622

Georgiades, N. J. and Phillimore, L. (1975) 'The Myth of the Hero-innovator and Alternative Strategies for Organisational Change' in C. C. Kiernan and F. P. Woodford (eds.), Behaviour Modification with the Severely Retarded, Associated Scientific Publishers, Amsterdam

Griffin, N. W. (1979) 'Training Parents of Retarded Children as Behaviour Modifiers: A Review', Australian Journal of Mental Retardation, 7, 18-26

Hall, J. (1983) 'Evaluation and Research: An Overview' in S. Simpson (eds.), Facing the Challenge, B.A.B.P., Rossendale

Hart, B. and Risley, T. R. (1976) Environmental Reprogramming: Implications for the Severely Handicapped, Unpublished paper, Center for Applied Behavior Analysis, Kansas

Hogg, J. (1975) Education of developmentally young mentally handicapped children: A programme of evaluated dissemination and research, Research application to the Department of Education and Science, Hester Adrian Research Centre, Manchester University

Hogg, J., Foxen T. H. and McBrien, J. A. (1979) Training staff responsible for profoundly retarded multiply handicapped children: An application of Kiernan and Riddick's staff training programme, Hester Adrian Research Centre, Manchester University

Hogg, J., Foxen, T. H. and McBrien, J. A. (1981) 'Issues in the Training and Evaluation of Behaviour Modification Skills for Staff Working with Profoundly Retarded Multiply Handicapped Children', Behavioural Psychotherapy, 9, 345-357

Houts, P. S. and Scott, R. A. (1975) Goal Planning with Developmentally Disabled Persons: Procedures for Developing an Individualised Client Plan, State University College of Medicine, Pennsylvania

Kiernan, C. C. (1975) 'Methodology of Behaviour Modification' in C. C. Kiernan and F. P. Woodford (eds.), Behaviour Modification with the Severely Retarded, Associated Scientific Publishers, Amsterdam

Kiernan, C. C. and Riddick, B. (1973) A draft programme for training in operant techniques: practical units, Thomas Coram Research Unit, University of London

Knight, G., Gale, E. and Pickerill, C. (1985) 'E.D.Y. in Health Service Settings' in P. T. Farrell (ed.), E.D.Y.: Its Impact on Staff Training in Mental Handicap, Manchester University Press, Manchester

Lange, D. N. (1971) 'An Application of Social Learning Theory in Effecting Change in a Group of Student Teachers Using Video Modelling Techniques', Journal of Educational Research, 65, 151-154

McBrien, J. A. (1985) 'Behavioural Training for Nurses in Mental Handicap: An Application of the E.D.Y. Course', Journal of Advanced Nursing, 10, 337-343

McBrien, J. A. and Edmonds, M. (1985) 'Evaluation of an E.D.Y. Training Course in Behavioural Techniques for Staff Working with Severely Mentally Handicapped Children', Behavioural

Psychotherapy 13, 202-217

McBrien, J. A. and Foxen, T. H. (1981a) The E.D.Y. In-service Course for Mental Handicap Practitioners: Instructor's Handbook, Manchester University Press, Manchester

McBrien, J. A. and Foxen, T. H. (1981b) Final Report on the E.D.Y. Project to the D.E.S., Hester Adrian Research Centre, University of Manchester

McBrien, J. A. and Thomas, M. (1980) Fourth Annual Report on the E.D.Y. Project to the D.E.S., Hester Adrian Research Centre, University of Manchester

McBrien, J. A. and Weightman, J. B. (1980) 'The Effect of Room Management Procedures on the Engagement of Profoundly Retarded Children', British Journal of Mental Subnormality, 26, 38-46

McClelland, D. C., Atkinson, J. W., Clark, R. A. and Lowell, E. L. (1953) The Achievement Motive, Appleton-Century-Crofts, New York

Mazza, J. and Pumroy, D. K. (1975) 'A Preview of Evaluation of Behavior Modification Programs', Psychological Record, 25, 111-121

O'Dell, S. (1974) 'Training Parents in Behavior Modification: A Review', Psychological Bulletin, 81, 418-433

Phillips, P. and Sapsford, A. (1985) 'Learning Together: A School Based Service for Severely Handicapped Pre-school Children and their Parents' in P. T. Farrell (ed.), E.D.Y.: Its Impact on Staff Training in Mental Handicap, Manchester University Press, Manchester

Piaget, J. (1951) Play, Dreams and Imitation in Childhood, Norton, New York

Porterfield, J., Blunden, R. and Blewitt, E. (1977) Improving environments for profoundly handicapped adults : establishing staff routines for high client engagement: Research report, Mental Handicap in Wales Applied Research Unit, Cardiff

Robinson, V. and Swanton, C. (1980) 'The

Generalisation of Behavioural Teacher Training', Review of Educational Research, 50, 486-498

Skinner, B. F. (1968) The Technology of Teaching, Appleton-Century-Crofts, New York

Stokes, T. F. and Baer, D. M. (1977) 'An Implicit Technology of Generalization' Journal of Applied Behavior Analysis, 10, 349-367

Uzgiris, I. and Hunt, J. McV (1975) Psychological Scales of Ordinal Development, University of Chicago Press, Chicago

Watson, L. S. (1972) How to use behavior modification with mentally retarded and autistic children: Programs for administrators, teachers, parents and nurses, Behavior Modification Technology, Alabama

Watson, L. S. (1975) How to design and implement therapeutic environments - an intensive training workshop, Behavior Modification Technology, Alabama

Watson, L. S. and Bassinger, J. F. (1974) 'Parent Training Technology: A Potential Delivery System', Mental Retardation, 12, 3-10

Chapter Ten

EXPANDING OPPORTUNITIES FOR STAFF TRAINING: A CONSIDERATION OF DISTANCE EDUCATION TECHNIQUES

K. Linfoot

Introduction

Changing attitudes to the needs of mentally handicapped people raises serious problems in the provision of sufficient well-trained teachers and other service delivery personnel. Access to educational opportunities, to 'normalised' residential services and to the typical employment and recreation facilities of local communities are coming to be seen as rights of all individuals, and consequently, as important areas for education and training for handicapped people.

If it is generally difficult to meet the need for appropriately trained personnel who can assist handicapped people in these areas of development, the challenge may be even greater in rural or other isolated communities and in older-established services where low staff turn-over has resulted in a low proportion of staff exposed to training programmes of recent development (Andrews, Elkins, Berry and Burge, 1979; Christie, Williams, Edelman, Hill, Fox, Fox, Sousie and York, 1977; McLeod, 1979; Fox, Williams and Fox, 1978). Indeed, Sontag (1980) noted in an address to a conference of special educators in the United States that many special classes in rural U.S. communities were without properly trained teachers while teacher unemployment was common among special educators in, for example, the large Californian coastal cities.

The present paper suggests that an examination of recent developments in the provision of off-campus (distance) training programmes by universities and colleges can lead to additional staff training opportunities for those who work with mentally handicapped people.

The Distance Education Approach

Various terms, for example, "correspondence teaching", "external study", "off-campus studies" and "open learning" are used to describe the situation where students do not pursue their studies mainly on the university or college campus. However, in the 1970s, increasing use of the term "distance education" became evident. In 1974, the Open University published a journal called Teaching at a Distance, while in 1980, the journal Distance Education was launched with an editorial board representing "distance educators" in five countries. It will appear then that observers of this particular body of literature can expect to see the term "distance education" used increasingly in the future.

In summarising various definitions of distance education, Rumble and Harry (1982) cite Keegan's identification of major elements which need to be present in an adequate definition of distance education:

- The separation of teacher and learner which distinguishes it from face-to-face lecturing;
- The influence of an educational organisation which distinguishes it from private study;
- The use of technical media, usually print, to unite teacher and learner and carry the educational content of the course;
- The provision of two-way communication so that the student may benefit from or even initiate dialogue, which distinguishes it from other uses of education technology;
- The teaching of students as individuals and rarely in groups, with the possibility of occasional meetings for both didactic and socialisation purposes;
- The participation in a more industrialised form of education (based on the view that distance teaching is characterised by division of labour, mechanisation, automation,

> application of organisational principles, scientific control, objectivity of teaching behaviour, concentration and centralisation). (pp.13-14)

Note: This last point suggests a mechanistic approach to the teaching relationship, which is not shared by the present writer.

International Developments in Distance Education

The practices involved in distance education are by no means new. For some time universities, colleges of education, technical colleges and school systems have attempted to use correspondence teaching methods to bring their educational programmes to students unable to attend on-campus classes. The Open University of the United Kingdom is perhaps the best known example of off-campus teaching, although Daniel and Stroud (1981) claim that correspondence courses had been offered in various forms for "nearly a century" before the commencement of the Open University programmes in 1970. For many school children living in isolated areas correspondence teaching has been used in many countries as a major format for providing educational services, while the School of the Air for children living in outback areas of Australia has provided distance education for many years. In recent times, those traditional distance education methods for schoolchildren have been supplemented by the establishment of regional study centres to allow for periodic visits by students for face to face teaching and for contact with other students. Additionally, the advent of domestic ownership of videoplaying facilities has meant that students are able to receive highly specialised lessons, specifically designed for their own needs and in their own homes.

Keegan and Rumble (1982) have indicated something of the 130 year history of distance education for technical and vocationally oriented courses and of the growth during the last century of correspondence tuition to prepare students for University of London examinations. From such beginnings, we now see a position where distance education methods are a part of the operations of many universities throughout the world. Indeed, there are other universities which have been established <u>solely</u> for the purpose of offering their courses by distance education techniques. The diversity of institutional models, which have been developed in various parts of the world, includes variations in the procedure for financial operations, for accreditation and examination purposes, for curriculum development and teaching methods, for student support services and for deciding which technological media are given importance in teaching.

Organisational variants have ranged from the highly centralised model of the Open University with local teaching centres controlled by an administrative headquarters, to a "service institution" model developing distance education projects for other institutions but not teaching students itself (Keegan and Rumble, 1982).

Keegan's typology of distance teaching approaches at university level (Figure 1) is an attempt to impose an organisational framework on the diversity which is apparent within distance education.

Such a typology is at best a simplification of the diversity of models and is achieved by identifying only major general dimensions of difference between various approaches. For example, within the "integrated" external studies department model of "mixed" institutions , we see, in Australasia:

- the case where a separate department both arranges and teaches the various courses (University of Queensland);

- another approach where both internal and external teaching is conducted by the same lecturing staff as in the University of New England model where the External Studies Department services an administrative function only; and

- the multi-institutional model typified by the Massey University in New Zealand, where students from any New Zealand university are able to take a Massey course instead of one from their own university but receive credit in their own institution (Bewley, 1984)

Indeed, it would not be surprising to see government demands in many countries for similar inter-university co-operation in the provision of courses

Figure 1: Keegan's typology of distance teaching at University level.

DISTANCE EDUCATION

Autonomous Institutions

Public and	Distance Teaching
Private	Universities
Correspondence	Autonomous
Schools and	multi-media distance
Colleges.	teaching universities
	("open" universities).

Mixed or Hybrid Institutions

Independent	Studia
"Integrated"	
Study Divisions	Zaochne
mode external	
of Extension	(in Poland)
studies	
Colleges of	Fernstudium
departments	
Universities	(DDR) and
(Australia).	
(In USA and	other socialist
Canada.)	consultation
	systems.

(Source: Keegan & Rumble, 1982;28)

to students. The advent of professional and well-resourced distance education courses does raise possibilities for conserving public expenditure on excessive duplication of expensive on-campus training programmes if co-operative teaching and accreditation arrangements involving the deliverers of high quality distance education programmes can be made. For individual students, there must be many advantages in being able to include in their programme of studies a distance education course in a specialised subject not available in their own university. Or, to be able to complete by part-time distance education methods, a course commenced by conventional studies. This will go a long way towards increasing the opportunities for participation in tertiary education for many people unable to undertake full-time study at university for a variety of reasons.

Those autonomous institutions involved exclusively in distance education, are described rather comprehensively in the recent publication of Rumble and Harry (1982). That discussion includes the variety of courses offered by this mode and also indicates the extent to which distance education has been embraced in developing countries.

Table 1 indicates those universities operating only in the distance education mode and which are described in some detail by Rumble and Harry (1982).

For a comprehensive discussion of the details of operations of those institutions and of the wide range of courses which are offered, the reader is referred to Rumble and Harry (1982).

Mixed Mode Institutions: The context for the introduction of special education courses by distance education.

In Australia, the University of Queensland and the University of New England (U.N.E.) at Armidale in New South Wales have been pioneers in teaching by external studies offering initially a wide range of courses within the Bachelor of Arts (B.A.) degrees. The scope of these universities' external programmes has gradually increased while other universities and colleges of advanced education (C.A.E.s' tertiary education institutions offering vocationally oriented courses mainly at diploma, first degree or graduate diploma levels) developed additional

Table 1: **Distance Teaching Universities**

Canada	Athabasca University
People's Republic of China	Central Broadcasting & Television University
Costa Rica	The Universidad Estatal a Distancia
Federal Republic of Germany	The Fernuniversitat
Israel	Everyman's University
Pakistan	The Allama Iqbal Open University
Spain	The Universidad Nacional de Educacion a Distancia
United Kingdom	The Open University
Venezuela	The Universidad Nacional Abierta

external studies courses which were initially based on the U.N.E. model. Presently, tertiary education courses are offered by distance education methods in such diverse areas as literature, modern languages, education, psychology, physical sciences (including experimental work), data processing, accountancy and in a range of fields related to business and public administration. Indeed, the scope of training courses which may be available by distance education methods is likely to increase as ways continue to be found to improve the quality of support given to students who undertake their studies away from the campus of their instructor.

Some support has been found for the effectiveness of the "mixed-mode" distance education model as a teaching medium. Records maintained by the University of New England's Division of External Studies (Mackenzie, Postgate and Scuphan, 1975; Rumble and Keegan, 1982) have consistently shown that external students' examination results show pass rates equal to or better than those obtained by on-campus students who were enrolled in the same courses. Not surprisingly, the quality of teaching and therefore the knowledge and skill of graduates are significant areas for critical attention in appraising distance education programmes. The U.N.E. records are especially interesting as evidence for the success of these programmes, at least in relation to examination performance. Smith (1979) has indicated that this achievement by the U.N.E. has been possible because of the cohesive and integrated teaching processes which emphasized a combination of independent study and face to face tuition at residential schools. Additionally, the involvement of the same academic staff in the teaching of internal and external courses has helped to provide a stronger academic programme at that university than at places where distance education operates separately from the university's other teaching. Nevertheless, a much broader evaluation of course effectiveness than examination results is also needed in judging outcomes. This is especially true of courses seeking to prepare personnel to work with handicapped people, where very practical and important human interaction skills also need to be developed.

Some Distance Education Programmes Dealing With Mental Handicap

Considerable growth occurred in Australia as in many

other countries during the 1970s, in the demand for and provision of training for teachers in special education. The growth was stimulated largely by the recommendations of an expert committee, the Interim Schools Commission to government (Karmel, 1973).

As a result of those recommendations, one-year courses of study in special education were developed for practising teachers by a number of C.A.E.s and by some universities. A small number of distance education courses in special education were also developed at that time. These courses arose because of the particular need in Australia to bring this form of training to teachers in isolated communities who were unable to attend colleges or universities in major centres. Similarly, teachers, in small or independent school systems were often unable to obtain release time to attend full time courses. The provision of a form of training which would allow part time enrolment and study at a distance from the student's own home emerged as an important need. In most Australian states, at least one C.A.E. responded with the provision of a course to be available by distance education methods.

Special education courses developed for practising teachers at this time were usually described as generalist courses providing students with skills of assessment, programming, knowledge of learning processes, of developmental disabilities, of parent counselling and school communication processes. These courses addressed needs of teachers working with children having a variety of developmental disabilities. The courses sought to provide information on special education principles which were appropriate for use in many situations (Andrews et al., 1979; Drummond, 1978).

Generalist courses were so described because they provided a non-categorical approach to service delivery to avoid or at least minimise the deleterious effects of labelling in service delivery.

Thus, staff may not be working in the shadow of minimal expectations of their clients' learning potential. Of course, non-categorical approaches to teaching may also be useful to a teacher whose pupils have other than intellectual handicaps. In particular, the generalist approach is helpful for children with learning disabilities affecting basic skills acquisition were a direct approach to assessment, pinpointing of difficulties, task analysis of new skills to be learned and their teaching have gained considerable recent support (Mercer, 1983; Smith, 1981). The student's newly acquired skills are intended to be generalisable to a variety of learning disabled and mentally handicapped populations.

The role of generalist courses in special education may be better understood against the background of the professional tasks performed by teachers who complete them. Most teachers involved in state school teaching in Australia are employed by large government employing authorities and, in theory at least, may find themselves transferred by their employer to a variety of teaching positions in a variety of geographical regions during their professional careers. Further, a teacher released from normal duties to engage in a full-time diploma course in special education may not necessarily be appointed, upon completing the course, to the particular form of special education facility in which the teacher specialised during training. Thus a trend developed in the special education courses introduced in the 1970s, to produce a curriculum which was generalisable for teachers across the areas of resource or remedial teaching, and of teaching mildly and moderately mentally handicapped people. It was this form of special education training which was also adopted by some tertiary institutions to presentation by distance education methods. (It should be noted that training courses for people who are hearing impaired, visually impaired and severely motorically impaired have remained as full-time on campus courses and have <u>not</u> been adapted for distance education methods.)

Other factors have also influenced the deployment of many "generalist" special education teachers. There has been recent widespread concern to promote integrated class placement of mentally handicapped children in regular school settings wherever possible. And with older populations, there is a movement towards deinstitutionalised arrangements for housing and training facilities. Pieterse and Center (1984) have shown that regular school enrolment is a practical alternative for Down's Syndrome children who have participated in appropriate early intervention programmes, while Hayes (1984) has recently renewed the call to Australian developmental disability service agencies to maintain the momentum towards least restrictive housing and training facilities for the developmentally disabled. Many states have recently presented reports to government in which such less restrictive service delivery arrangements have been recommended (e.g. Doherty, 1982; Richmond, 1983).

A later section of this chapter will outline some Australian distance education programmes which illustrate the development of generalist special education courses for teachers and also for staff working with adult mentally handicapped people in rehabilitation or vocational training settings.

Finally, it should be acknowledged that Australian distance education courses in special education have been modelled on existing full-time on-campus courses. The same academic staff have been involved in both on- and off-campus presentations of the course. Teaching and student assessment methods have been largely identical in both presentation modes. In recent times, some colleges have concentrated their efforts on the presentation of the off-campus version of the course in response to student demand. However, in almost all cases, the distance education (often called "external studies") course has developed initially as an alternate means of presenting a course originally designed for full-time teaching on the college campus.

Distribution of Australian Special Education In-Service Course Offered By Distance Education Methods

The Australian Directory of Higher Education Courses 1984 includes information on those award courses dealing with special education, including mental handicap. Table 2 summarises the information from that source which is concerned with distance education courses.

CHARACTERISTICS OF ONE COLLEGE'S DISTANCE EDUCATION COURSES IN SPECIAL EDUCATION

The design and planning procedures for all courses taught in Australian CAEs involve complex processes of external advice to the College planning team. Assessment of courses is undertaken by committees appointed or approved by state coordinating bodies. This approach, together with the strong link with full time versions of the same courses where they

Table 2

Institution	Award Course	Availability
Bendigo CA Victoria	G.Dip. Special Assistance Teaching	PT, E
Darling Downs IAE Toowoomba, Qld	G.Dip Teaching (Exceptional Children)	E
Melbourne CAE Victoria	G.Dip Special Education	PT, FT, E
Mitchell CAE Bathurst NSW	1. Diploma in Special Education	E
	2. Graduate Diploma in Educational Studies (Special Education)	E
	3. Associate Diploma in Arts* (Vocational Rehabilitation)	E
South Australian CAE Adelaide, SA	Part of B.Ed. Conversion Course	Partly E
Tasmanian CAE Launceston Tas.	G.Dip Special Education	E
Western Australian CAE, Mount Lawley Western Australia	G.Dip Special Education	PT, FT, E

Code G.Dip = Graduate Diploma course,

FT = Full time on campus,

PT = Part time but on campus, and

E = Mainly off campus, and at part time rate.

* Not indicated in Directory of Higher Education Courses, 1984.

The above table indicates that distance education courses in special education are available from colleges in all Australian states. Teachers in the Northern Territory enrol in courses offered by institutions in the states.

exist, ensures that distance education courses are offered at appropriate standards and are reasonably well resourced. It also assists in achieving parity of standards and cohesion with on-campus courses, an important feature referred to by Smith (1979), and described earlier in this discussion.

Mitchell CAE in Bathurst, NSW, first presented a distance education course in special education in 1976. That course sought to present the same content as an on-campus full-time course taught at that College in 1974 and 1975. The same staff were involved in both courses, and similar student assessment procedures were used. An attempt was also made to present the same practicum experience to off-campus students as internal students had experienced.

Various characteristics of Mitchell CAE external courses in special education can be identified:

1. Academic staff are responsible for all aspects:

   - planning courses,

   - writing materials for individual subjects,

   - teaching subjects through combination of prescribed reading and lectures at residential schools,

   - assessing students through assignments and formal examinations.

2. Students meet with academic staff at least once during each semester for weekend or week-long residential schools.

3. Deliberate efforts are made to design course study materials according to established principles of instructional design. An instructional design unit cooperates with academic staff to ensure that materials are presented in clear, unambiguous formats.

4. Printed course materials have been supplemented where appropriate:

   - with telephone tutorials from academic staff to groups of students;

- with videotapes sent to students' homes on loan where a practical demonstration of, e.g., an assessment procedure, is appropriate;

- with lecturer visits to students' workplaces for particular subjects where on-the-spot advice is considered necessary to assist students to implement practical programming with handicapped individuals.*

* Subject to review. Logistics of this procedure over widely dispersed areas make the practice difficult to maintain.

1. Associate Diploma in Arts (Vocational Rehabilitation)

This course has been devised to cater for the needs of personnel employed in sheltered workshops, activity centres and other settings where training programmes are offered to adults handicapped in an important developmental domain.

Admission to the course is on the basis of completion of the Higher School Certificate Examination. However, most entrants to the course are eligible for adult admission to the College and are often people who have not completed the later years of secondary school education.

The course normally takes four years to complete by external study as it is offered at the equivalent of half the workload of a full-time course.

Subjects of the course include two, in the first semester, which are designed to enhance the students' own efficiency in study skills, recognising that many students may not have been engaged in academic study for some years.

Subjects

Semester 1	Research Skills and Report Writing Reading and Study Skills
Semester 2	Introduction to Psychology Understanding Work Organisations
Semester 3	Exceptionality and Special Education Psychology of Training

Expanding Opportunities

Semester 4	Managing Rehabilitation Facilities Programme Development in Special Education
Semester 5	Counselling 1 Personnel Management
Semester 6	Introduction to Welfare Studies Option
Semester 7	2 options
Semester 8	2 options

Optional Studies

The optional studies are drawn from a list including studies in Learning Theory; Statistics in Social Research; Social Psychology; Disadvantaged Person and the Law; Recreation for Disadvantaged People; Gross Motor Development; and other approved units.

Teaching processes used in this course share those characteristics described earlier in this paper. However, it is important that students are brought into contact with the clients they are being trained to help. This is, of course, a key problem facing all institutions involved in personnel preparation in special education. It is especially important if distance education methods are used.

In the present case, students are given assignments in the various subjects which place gradually increasing demands upon them in working with handicapped people. These demands range from case study descriptions including details of the client's functional behaviours over 24-hour periods, to the planning and implementation of a comprehensive training programme in a functional area of relevance to the client.

Lecturer assistance to students in completing these projects has been provided through:

- face to face contact during student residential schools at college;

- telephone consultations;

- lecturer advice to students in relation to

preliminary assignments on the project; and

- lecturer visits to students' work settings at the time of programme implementation.

Ways are currently being explored in the present course to increase the amount of lecturer advice to students in their work settings.

While not providing the ideal support system for students working with the adult people with handicap, this Associate Diploma Course has taken a first step in providing training support for many individuals who would otherwise continue their jobs in various facilities for the adult people with handicap without access to training support at all. Evaluative comments on the course from students and their employers have strongly supported the course's contribution and encouraged its continuation.

2. Diploma in Special Education

This course was designed for practising teachers and was first offered in 1976. The course also serves as an up-grading course for teachers whose initial training was of two years' duration, enabling those teachers to obtain a three-year equivalent Diploma Award.

The course is offered over two years of external study and shares the same general teaching method characteristics as have been already described. The course was developed as a 'generalist' course in special education, seeking to serve the needs of teachers in remedial education as well as those working with mildly and moderately mentally handicapped children. Subjects include the following areas:

Background theory

- Exceptionality and Special Education
- Communication, Learning and Teaching
- Study of Atypical Groups

Diagnosis/Assessment

- Diagnostic Remediation Process

School Curriculum Components

- The Teaching of Reading
- Curriculum for Special Class: Mathematics
  Curriculum for Special Class: Creative Arts

Communication Skills

- Resource Teacher as Leader
- Teacher and Group Dynamics

Programme Development

- Programme Development for People with Handicaps
- Study of Atypical Group B
- Case Studies of Children with Handicaps

Evaluation of Course Outcomes

This is an especially important issue in courses where it is hoped that outcomes will include the development of practical skills on the part of course participants. Evaluation of changes in students' practical skills alone is a complex if not impossible task.

One approach to course evaluation which is possible in this context is to survey the opinions of students who have completed the course. That procedure has been followed in relation to the Diploma in Special Education course on a number of occasions and the results of such a survey are now described. That survey was conducted and analysed independently of the College academic staff.

The following summary by T. A. Fishburn, the Senior Research Officer, describes responses to the survey:

1979 Opinion Survey of Diploma in Special Education

"A mailed questionnaire survey of graduates and those currently enrolled in the college's Diploma in Special Education areas was conducted in November 1979. Of the ninety-three surveyed, 52.7 per cent responded within two weeks and a total of ninety-four (68.8 per cent) responded.

Overall, the response was supportive of the course. Agreement that the course had achieved or would achieve its aim ranged between 90.6 per cent and 98.4 per cent of the responses. A little more than two thirds (67.2 per cent) of the respondents had no reservations regarding the appropriateness of external teaching for this course; a further 28.1 per cent (to a total of 95.3 per cent) considered internal teaching generally appropriate but with certain restrictions. Of the components of the curriculum, the majority were considered to be very important or valuable to the teaching function, ranging down from 98.2 per cent agreement to 93.8 per cent, apart from resource teacher skills which rated only 78.1 per cent agreement.

A little less than three quarters of those responding (71.9 per cent) expressed interest in further study in special education at Mitchell."

Another index of some aspects of the course's operation may be obtained by reference to course graduation rates. This and the related issue of course drop-out rates have been noted by Keegan and Rumble (1982) as significant matters of concern in many distance education programmes.

Table 3 sets out details of course graduation withdrawal rates for the period 1976-1982.

Table 3

Summary of Student performance: 1976-1982

	No	Per cent
Total enrolments (intakes of approx. 34 students each year)	234	-
Withdrawals	67	29
Graduate in minimum time (2 years)	85	36
Grad min time + 1 year	18	8
Grad min time + 2 years	1	-
Grad min time + 4 years	1	-
Current students	62	27

Source: Mitchell College of Advanced Education, **Diploma a in Special Education: Stage IV Review**, Bathurst, NSW, 1982.

Direct comparison of these figures with those for similar courses is difficult to make as few comparable data are available. Comparison with graduation/drop out rates for traditional college attendance is not helpful since distance education students are usually mature age students, often in full-time employment and with family responsibilities in addition to their studies.

Some comparison may be useful with data offered by Keegan and Rumble (1982) on time taken to graduate by Open University students of the United Kindom. They indicated "even one in three" of the OU's first cohort group did graduate in the minimum time of three years.

Table 3 above shows that 36 per cent of all those commencing the Diploma in Special Education course by distance education methods to 1982 also graduated in minimum time. Further, Keegan and Rumble (1982) have reported drop-out rates in many university distance education programmes as high as 70 per cent. In that context, the data on Diploma in Special Education withdrawals in Table 3 (29 per cent) is very encouraging.

While not yet answering the question of how successfully course graduates undertake their work with children with mental handicap, the above data do suggest that teachers' experience in the course does encourage them to maintain their studies and that they are generally satisfied that their time has been usefully spent. School systems have also encouraged new teachers to enroll in the course, as indicated by its generally stable pattern of enrolments since the course's inception. Finally, the limited data so far available on drop out and graduation patterns in distance education programmes suggest that the performance of this particular course may have been quite good.

3. Graduate Diploma In Educational Studies (Special Education)

The third of the courses incorporating material for staff training in mental handicap which is offered by Mitchell CAE is the Graduate Diploma course for practising teachers. In the Australian CAE sector, Graduate Diploma courses for teachers are post-graduate awards which are based upon initial teacher training. This characteristic of their evolution and administrative control by the Australian Council for Awards in Advanced Education has the possibly unfortunate consequence of excluding from training other professionals who work with people with mental handicap including psychologists, speech pathologists, graduate nurses and others whose basic training was other than in education. Unfortunately, we are unable to offer post-graduate diplomas in special education by distance education methods to professionals other than teachers.

The present Graduate Diploma course for teachers has recently undergone a review process similar to that described above for the Diploma course. Subjects originally offered in the Graduate Diploma course include:

- Communication, Learning and Teaching (Special Education)
- Applied Behaviour Analysis in Special Education
- Language and Language Learning
- Disorders of Child Development
- Assessment and Evaluation in Special Education
- Reading Methods for Handicapped Learners
- Creative Arts for the Exceptional Child
- Developmental Approaches to Mathematics
- School Programming for Children with Handicap
- Special Education Dissertation.

This course has also recently undergone a reaccreditation review.

Course evaluation processes used in the review of this course included:

survey questionnaire to past and present students;

advisory committee meetings involving practising teachers, employers and course graduates;

formal review/assessment process conducted by an external committee appointed by the NSW state government's higher education coordinating body.

A useful addition to course evaluation processes in general might be the introduction of a methodology to consider the effect of such courses on teacher performance. Unfortunately, such a possibility does not exist at this stage, with no opportunity available to obtain reliable pre-course measures of a teachers' performance. Naturally, this course does provide the opportunity to ensure that all students achieve competency in a practical teaching project forming part of one of the course's subjects. However, this is a simpler issue than using measures of teacher performance to make course evaluation judgements. At this stage, there appears no possibility for evaluating course effects on teachers' pre-course and post-course classroom performance.

Results Of Student Surveys

Thirty-six past or continuing students of the Graduate Diploma in Education Studies (Special Education), representing 48 per cent of possible respondents, returned completed survey instruments. Students were invited to use a Likert-type five-point rating scale format to convey their opinions of the course as a whole and of individual subjects (units). Replies to the question on reactions to the course as a whole indicated support for all aspects of the course, with mean rating-scale scores ranging from 2.1 to 2.6 (where 1 represents strong support and 5, lack of support) for the five categories in the question. The largest mean and thus the one closest to a negative reaction to the course was 2.6, in response to the "contains a reasonable workload". The organisation and teaching aspects of the course attracted mean scores of 2.1. Support was also shown for the value of residential schools, with scores of 1.5 to 2.1. Most support for residential schools concerned their value in enabling personal contact with staff and with other students.

Other analyses were concerned with attitudes to individual units and their presentation. Generally strong support was shown for most units, with typical mean scores of from 1 to 2 (strong support) for the unit statements on the evaluation form.

One area which received adverse comment on a number of occasions was the matter of course workload. Many students complained that for some subjects and for the course as a whole, the amount of material expected to be studied and the scope of required assignments was in excess of a reasonable workload for part-time students who needed to combine the time for their studies with a number of other commitments, often including full-time employment. Indeed, distance education programmes are likely to continue to accept this criticism as they aim to serve students usually unable to have access to full-time study.

Nevertheless, a conscientious effort needs to be made in designing these programmes to resolve what conflicts may arise between compassion for the busy part-time student and the need to provide appropriate learning experiences for students which will result in a proper understanding or mastery of the topics being treated.

Student responses to the survey instrument also included favourable comments on the administrative arrangements involved in presenting the course, and also on the quality of the printed lecture materials and subject information which students receive from the College.

Course Outcomes: Student completion rates

Table 4 indicates rates of student progress through this course, allowing direct comparison with Table 3, showing completion rates for the Diploma in Special Education course. A slightly lower proportion of students has completed the post-graduate course than was found for the Diploma course. Neverthless, the present Table still indicates a course completion rate close to the "one in three" for Open University students, noted by Keegan and Rumble (1982). Those authors have indicated that high course drop-out rates are not uncommon in distance education programmes in general. Indeed, it may well be that professionals involved in full-time employment in service delivery with people having special disabilities and/or handicaps may well have difficulty in sustaining active participation in a part-time course of study, whether by distance education or by evening lectures at a university.

Table 4

Summary of Student Performance: 1981-1984

	No	per cent
Total enrolments	114	-
Withdrawals	49	43
Grad in min time 2 years	33	29
Grad in min time + 1 year	7	6
Current students	25	22

Source: Mitchell College of Advanced Education, **Graduate Diploma in Education Studies (Special Education): Stage IV Review** Bathurst, NSW, 1984.

An examination of the letters which students submit when deciding to withdraw from these distance education courses usually reveals "pressures of work", "changed family circumstances", "unexpected additional work commitments", "onset of illness" and similar reasons for students' decisions to withdraw from the course. On a different dimension, the realisation by some students that the course does not deal with topics they anticipated when enrolling in the course, or that the workload for the course turned out to be greater than they had anticipated are reasons for withdrawal. For course planners, the matter of student withdrawal is a serious one as considerable resources go into the creation of those student enrolments which may not ultimately continue to graduation. At present, it would appear that drop-out rates from distance education programmes are likely to be generally higher than for full-time enrolments in similar courses.

It remains important however for those involved in this mode of course presentation to ensure that optimum levels of student advice and support are provided both before and after enrolment. This support, together with emphasis on the clear presentation of teaching materials utlilising instructional design principles in their development, should result in useful strategies for assisting the student unfamiliar with studying "at a distance".

Concluding Comment

Staff training opportunities for those working with people with mental handicap have increased in recent times. However, there are still many people who work with those who are handicapped without the benefit of practical training in the skills needed to present a developmental rather than custodial approach to their clients.

The high costs and often practical inconvenience involved in providing access to training to these many people who are often geographically or financially isolated from training centres is likely to mean that access to staff training would remain a problem for many people if only full time courses are employed.

Early efforts in the use of distance education methods to provide staff training for workers with people with handicaps have resulted in courses for teachers and a course for staff of sheltered workshops, activity centres and some other rehabilitation agencies.

Completion rates in these courses have been comparable with other courses offered by distance education methods, while student opinion has generally supported the courses and their outcomes. The rapid growth in the quantity and variety of courses being offered by distance education techniques worldwide (Rumble and Harry, 1982) in recent years suggests that as some of the inherent difficulties of this approach are satisfactorily overcome, courses for staff assisting people with mental handicap may continue to be developed to reach workers at other parts of the service delivery network. It is suggested that the experience gained in presenting the three courses described in this paper would argue strongly for the further development of courses in distance education for staff working with people with handicaps.

References

Andrews, R. J., Elkins, J., Berry, P. B. and Burge, J. A. (1979) A Survey of Special Education in Australia, University of Queensland, Brisbane

Bewley, D. (1984) 'New Zealand: Complementary 'Qualified Monopolies"' in K. Smith (ed.), Diversity Down Under in Distance Education, Darling Downs Institute Press, Toowoomba, W.

Christie, L. Williams, W. Edelman, S., Hill, M., Fox, T., Fox, W., Sousie, S. and York, R. (1977) A master's level training program to prepare teachers serving learners in need of intensive special education, Unpublished paper, Center for Development Disabilities, University of Vermont, Burlington

Daniel, J. S. and Stroud, A. (1981) 'Distance Education: A Reassessment for the 1980s', Distance Education, 2,2

Department of Education and Youth Affairs (1983) Directory of Higher Education Courses 1984, Australian Government Publishing Service, Canberra

Doherty, P. J. (1982) Strategies and Initiatives for Special Education in New South Wales, Government Printer, Sydney, NSW

Drummond, N. W. (1978) Special Education in Australia, Royal Far West Children's Health Scheme, Sydney, NSW

Fishburn, T. A. (1979) 1979 Opinion Survey on Diploma in Special Education, Unpublished paper, Mitchell College of Advanced Education, Bathurst, NSW

Fox, W. L., Williams, W. and Fox, T. J. (1978) 'Program Planning and Development for the Multihandicapped in Rural Areas: Vermont's Service Delivery Model' in A. Rehman, (ed.), Special Education Leadership Series, University of Minnesota Press, Minneapolis, Minnesota

Hayes, S. C. (1984) 'Out of the Frying Pan - Making De-Institutionalisation Work', Australian and New Zealand Journal of Developmental

Disabilities, 10, 187-190

Karmel, P. (1973) Schools in Australia: Report of the Interim Committee of the Australian Schools Commission, Australian Government Publishing Service, Canberra

Keegan, D. and Rumble, G. (1982) 'Distance Teaching at University Level' in G. Rumble and K. Harry, (eds.), The Distance Teaching Universities, Croom Helm, London and Canberra

Mackenzie, N., Postgate, R. and Scuphan, J. (1975) Open Learning, The UNESCO Press, Paris

McLeod, J. (1979) The Saskatoon Region Project: Provision of education services in rural and sparsely populated areas for children with special needs, Transcript of address to seminar to Post-Graduate Medical Institute, Department of Pediatrics, Prague, Czechoslovakia

Mercer, C. D. (1983) Students with Learning Disabilities: 2nd Edition, Merrill, Columbus, Ohio

Mitchell College of Advanced Education (1982) Stage IV Review: Diploma in Special Education, Mitchell C.A.E., Bathurst, NSW

Pieterse, M. and Centre, Y. (1984) 'The Integration of Eight Down's Syndrome Children into Regular Schools', Australian and New Zealand Journal of Developmental Disabilities, 10, 11-20

Richmond, D. (1983) Inquiry into Health Services for the Psychiatrically Ill and Developmentally Disabled, Government Printer, Sydney, NSW

Rumble, G. and Harry, K. (1982) The Distance Teaching Universities, Croom Helm, London and Canberra

Rumble, G. and Keegan, D. (1982) 'General Characteristics of the Distance Teaching Universities' in G. Rumble, and Harry, K. (eds.), The Distance Teaching Universities, Croom Helm, London and Canberra

Smith, K. C. (1979) External Studies at New England - A Silver Jubilee Review 1955-1978, The University of New England, Armidale NSW

Smith, D. D. (1981) Teaching the Learning Disabled, Prentice-Hall, Englewood Cliffs, N.J.

Sontag, E. (1980) An address on the implementation of PL 94-142, The Oregon Conference, University of Oregon, Eugene, Oregon

INDEX